"This is a theoretically robust and bold work that is well positioned to provoke debate, productive thinking, and practical responses."

Lisa M. Mitchell,
University of Victoria, Canada

BIRTHING TECHNO-SAPIENS

This ground-breaking book challenges us to re-think ourselves as *techno-sapiens*—a new species we are creating as we continually co-evolve ourselves with our technologies. While some of its chapters are imaginary, they are all empirically grounded in ethnography and richly theorized from diverse disciplines.

The authors go far beyond a techno-optimism vs. techno-pessimism stance, stretching our thinking about birthing techno-sapiens to consider not only how our cyborgian reproductive lives are constrained and/or enabled by technology but are also about emotions and spirit. The world of reproductive health care and particularly that of genetic engineering is developing exponentially, and current challenges are vastly different from those of a decade ago. The book is provocative, intended to generate debate, ideas, and future research and to influence ethical policy and practice in human techno-reproduction. It will be of interest across the social sciences and humanities, for reproductive scholars, bioethicists, techno-scientists, and those involved in the development and delivery of maternity services.

Robbie Davis-Floyd, Adjunct Professor, Department of Anthropology, Rice University, is author of *Birth as an American Rite of Passage* (2003) and *Ways of Knowing about Birth: Mothers, Midwives, Medicine, and Birth Activism* (2018). She has served as lead editor for 15 volumes, including *Cyborg Babies: From Techo-Sex to Techno-Tots* (1998) and *Birth in Eight Cultures* (2019).

Social Science Perspectives on Childbirth and Reproduction

Series editor: Robbie Davis-Floyd (Rice University)

This series focuses on issues relating to childbirth and reproduction from social science perspectives. It includes single-authored, co-authored, or edited books concerned both with people's reproductive experiences and with birth practitioners such as midwives (both professional and traditional), obstetricians, nurses, doulas, and others. It seeks to provide new viewpoints on functional and sustainable birth models and the challenges to their creation and maintenance, as well as on obstetric violence, disrespect, and abuse and their root causes. Single-case or comparative ethnographies on birth and other reproductive issues are featured, from high-tech conceptions to normal pregnancy and birth, including reproductive politics and human-rights issues in reproduction worldwide.

Birthing Models on the Human Rights Frontier
Speaking Truth to Power
Edited by Betty-Anne Daviss and Robbie Davis-Floyd

Midwives in Mexico
Situated Politics, Politically Situated
Hanna Laako and Georgina Sánchez-Ramírez

Birthing Techno-Sapiens
Human-Technology Co-Evolution and the Future of Reproduction
Edited by Robbie Davis-Floyd

https://www.routledge.com/xxxx/book-series/SSPCR

BIRTHING TECHNO-SAPIENS

Human-Technology Co-Evolution and the Future of Reproduction

Edited by Robbie Davis-Floyd

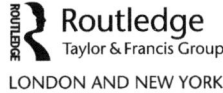

Routledge
Taylor & Francis Group

LONDON AND NEW YORK

First published 2021
by Routledge
2 Park Square, Milton Park, Abingdon, Oxon OX14 4RN

and by Routledge
52 Vanderbilt Avenue, New York, NY 10017

Routledge is an imprint of the Taylor & Francis Group, an informa business

British Library Cataloguing-in-Publication Data
A catalogue record for this book is available from the British Library

Library of Congress Cataloging-in-Publication Data
Names: Davis-Floyd, Robbie, editor.
Title: Birthing techno-sapiens : human-technology co-evolution and the future of reproduction / edited by Robbie Davis-Floyd.
Description: Milton Park, Abingdon, Oxon ; New York, NY : Routledge, 2021. | Series: Social science perspectives on childbirth and reproduction |
Identifiers: LCCN 2020045042 | ISBN 9780367535445 (hardback) | ISBN 9780367535438 (paperback) | ISBN 9781003082422 (ebook)
Subjects: LCSH: Human reproductive technology--Social aspects. | Human reproductive technology--Moral and ethical aspects.
Classification: LCC RG133.5 .B573 2021 | DDC 618.1/7806--dc23
LC record available at https://lccn.loc.gov/2020045042

ISBN: 978-0-367-53544-5 (hbk)
ISBN: 978-0-367-53543-8 (pbk)
ISBN: 978-1-003-08242-2 (ebk)

Typeset in Bembo
by Deanta Global Publishing Services, Chennai, India

Robbie Davis-Floyd dedicates this book to Beverley Chalmers, who has long been an effective champion of family-centered perinatal care and who was with me every step of the way as we co-created this book. For serving as my de-facto co-editor and for your outstanding and directly applicable work in the world, my eternal gratitude, Beverley!

Beverley Chalmers dedicates this book to Bernie and to our daughters Carmen, Dana, and Tandy, with grateful thanks for teaching us about birth, babies, and parenthood.

CONTENTS

FIGURES

CONTRIBUTORS

Beverley Chalmers DSc(Med), PhD (Canada), has two doctoral degrees: a PhD in Psychology and a DSc (Med) in Multicultural Childbirth. Her research examines birth experiences of women in difficult religious, social, political, and economic situations. She has over 300 publications including 57 book chapters and 10 books. She has given over 460 conference presentations globally and has undertaken 141 international health promotion activities in 26 countries. Her book *Family-Centred Perinatal Care: Improving Pregnancy, Birth and Postpartum Care* (UK: Cambridge University Press, 2017) integrates her decades of work in perinatal care. Her books, *Birth, Sex and Abuse: Women's Voices under Nazi Rule* (2015) and *Betrayed: Child Sex Abuse in the Holocaust* (2020) have together won 15 book awards. They expose neglected and often taboo topics in Holocaust studies. Other publications include *African Birth: Childbirth in Cultural Transition* (1990); *Female Genital Mutilation and Obstetric Care* (2003); *Humane Perinatal Care* (2001); and *Pregnancy and Parenthood: Heaven or Hell* (1990).

Melissa Cheyney, PhD, LDM, CPM, is Associate Professor of Clinical Medical Anthropology at Oregon State University (OSU) and a community midwife. She co-directs *Uplift*—a research and reproductive equity laboratory at OSU, where she serves as the Primary Investigator on more than 20 maternal and infant health-related research projects. She is author of *Born at Home* (2010), co-editor with Robbie Davis-Floyd of *Birth in Eight Cultures* (2019), and author or co-author of more than 60 peer-reviewed articles. In 2019, she served on the National Academies of Science, Engineering, and Medicine's *Birth Settings in America Study* and in 2020 was named Eminent Professor by OSU's Honors College and received OSU's prestigious Scholarship Impact Award. She is the Editor-in-Chief of the journal *Birth: Issues in Perinatal Care* and the mother of a daughter born at home on International Day of the Midwife in 2009. Melissa.Cheyney@oregonstate.edu.

Margaret Eby is a PhD student in Sociology at the University of California, Berkeley. Her work traces the evolution of eugenics from early reproductive control through contemporary genetic technologies, particularly feminist-led reproductive control movements in the first half of the 20th century. Margaret previously worked in public health researching socioeconomic disparities in dietary decisions and systemic barriers to health equity. margaret_eby@berkeley.edu

Suki Finn, PhD, Lecturer, Dept. of Philosophy, Royal Holloway University of London, is an analytic philosopher with research interests in metaphysics and logic who has published work in many journals and books on the topics of the metaphysics of pregnancy and the epistemology of logic. Website: www.sukifinn.com

Marcia C. Inhorn, PhD, MPH, is the William K. Lanman Jr. Professor of Anthropology and International Affairs at Yale University, where she serves as Chair of the Council on Middle East Studies. A medical anthropologist specializing in Middle Eastern gender, religion, and reproductive health issues, Inhorn has conducted research on the social impacts of infertility and assisted reproductive technologies in Egypt, Lebanon, the United Arab Emirates, and Arab America over the past 30 years. She is the author of six books on the subject, including her latest, *America's Arab Refugees: Vulnerability and Health on the Margins* (2018). Inhorn is Past President of the Society for Medical Anthropology and is co-PI with Prof. Sarah Franklin (University of Cambridge) on a Wellcome Trust grant entitled "Changing (In)Fertilties." Most recently, she completed a US National Science Foundation funded study of oocyte cryopreservation (egg freezing) for fertility preservation. marcia.inhorn@yale.edu

Rebecca Irons holds a PhD in Medical Anthropology from University College London. Her doctoral work investigated Quechua women's use of biomedical contraceptives and family planning in the Peruvian Andes, examining how state health care interacts with Indigenous subjectivities, race, kinship, gender, and citizenship. Her latest projects include a study on Venezuelan migrant reproductive and sexual health and the effects of the COVID-19 pandemic on the NHS in the UK. Her work is funded by the Wellcome Trust. rebecca.irons@ucl.ac.uk

Sasha Isaac is a doctoral student in sociology at the City University of New York. Her research focuses on issues in reproductive sociology and reproductive ethics, with a particular focus on their emergence in the development context. sashagisaac @gmail.com

Kelly Kara, RM, PGDipHealth, is a Senior Academic Staff Member in the Bachelor of Midwifery program at Ara Institute of Canterbury in Aotearoa New Zealand and an experienced midwife who has practiced across the full range of maternity settings, from home births and remote rural locations to high-technology urban hospitals. She is passionate about the provision of midwifery care that is holistic and empowering, sustainable for midwives, and works to support and promote the physiological processes of pregnancy, labor, and birth. Kelly is currently researching the experiences of women with complex pregnancies who make the choice to use water immersion for birth in a hospital setting. kelstommo@gmail.com

Amarpreet Kaur is a PhD Student in the Department of Sociology at the University of Cambridge. Her research focuses on the parameters of human germline genome editing in the United Kingdom in relation to disease and reproduction. Amarpreet's research activity can be followed on Twitter @lioness1992.

Sarah Melancon, PhD, is a sociologist and Clinical Sexologist. Her research interests center on the intersection of trauma, the autonomic nervous system, sexuality, birth, and intimate relationships. sarahilenemelancon@gmail.com

Noémie Merleau-Ponty, PhD, is a researcher at the French National Center for Scientific Research. As an anthropologist, she develops interdisciplinary feminist practices to study and question the making of reproductive technologies. Noemie .MERLEAU-PONTY@cnrs.fr

Suzanne Miller, PhD, RM, is a Principal Lecturer, Postgraduate Programme Leader, School of Midwifery, Otago Polytechnic, Aotearoa, New Zealand and a homebirth midwife. Her research interests include place of birth and its impact on birthing women and midwifery practice. Suzanne.Miller@op.ac.nz

Tessa Moll, PhD, is a Postdoctoral Research Fellow at the Alfred Deakin Institute for Citizenship and Globalization at Deakin University, Australia. Her research interests include the anthropology of reproduction; medicine, science, and technology; and racialization in post-apartheid South Africa. She is currently researching the circulation and translation of epigenetic knowledges in the Global South and completing a monograph on reproductive technology in South Africa. tessamoll@ gmail.com

Meghna Mukherjee is a doctoral candidate and Regents' Fellow in the Department of Sociology at the University of California Berkeley, where she studies the social inequalities arising alongside emerging fertility and genetic technologies. She is particularly interested in understanding how medicalized spaces are reinforcing social hierarchies and reconstituting health and family-building. Meghna graduated Magna Cum Laude from Columbia University with a BA in Sociology (Honors) and Human Rights. meghna_mukherjee@berkeley.edu

Anna Ozhiganova, PhD, is an anthropologist and senior researcher at the Institute of Ethnology and Anthropology, Russian Academy of Sciences. Her research interests concern the intersections of religion, health, reproduction, and alternative social movements. She is currently researching the Russian homebirth movement and changing obstetrics in Russia. Anna is the co-author (with Yuri Filippove) of *New Religiosity in Modern Russia: Teachings, Forms and Practices*, 2006. anna-ozhiganova@yandex.ru

George Parker, PhD, MPhil, RM, is a Lecturer in the Postgraduate Program, School of Midwifery, Otago Polytechnic, Aotearoa New Zealand. George also lectures in the medical humanities program at the School of Medicine at the University of Auckland. Their research interests include the politics of women's health; reproductive justice and health equity; and gender-inclusive health care. George.Parker@op.ac.nz

Emaline Reyes is a childbirth researcher and Medical Anthropology PhD student at Temple University. She is also a trained childbirth doula through Birth Arts International. Her research has been published in the *American Journal of Human Biology*, and she has forthcoming publications in the *Journal of Mother Studies* and *Frontiers in Sociology*. emalinereyes@gmail.com

Annekatrin Skeide, PhD, is a medical anthropologist with a special interest in reproductive technologies, bodies, health, and care. Her research draws on feminist science and technology studies and empirical philosophical approaches. a.skeide@uva.nl

Dana Solomon, PhD, is the Knowledge Translation specialist at the Birth Place Lab, University of British Columbia. She has an MA and PhD in interdisciplinary studies focusing on genocide prevention and countering prejudice and discrimination. She is the author of *Ideological Battlegrounds: Entertainment to Disarm Divisive Propaganda,* in which she developed the theory and practice of Ideologically Challenging Entertainment (ICE). Dana owns her own business, D-Editions & Chalmers-Solomon Solutions, through which she creates ICE productions and provides research and publication support. danalori@gmail.com

Lucy van de Wiel is a Research Associate in the Reproductive Sociology Research Group (ReproSoc) at the Department of Sociology, University of Cambridge. She is also a Turing Fellow at the Alan Turing Institute in London. She is the author of *Freezing Fertility: Oocyte Cryopreservation and the Gender Politics of Aging* (2020) and has published in journals such as *New Genetics and Society* and *Sociology of Health and Illness*. Her work on egg freezing has been recognized with an ASCA Award and the Erasmus Research Prize. lucy.vandewiel@gmail.com

ABOUT THE EDITOR

Robbie Davis-Floyd, PhD, Adjunct Professor, Department of Anthropology, Rice University and Fellow of the Society for Applied Anthropology, is a well-known medical anthropologist, international speaker, and researcher in transformational models in childbirth, midwifery, and obstetrics. She has given over 1000 presentations globally, and is author of over 80 journal articles and 24 encyclopedia articles and of *Birth as an American Rite of Passage* (1992, 2003) and *Ways of Knowing about Birth: Mothers, Midwives, Medicine, and Birth Activism* (2018); coauthor of *From Doctor to Healer: The Transformative Journey* (1998) and *The Power of Ritual* (2016); and lead or co-editor of 15 collections, including the award-winning *Cyborg Babies: From Techno-Sex to Techno-Tots* (1998) and *Childbirth and Authoritative Knowledge: Cross-Cultural Perspectives*; the "seminal" *Birth Models That Work* (2009); and *Birth in Eight Cultures* (2019). She served as co-editor with Betty-Anne Daviss of *Birthing Models on the Human Rights Frontier: Speaking Truth to Power* (2021) and with Kim Gutschow and Betty-Anne Daviss of *Sustainable Birth in Disruptive Times* (2021). In process is a co-edited Special Issue of *Frontiers in Sociology* on "The Global Impact of COVID-19 on Maternity Care Practices" and the complete revision and update of her first book, *Birth as an American Rite of Passage*. Also in process is a 3-volume collection on *The Anthropology of Obstetrics and Obstetricians: The Practice, Maintenance, and Reproduction of a Biomedical Profession*, to be co-edited with perinatologist Ashish Premkumar. She currently serves as Lead Editor for the Routledge series "Social Science Perspectives on Childbirth and Reproduction," as Senior Advisor to the Council on Anthropology and Reproduction, and as a Board Member of the International MotherBaby Childbirth Organization. Robbie is a lifelong birth activist and doula and midwifery advocate. Many of her published articles are freely available on her website www.davis-floyd.com. davis-floyd@outlook.com

INTRODUCTION:

Birthing *Techno-Sapiens*

Robbie Davis-Floyd and Beverley Chalmers

Cyborgs and Techno-Sapiens

Following on from the award-winning *Cyborg Babies: From Techno-Sex to Techno-Tots* (Davis-Floyd and Dumit 1998), this present volume addresses the futuristic implications of our current and ongoing co-creation of a new species, *techno-sapiens*, as we humans continually co-evolve ourselves with our technologies, and the implications of that co-evolution for our reproductive futures. Robbie had originally thought that she coined this term herself, but an internet search revealed that it already existed, and is defined in the *Urban Dictionary* (2020) as:

> A new intelligent species resulting from Homo sapiens' integration with technology. Techno sapiens are physically different from previous human groups through the use of technology assisted genetic and physical modification. Techno sapiens evolution is technology driven and its genome will be different from Homo sapiens' genome in ways never before imagined possible through natural evolution.

Some of the chapters in this book directly address such potential transformations in the human genome. And whether those transformations in our genome actually occur in the future or not, even without them we are already far along the road of becoming techno-sapiens, for as Donna Haraway (1991:150) famously said years ago, "We are all…theorized and fabricated hybrids of machine and organism; in short, we are cyborgs." Dictionary.com defines a "cyborg" as "a person whose physiological functioning is aided by or dependent upon a mechanical or electronic device"; its original use was as a shorthand for "cybernetic organism"—a fusion of human and machine. The word first appeared when scientist Manfred Clynes (Clynes and Kline 1960) used it to describe imagined beings with both artificial and biological parts; one of the first astronauts soon used it to describe the symbiotic, interdependent relationship of himself as a human and the space capsule he inhabited—neither could function without the other. The imaginary Borg of *Star Trek* have long constituted the most extreme examples of cyborgs, yet indeed, billions of humans carry technologies—including pharmaceuticals and prostheses—inside their bodies and/or are entirely dependent on technologies to function in their lifeworlds. And as the many aerospace engineers Robbie (Davis-Floyd 2000) interviewed back in the 1990s often repeated, "There are *no limits* to where technology can take us." From that perspective, it seems that those potential transformations in the human genome, which would be evolutionarily passed on to future generations, are not only entirely possible, but also appear to be inevitable, given what Robbie (Davis-Floyd 2003) has long called *the technological imperative*—the notion that if it *can* be done with technology, it must and *will* be done with technology.

In this book, we take as a given that human-technology co-evolution is a happening thing. We aim to deal with the following questions it raises: What shapes and forms are human-technology co-evolution now taking in regards to reproduction? How do we deal ethically with the endless possibilities it presents? Will we create genetically enhanced meta-humans? If so, will they be superheroes, or monsters? What does the male/female population imbalance created in some countries by aborting female fetuses (identified as such via ultrasound technology) project for our techno-sapiens future? What are its implications for women, and for men? (See Conclusions.) Will our ethical or religious guidelines eventually allow us to clone a human—as we have already cloned animals—or grow a baby in an artificial womb, bathing in artificial hormones? Would that baby know how to love? What are we doing to ourselves as we rush up the ladder of techno-progress? Who benefits? Who loses? The horrific social stratification of reproduction, by race, class, and gender, and the consequent inability of many to access desired reproductive technologies such as egg freezing and in-vitro fertilization are essential issues dealt with herein.

And what happens to spirituality, psychic communication with our unborn babies, "calling the baby" to call in its spirit when it is born but not breathing, as many midwives ask the parents to do? (Davis-Floyd and Davis 2018; Davis-Floyd et al. 2018). Can we develop our spiritual, intuitive, holistic capacities along with our technological ones? Or will our technological creativity drown out aspects of our humanity? Herein, we insist that cyborgs—cybernetic organisms—can be as organic as they are technological, as holistic and spiritual as they are mechanistic, as *Cyborg Babies* clearly showed.

From the cyber-dazzle of the burgeoning numbers of "artificial" or "assisted" reproductive technologies (ARTs), the current global cesarean epidemic, and the possibilities for gene selection and a new eugenics, to the racialized stratification of reproductive possibilities, the chapters in this book examine the dark and dire implications of futuristic reproductive technologies, their ethical and unethical uses, and the remarkable optimistic options they hold for increasing fertility and for better birthing. The theoretical framings of our chapters—evolutionary, futuristic, metaphysical, organic-technological-spiritual—are innovative, robust, and rooted in examples from a wide variety of cultural contexts. The database for our chapters is rich; it includes observations in homes, labs, and clinics; individual narratives drawn from interviews and birth stories; larger scale surveys; and analyses of scientific and popular culture and policy. The technologies our chapters discuss are also varied: they include current realities and imaginaries of widely used IVF, egg freezing, embryo selection, human germline genome editing via CRISPR-Cas9, gametogenesis, ectogenesis, human enhancements, cesarean births[1], cloning, the incubation of "monsters" brought about by the contraceptive Depo-Provera, and the relatively "low tech" practices of water birthing, home birthing, touch/physical contact, and emotional support.

Reproduction in the Technocracy: The Technocratic, Humanistic, and Holistic Paradigms of Birth and Health Care

Robbie (Davis-Floyd 2003) has long defined a *technocracy* as a capitalistic, hierarchical, bureaucratic, institution-laden, and (still) patriarchal society organized around an ideology of ongoing progress through the development of ever-higher technologies and the global flow of information via those technologies. In Chapter 1, she and Melissa Cheyney identify technocracies as the *6th subsistence strategy*, very different from the industrial societies that preceded them. Two decades ago, Robbie named and placed on a spectrum "the technocratic, humanistic, and holistic paradigms (or models) of birth (Davis-Floyd 2001, 2018). Her identification of these ideologies and their effects on practitioners and childbearers has been widely referenced, has stood the test of time, and has been utilized by many practitioners to help them understand the huge influence of ideology and to make conscious choices about which paradigm they wish to put into practice. Many have worked hard to make intentional paradigm shifts from technocratic to humanistic or holistic ideologies and practice (see Davis-Floyd and Georges 2018).

To briefly summarize: in the technocratic model, the body is metaphorized as a machine, and the laboring body as a dysfunctional machine in constant need of technological surveillance and intervention. This ideology is encapsulated in Reynold's (1991) theory of the "1-2 Punch" of the technocracy. Punch 1: Technologically intervene in a natural process to improve it, thereby mutilating it

---

1 Please note that throughout this book, we will not be using the commonly employed term "cesarean section" but rather "cesarean" or "cesarean births" (CBs), to index the fact that these are births, and that those who experience cesareans are not simply passive but actively cope with what is happening to them on the operating table. According to Melissa Cheyney, current editor of *Birth: Issues in Perinatal Care*, this change in terminology reflects the rapid changes in the social sciences of reproduction that often stem from consumer demand (personal communication, August 2020).

and causing harm. Punch 2: Prosthetically fix the damage done with more technology (see Chapter 1). In this 1-2 Punch of mutilation and prosthesis, Reynolds insisted that *Punch 2 is the point*: we believe that we improve on a natural process, such as childbirth, when we fix its perceived dysfunctions with technology; hence the large numbers of technological interventions in labor and birth.

In the humanistic paradigm, the body is viewed as an organism, the focus is on the birthing woman, and kind and compassionate, relationship-based care prevails. Robbie (Davis-Floyd 2001, 2018) is careful to distinguish between *superficial humanism*, in which many interventions are still performed but with a compassionate overlay, and *deep humanism*, in which the normal physiology of birth is facilitated and the childbearer's emotional needs are addressed.

The holistic model goes deeply into the realm of the spiritual and the intuitive: the body is viewed as an energy field in constant interaction with the other energy fields around it, and the outcome of a birth can be facilitated by paying attention to the energy surrounding it and changing that energy if needed—for example, by sending someone with "negative" energy out of the birthing room, or helping the laboring person to dance, to laugh, to cry if needed, or to chant or sing. Most homebirth midwives in the US perceive an energetic connection between the throat and the cervix—if the throat is tight and closed, the cervix will be too. So they encourage the laboring person to chant or make deep guttural sounds that open the throat so the cervix can follow (Davis-Floyd et al. 2018; Chapter 13). It is within this holistic paradigm that "calling the baby" makes sense: many midwives believe that when a baby does not immediately breathe after birth, its spirit or soul is hovering on the brink, trying to make the decision to come into the body or remain on the other side. Many midwives believe that having the parents immediately call the baby before or during resuscitation can make all the difference in that choice. Robbie (Davis-Floyd 2018) shows that holism in birth, which mainly characterizes births at home or in freestanding birth centers where the midwifery model of care—a combination of the humanistic and holistic models—can prevail, is highly economically and racially stratified, as most such care has to be paid for out of pocket, and thus remains inaccessible to many—unless the community midwives in question are covered by insurance, as indeed they all should be.

These three paradigms—technocratic, humanistic, and holistic—though not necessarily mentioned in all chapters, set the ideological tone of our book, as the chapters in Part I are generally grounded in the technocratic approach to birthing techno-sapiens, while those in Part II are more grounded in the humanistic and holistic approaches to creating this new planetary species in the Anthropocene Era.

Eco-Obstetrics or the Technological Imperative?

Thus herein we ask such questions as: What will be midwives' roles in the future of birth? Will they become the primary attendants for the vast majority of births, with obstetricians reserved for the truly high-risk cases—as the scientific evidence would demand? (Chalmers 2017:156). Can technocratic obstetrics be transformed into eco-obstetrics, or holistic obstetrics, or at least humanistic obstetrics, as the authors envisage in Chapters 13 and 14? What will we do with our knowledge and ability to perform cesareans (Chapter 9)? Will we replace these with practices that honor water birth or vagal nerve stimulation (Chapters 12–13)? Will home birth again take a place of prominence as statistics continue to demonstrate its safety? (See Cheyney et al. 2014; de Jonge et al. 2009, 2015). This question is especially pertinent in light of the recent coronavirus pandemic, during which homebirth rates rapidly rose in many countries, along with births in freestanding birth centers, as women sought to avoid the contagion of the hospital and separation from their partners and doulas (see Davis-Floyd, Gutschow, and Schwartz 2020). Will that trend continue as more women come to realize the advantages of avoiding the non-evidence-based technological surveillance and frequent interventions in labor and birth that characterize hospital birth "management"? Can more women learn to let go of their fear of birth (described in Chapters 9 and 13) and simply flow with the physiologic process, supported by midwives and doulas?

Or must we continue to follow the technological imperative—*if you can do it with technology, you must and will do it with technology* (Davis-Floyd 2003)—ending up with normal vaginal birth a distant species memory? Who will we be then? We keep climbing up the technological ladder, clearing more and more land to build our cities and towns and polluting our environments with pesticides and chemicals, with disastrous consequences to our own health, massive species extinctions (Wallace-Wells 2020), and the Climate Crisis (see Chapter 16 and Conclusions)—so we wonder, can we find "a prosperous way down," as Odem and Odem (2001) suggest?

We also ask, how will our newly emerging knowledge of assisted reproduction impact religion, science, society, kinship, and family life? What does egg freezing mean to us today and tomorrow? Will it liberate women to achieve their career goals before having children, and/or will it result in more cesarean births for women coded as "high-risk" because of their advanced age? Regarding genetic editing, which is increasingly becoming possible (Chapters 4, 6, 7), will it only be used benignly to eliminate devastating hereditary diseases? Or for other purposes, such as creating enhanced humans? Where do we draw the line on that?

As shown in Chapter 7, the academic "assumed consensus" on refraining from creating actual pregnancies from genetically edited embryos was broken by a Chinese scientist in 2018, resulting in the births of cyborgian twins. His work was roundly condemned and he was imprisoned, yet if the technological imperative holds, others, somewhere, someday, will do the same. And then where will the line be drawn? Will political systems manipulate genes to achieve genocidal goals, or implement ethnic cleansing, as happened in the Nazi era—as exposed in Beverley's multiple-award-winning book *Birth, Sex and Abuse: Women's Voices under Nazi Rule* (Chalmers 2015)? Could fearful perceptions in some societies that have suffered from mass sterilizations make people believe these are still happening, as in the Quechua of Peru (Chapter 10)? Or, as discussed in Chapter 17, will we be able to learn from utopian reproductive creations such as those shown in the *Star Trek* film and television series and emerge as better people? We are asking these questions here as binaries, yet our chapters provide nuanced answers. Herein we provide fantastical yet achievable imaginaries based on current understandings of the normal physiology of birth that should, in fact, come to pass, and make recommendations for how that can happen (Chapters 11–17).

Background: A Brief Review of Relevant Literature

We are not the first or only authors to address these issues; in fact, so many have that it is impossible to address all of them here. Many such books are case studies of individual reproductive phenomena or of reproduction in particular countries or sites. We focus here on the broader, more popular works in the public field, and particularly on *Cyborg Babies: From Techno-Sex to Techno-Tots* (Davis-Floyd and Dumit 1998), as that was our takeoff point for this present volume. This scholarly work found its own popular audience: it was voted one of the Top 25 Books of 1998 by the *Village Voice*. *Cyborg Babies* mixes many considerations and treatments of technology to describe and analyze the increasing cyborgification of the American child, from conception through birth and beyond, and also considers a possible spiritual, holistic future, demonstrating, as previously noted, that cyborgs can be as organic as they are technological.

Robbie's chapter in *Cyborg Babies*, "Reflections on the Emergent Discourse of a Holistic Anthropologist," illustrates her struggle with the paradigmatic dilemmas posed by her personal engagements with cyborg anthropology and the resistance to the cyborgification of birth embodied by the midwives and homebirthers with whom she is ideologically aligned. Robbie's first birth, in 1979, was via a medically unnecessary cesarean; during the operation, numbed by an epidural, she experienced herself as a disembodied head. In her *Cyborg Babies* chapter, she details this experience and laments that she was not then familiar with the concept of the cyborg, as she thinks that had she been, during the operation, instead of feeling totally disempowered, she could have empowered herself by intellectually musing on the cyborg she had clearly become. Yet the experience, though traumatic for Robbie, showed her that in fact she lived too much in her head, in disconnection from her body. So she spent the next 4 years learning various techniques of mind-body integration, and then in 1984 gave birth at home to a 10-pound baby boy, Jason. So much for the "cephalo-pelvic disproportion" she was diagnosed with during her first birth—that cyborg baby born via CS, her daughter Peyton, weighed only 7 pounds. Given her move into a more holistic way of life, in her chapter she ponders her ongoing fascination with Science and Technology Studies (STS) and her move into Cyborg Anthropology, which led to her conceiving the concept to create *Cyborg Babies*, along with Joe Dumit, when they happened to find themselves in the same, highly engaging session at an STS conference.

In the Introduction to *Cyborg Babies* (Dumit and Davis-Floyd 1998:8) and in Robbie's chapter (Davis-Floyd 1998:273), Robbie and Joe identify 6 types of uses of the concept of cyborgs at work:

1. The cyborg as positive technoscientific progress;
2. The cyborg as mutilator of natural processes;
3. The cyborg as neutral analytical tool and metaphor for all human-techno-logical inter-relationships;
4. The cyborg as signifier of contemporary, postmodern times in which human relations with technoscience have changed for better and for worse;
5. The cyborg as oppressor;
6. The cyborg as liberator.

In this present volume, all of these concepts are relevant. The chapters in Part I focus more on 1, 2, 3, and 5, while the chapters in Part II focus more on 4 and 6. All chapters use 3—the cyborg as analytical tool and metaphor—though we substitute the term "techno-sapiens" for "cyborg"—as "techno-sapiens" indicates that we are creating an entirely new species, which is our major point in this book, along with illustrating the many and varied ways in which that is happening and their present and futuristic meanings and implications.

Of course, other texts and events have contributed to our development of the techno-sapiens concept. In the mid-1990s, the international community pronounced prenatal sex selection via abortion an "act of violence against women" and "unethical" (Avakyan 2015). At the same time, new developments in reproductive technology in the US led to a method of preconception sex selection, which occurs just after fertilization, by means of IVF combined with pre-implantation genetic diagnosis (PGD), and aiming at a selective transfer of an embryo of the desired sex (Wert and Dondorp 2010). Its US inventor marketed the practice as "family balancing" and defended it with the rhetoric of "freedom of choice." In *Gender before Birth: Sex Selection in a Transnational Context* (2018), Rajani Bhatia takes on the double standard of how similar practices in the Global North and Global South are divergently named and framed.

In 2002, Gregory Stock published the highly popular *Redesigning Humans: Choosing our Genes, Changing our Future*. He posited that as scientists rapidly improve their ability to identify and manipulate genes, people will want to protect their future children from genetically transmitted diseases, help them live longer, and even influence their looks and abilities. Stock insisted that neither governments nor religious groups will be able to stop the coming trend of choosing an embryo's genes. While his predictions have not yet reached fruition, abundant signs and some of the chapters in our book suggest they are well on their way. Recent developments in biotechnology and genetic research are raising complex ethical questions concerning the legitimate scope and limits of genetic intervention. In *The Future of Human Nature* (Polity 2003), Jurgen Habermas showed that as we begin to contemplate the possibility of intervening in the human genome to prevent diseases, we cannot help but feel that the human species might be able to take its biological evolution into its own hands. "Playing God" is the metaphor commonly used for this self-transformation of the species, which, it seems, might eventually be within our grasp.

A decade after his now-famous pronouncement of "the end of history," Francis Fukuyama argues in *Our Post-Human Future: Consequences of the Biotechnology Revolution* (2003) that as a result of biomedical advances, we are facing the possibility of a future in which our humanity will be altered beyond recognition. Fukuyama sketches a brief history of man's changing understanding of human nature: from Plato and Aristotle to modernity's utopian and dystopian dictators who sought—and seek—to remake humankind for ideological ends. Fukuyama argues that the ability to manipulate DNA will have profound, and potentially terrible, consequences for our political order, even if undertaken with the best of intentions. He describes how genetic "enhancement" could seriously challenge the foundation of democracy: the belief that human beings are equal by nature.

Also in 2003, a report by the President's Council on Bioethics, *Beyond Therapy: Biotechnology and the Pursuit of Happiness* revealed the promises and perils of biotechnology for the future of American society. Biotechnology offers exciting prospects for healing the sick and relieving suffering. But because our growing powers also enable alterations in the workings of the body and mind, they are becoming attractive to healthy people who would just like to look younger, perform better, feel happier, or become more "perfect." With frequency, news appears of novel methods for screening genes and testing embryos, choosing the sex and modifying the behavior of children, enhancing athletic performance, slowing aging, blunting painful memories, brightening mood, and altering basic temperaments. But this report also asks the fundamental question: Should we be turning to biotechnology—or biohacking (see Chapters 7 and 10)—to fulfill our deepest human desires?

Some of these issues are further examined by Ronald Green in his book *Babies by Design: The Ethics of Genetic Choice* (2007). Noting that ARTs now enable parents to select some genetic traits for their children, Green argues, as we do, that soon it will be possible to intentionally shape ourselves as a species. Yet Green goes further, insisting that we will—and should—undertake the direction of our own evolution. Green maintains that fears of a terrible "brave new world" or a new eugenics movement are overblown, and that in the more likely future, genetic modifications may not only improve parents' ability to enhance children's lives but may even be able to promote social justice.

This more optimistic view of "cyborgs as technoscientific progress" (Davis-Floyd and Dumit 1998:8) is reinforced by Lee Silver's (2007) *Remaking Eden: How Genetic Engineering and Cloning Will Transform the American Family*, which takes a cautiously optimistic look at the scientific advances that will allow us to engineer life in ways that were unimaginable just a few short years ago—indeed, in ways that go far beyond cloning. In the same year, an even more cautious argument was put forward by Michael J. Sandel (2007) in *The Case against Perfection: Ethics in the Age of Genetic Engineering*. He acknowledged both the promises and predicaments of genetic engineering, which include preventing genetic diseases and dealing with our potential will to enhance our genetic traits and those of our children. Sandel contends that the genetic revolution will change how philosophers discuss ethics and will force spiritual questions back onto the political agenda.

Evolutionary biologist Scott Solomon (2016) draws on the explosion of discoveries in recent years to examine *Future Humans: Inside the Science of Our Continuing Evolution*. Combining knowledge of our past with current trends, Solomon offers convincing evidence that evolutionary forces still affect us today, asking how will modernization—including longer lifespans, changing diets, global travel, and widespread use of medicine and contraceptives—affect our evolutionary future? Drawing on fields from genomics to medicine and the study of our microbiome, Solomon discusses topics ranging from the rise of online dating and cesareans to the spread of diseases such as HIV and Ebola, and suggests that we are entering a new phase in human evolutionary history—one that makes the future less predictable, more interesting, and more dangerous than ever before. And indeed, the 2020 coronavirus pandemic has proven this to be true.

In perhaps the most powerful of the books we briefly address here, *A Crack in Creation: Gene Editing and the Unthinkable Power to Control Evolution* (2017), Doudna and Sternberg address the most up-to-date concerns regarding gene editing. Not since the atomic bomb has a technology so alarmed its inventors that they warned the world about its use. But in 2015, biologist Jennifer Doudna, who later won a Nobel Prize for her work, called for a worldwide moratorium on the use of the gene-editing tool CRISPR—a revolutionary new technology that she helped create to make heritable changes in human embryos. The cheapest, simplest, most effective way of manipulating DNA ever known, CRISPR may well give us the cure to HIV, genetic diseases, and some cancers. Yet, as noted above, even the tiniest changes to DNA could have myriad, unforeseeable consequences. Writing with fellow researcher Sam Sternberg, Doudna shares the story of her discovery and describes the enormous responsibility that comes with the power to rewrite "the code of life." Interestingly, Doudna acknowledges her appreciation of lessons from *Star Trek*, which are addressed in this volume's final chapter.

A Brief Overview of the Contents of This Volume

Part I, "From Biocultural Evolution to Human-Technology Co-Evolution," focuses on the technological aspects of human-technology co-evolution and their futuristic implications. Key topics in Part I include the transition from human biocultural evolution to human-technology co-evolution; the futuristic implications of the global cesarean epidemic; ectogenesis—growing babies in artificial wombs; egg freezing, cyborg eggs, and embryos; *culturing technology* via in vitro gametogenesis—studying stem cells as a future assisted reproductive technology (ART); the possibilities for editing the human genome and their futuristic implications; and Indigenous views of biomedical contraceptives as producing futuristic "monsters."

Taking as a given that cyborgs can be as organic as they are technological, Part II, "Imagining Techno-Holistic Reproductive Futures," builds on the holistic, emotional, psychological, and spiritual possibilities of the future of techno-sapiens. Key topics addressed in Part II include adapting obstetric technologies for better birth; water as a futuristic birthing technology; the Soviet water birth movement's efforts to create a new, more intelligent, intuitive, and spiritual meta-human/dolphin being; family-centered, evidence-based, psychosocially sensitive, culturally respectful futuristic maternity care; reconceptualizing risk to imagine home birth as the futuristic norm, made essential by the Climate Crisis and the increasing (un)natural disasters that accompany it; the human nervous system, polyvagal theory, and co-regulation: the futuristic importance of making women feel safe and supported during labor and birth; and *Star Trek* birth: surrogacy, androids, holograms, genetic engineering, cloning, selective breeding, and reproducing artificial intelligence. Technological innovation regarding reproduction is fascinating in *Star Trek*, but even more important is the humanism and holism that supersedes such technologies in the *Star Trek* creations.

In addition to summarizing what we have learned from our chapters, our Conclusions also address the devastating male-female population imbalance in some countries resulting from aborting female fetuses, and the futuristic implications of the Climate Crisis for birthing and living as techno-sapiens.

In sum, the world of reproductive health, and particularly that of genetic engineering, is developing exponentially, and current challenges are vastly different from those of a decade ago. Most available books specialize in one aspect of the future of reproduction; ours is multidisciplinary, encompassing not only science and medicine, but also philosophy, psychology, sociology, anthropology, and politics. Most books in this field are decidedly US-centric or Global North-centric, while this book encompasses a global perspective that includes South Africa, Russia, Canada, the UK, the Netherlands, India, New Zealand, and the US. Our inclusion of a diversity of cultural settings is a particular strength of this collection, forming an important corrective. In addition, no other books in this field, with the exceptions of *Cyborg Babies* and *The Case Against Perfection*, address futuristic possibilities for holistic or spiritual evolution, or for more humanistic and organic means of reproduction, while half of our book is about such possibilities. Our chapters go far beyond a techno-optimism vs. techno-pessimism stance to address the nuances and complexities of thinking about techno-sapiens. In this book, like the Starship Enterprise, we seek to "boldly go where no one has gone before."

Acknowledgment

Robbie Davis-Floyd sincerely thanks her colleague Beverley Chalmers for her careful editing of each chapter, the speed with which she turned them around, and her overall support of this joint project. Beverley did not wish to be listed as my official co-editor, but in fact she generously served as such throughout the creation of this volume, and I am deeply grateful! Together we thank our chapter authors for their brilliance, dedication, and futuristic thinking.

References

Avakyan Y. 2015. "Prenatal Sex Selection: A Problem of Violence against Women." https://berkleycenter.georgetown.edu/posts/prenatal-sex-selection-a-problem-of-violence-against-women.

Bhatia R. 2018. *Gender before Birth: Sex Selection in a Transnational Context*. Seattle: University of Washington Press.

Chalmers B. 2015. *Birth, Sex and Abuse: Women's Voices Under Nazi Rule*. United Kingdom: Grosvenor House Publishers.

Chalmers B. 2017. *Family-Centred Perinatal Care: Improving Pregnancy, Birth and Postpartum Care*. Cambridge: Cambridge University Press.

Cheyney M, et al. 2014. "Outcomes of Care for 16,924 Planned Home Births in the United States: The Midwives Alliance of North America Statistics Project, 2004 to 2009." *Journal of Midwifery & Women's Health* 59(1):17–27.

Clynes M, Kline N. 1960. Cyborgs and Space. *Astronautics* 14(9):26–27.

Davis-Floyd R. 2003 [1992]. *Birth as an American Rite of Passage*, 2nd edition. Berkeley: University of California Press.

Davis-Floyd R. 1998. "Reflection on the Emergent Discourse of a Holistic Anthropologist." In: *Cyborg Babies: From Techno-Sex to Techno-Tots*. Eds. Davis-Floyd R, Dumit J. New York: Routledge, 255–284.

Davis-Floyd R. 2000. "Commercializing Outer Space: The SATWG Stories." In: *Late Editions VII, Para-Sites*. Ed Marcus G. Chicago: University of Chicago Press.

Davis-Floyd R. 2001. "The Technocratic, Humanistic, and Holistic Models of Birth." *International Journal of Gynecology & Obstetrics* 75(Supplement No. 1):S5–S23.

Davis-Floyd R. 2018. "The Technocratic, Humanistic, and Holistic Paradigms of Birth and Health Care." In: *Ways of Knowing about Birth: Mothers, Midwives, Medicine, and Birth Activism* by Davis-Floyd R Long Grove, IL: Waveland Press, 3–44.

Davis-Floyd R, Davis E. 2018. "Intuition as Authoritative Knowledge in Midwifery and Homebirth." In: *Ways of Knowing about Birth: Mothers, Midwives, Medicine, and Birth Activism* by Davis-Floyd R. Long Grove, IL: Waveland Press, 189–220.

Davis-Floyd R, Dumit J, eds. 1998. *Cyborg Babies: From Techno-Sex to Techno-Tots*. New York: Routledge.

Davis-Floyd R, Georges E. 2018. "The Paradigm Shift of Humanistic and Holistic Obstetricians." In: *Ways of Knowing about Birth: Mothers, Midwives, Medicine, and Birth Activism* by Davis-Floyd R. Long Grove, IL: Waveland Press, 141–164.

Davis-Floyd R, Gutschow K, Schwartz DA. 2020. "Pregnancy, Birth, and the COVID-19 Pandemic in the United States." *Medical Anthropology* 39(5):413–427.

Davis-Floyd R, Matsuoka E, Horan H, Ruder B, Everson CL. 2018. "Daughter of Time: The Postmodern Midwife." In: *Ways of Knowing about Birth: Mothers, Midwives, Medicine, and Birth Activism* by Davis-Floyd R. Long Grove, IL: Waveland Press, 221–264.

de Jonge A et al. 2009. "Perinatal Mortality and Morbidity in a Nationwide Cohort of 529,688 Low-Risk Planned Home and Hospital Births." *BJOG: An International Journal of Obstetrics & Gynecology* 116(9): 1177–1184. doi:10.1111/j1471-0528.2009.02175.x/full.

de Jonge A et al. 2015. "Perinatal Mortality and Morbidity up to 28 Days after Birth among 743,070 Low-Risk Planned Home and Hospital Births: A Cohort Study Based on Three Merged National Perinatal Databases. " *BJOG: An International Journal of Obstetrics & Gynecology* 122(5):720–728.

Doudna JA, Sternberg SH. 2017. *A Crack in Creation: Gene Editing and the Unthinkable Power to Control Evolution.* New York: Houghton Mifflin Harcourt.

Dumit J, Davis-Floyd R. 1998. "Cyborg Babies: Children of the Third Millennium." In: *Cyborg Babies: From Techno-Sex to Techno-Tots.* eds. Davis-Floyd R, Dumit J. New York: Routledge, 1–20.

Fukuyama F. 2003. *Our Post-Human Future: Consequences of the Biotechnology Revolution.* Picador.

Green R. 2007. *Babies by Design: The Ethics of Genetic Choice.* New York: Yale University Press.

Habermas J. 2003. *The Future of Human Nature.* New York: Polity.

Haraway D. 1991. "A Cyborg Manifesto." In: *Simians, Cyborgs, and Women: The Reinvention of Nature* by Haraway D. New York: Routledge, 149–182.

Odem EC, Odem H. 2001. *A Prosperous Way Down: Principles and Policies.* Boulder: University of Colorado Press.

Reynolds PC. 1991. *Stealing Fire: The Mythology of the Technocracy.* Palo Alto: California Iconic Anthropology Press.

Sandel M. 2007. *The Case Against Perfection: Ethics in the Age of Genetic Engineering.* Cambridge: Belknap Press.

Silver L. 2007. *Remaking Eden: How Genetic Engineering and Cloning Will Transform the American Family.* New York: HarperCollins Books.

Solomon S. 2016. *Future Humans: Inside the Science of Our Continuing Evolution.* New Haven: Yale University Press.

Urban Dictionary. 2020. *Definition of Techno Sapiens.* www.urbandictionary.com/define.php?term=Techno.

Wallace-Wells D. 2020. *The Uninhabitable Earth: Life after Warming.* New York: Tim Duggan Books.

Wert G, Dondorp W. 2010. "Preconception Sex Selection for Non-Medical and Intermediate Reasons: Ethical Reflections." *Facts Views Vis Obgyn* 2(4):267–277. PMCID: PMC4086011. PMID: 25009714.

PART I

From Biocultural Evolution to Human-Technology Co-Evolution

1

BIRTH AND THE BIG BAD WOLF:

Biocultural Evolution and Human Childbirth

Melissa Cheyney and Robbie Davis-Floyd

Introduction: Let Us Tell You a Story

Folklorists, anthropologists, and oral historians have long understood that myths and folktales can condense millennia of historical events into stories that are transmitted from one generation to the next; they are, in essence, forms of stored and transmittable collective memory. Many myths are creation or origin narratives that explain—for the people who experience their cultural lives in terms of those stories—who they are, where they came from, what values they hold, and how they are to live their lives. Myths give coherence and meaning to the lives we live by situating our existence within a larger, cosmological context (Davis-Floyd and Laughlin 2016).

For example, Robbie, trained in both anthropology and folklore, figured out many years ago that the Genesis creation myth could be interpreted as an encapsulation of the transitions made by many human groups from foraging to large-scale agriculture. In *The Power of Ritual* (Davis-Floyd and Laughlin 2016), she argued that this myth conveys the stories of hunters and gatherers who, metaphorically speaking, lived in the Garden of Eden—an abundant natural environment. Eventually hunter-gatherers over-foraged in some areas, thereby straining their environmental carrying capacities, so adapted by cultivating, planting, and plowing. This much more labor-intensive agricultural lifestyle is metaphorized in the story of Adam and Eve being "cast out of the Garden," with Adam then having to live "by the sweat of his brow" as he planted the fields, while Eve was forced to give birth in pain as punishment for her "original sin" of eating fruit from a forbidden tree. Eve's story reflects the intensely patriarchal structure of early Hebrew society, passed down through millennia, and of other subsequent similarly powerful and patriarchal religions.

Because myths and stories/folktales have played central roles in human cultural development, we begin our exploration of evolutionary perspectives on childbirth with a creative re-telling of a well-known folktale, "The Three Little Pigs and the Big Bad Wolf." We use this story to convey the major cultural transformations in human subsistence strategies that have occurred around the world over time, and thus were encoded in collective memory and preserved through storytelling. Below in our own re-imagining of the "Three Little Pigs," we place particular emphasis on the role of the Wolf, whom we have employed as a metaphor for the uncontrollable, and therefore often frightening, aspects of the natural world that ritual, storytelling, and technological innovation attempt to keep at bay. We have gendered the Wolf as male in keeping with how he is traditionally depicted, but also to challenge the powerful cross-cultural binary that often equates women with nature and submission, and men with culture and dominance (Martin 1987; Ortner 1974). Events attributed to nature such as diseases, floods, droughts, storms, and normal healthy processes like childbirth can all be experienced as challenges or threats "knocking at our doors." Human culture shapes how we respond to and attempt to understand and control unpredictable and uncontrollable aspects of our natural world, and these attempts have implications not only for how we subsist, but also for how we give birth.

Our re-telling of this ancient folktale diverges from the traditional story in that we describe *six* little groups of pigs who represent each of the basic subsistence strategies engaged in by humans: (1) foraging/hunting-gathering; (2) horticulture; (3) agriculture; (4) pastoralism; (5) industrialism; and (6) technocracy—all of which have to deal with the Big Bad Wolf/Nature as their members navigate their daily needs and give birth to the children upon whose existence their future depends. We base our re-imagined story on anthropological findings about the lives of people engaged in these subsistence strategies. While many anthropologists might list only the first five, we have included the post-industrial technocratic societies many live in today as a sixth subsistence strategy because we believe they are qualitatively different from earlier periods or stages of industrialism. We do take some liberties with over-simplifications and over-generalizations, as our aim in this retelling is not to covey the complex and context-dependent details of global subsistence transitions, but rather to highlight the dramatic shift in birthing practices that accompanied the Industrial Revolution and further intensified as technocratic societies emerged. So please, sit back, and let us tell you a story.

The Six Little Pigs and the Big Bad Wolf: An Anthropological Tale

Once upon a time, many millennia ago, there was a small band of little pigs somewhere in Africa who set out to seek their fortunes. As they journeyed, they picked the fruit from the trees, the grains from the ground, the fish from the rivers and seas, and followed the big game animals in their seasonal migrations. Each night, no matter how tired they were from walking, they built houses of straw to have a home base, sometimes staying in the same place for a while, sometimes moving on rapidly. To these temporary homes they brought the results of their 3–5 hours of foraging, for that was usually all it took to find plenty of food for the day. The female pigs fished, trapped small animals, and gathered wild grains, tubers, edible insects, and fruits, so that food was available even if the males' hunting failed. Although the first little pigs didn't much like to admit it, the female pigs brought in 70%–80% of the diet, and often helped with the hunting as well, since any strict sexual division of labor often broke down out of necessity.

Giving birth went smoothly most of the time, but when labor was difficult, midwives were available to assist. They passed their skills on to others, so each new generation learned from elder midwives, as well as from birth itself. The first little pigs were feeling content, for they had wished to find an environment that could sustain their small band of 25–30 kin pigs, and they had.

Sure, these bands experienced high infant mortality rates and a resulting mean life expectancy of around 35 years, as well as high death rates from endemic disease and accidental death, and, occasionally, from problems in birth. However, as they discussed frequently in their abundant leisure time (in between the long stories they loved to tell, many of which were later written down by anthropologists fascinated by foraging societies), these concerns were offset by their varied and nutritious diets, low population densities, and high mobility, which made sanitation and infectious disease transmission non-issues. They simply moved away when waste began to accumulate. Life was good, always interesting, and gender relationships were mostly, but not always, egalitarian.

The first little pigs were so successful at their hunting and gathering that after a couple hundred thousand years, under growing population pressure, necessity was combined with the knowledge of plant life cycles developed during millennia of gathering to create a new subsistence strategy—small-scale horticulture. Since they already knew that they could plant food where they wanted it to grow, the second group of little pigs headed along the human subsistence transition road and began to fell trees and to plant gardens to supplement foods that could still be foraged. Rather than just finding food, they also began to produce it.

Subsistence work was harder and longer; it took 5–6 hours a day, though there was still plenty of leisure time. The female horticultural pigs did much of the work—planting, cultivating, harvesting, and processing the food they grew. They generally birthed their babies communally, benefiting like their predecessors from the knowledge of their midwives. They also chopped wood and carried water, while the male pigs generally spent their time hunting and performing the rituals that connected them to their ancestors and assured them that all would remain well. They built their houses of sticks because they were semi-nomadic, moving their villages every five years or so as garden soil and large game populations were depleted. Their diet was highly varied and population densities still low enough to keep infectious disease in check. While the seeds of gender inequality and patriarchy were sown along with the first domesticated plants, for the most part, life was good for the horticultural groups.

Eventually, along came the third little pigs, who were horrified at their ancestor pigs' lack of industriousness. They knew the danger these tribes were facing from the Big Bad Wolf, and that houses made of straw and sticks stood no chance should the Wolf try to huff and puff and blow their houses down. So they moved further away from the Wolf's territory, until they found a nice flat field good for planting, near a large river. They set to work building themselves sturdy houses of wood and stones that the Wolf could not blow down, and digging irrigation canals to water the large fields they planted, which they would have to work 8–10 hours per day "by the sweat of their brows." Soon they planted more food than their families needed so they could barter or sell it, eventually developing a cash economy and paying or bullying pigs farther down in the emerging social hierarchy to work the fields.

Sure, there was less variability in what they had to eat, as they could focus only on a few staple crops such as barley, soy, rice, wheat, or corn. However, with the availability of safe weaning foods, female pigs could nurse for shorter periods of time, allowing for shorter interbirth intervals so more little pigs could be born to work the fields and build communities.

Unfortunately, standing water in the irrigation canals became a vector for mosquito-borne diseases like malaria, and lack of sanitation and its accompanying epidemics of infectious disease became major problems. The occasional crop failures could mean starvation for many. Yet agriculturalist pigs could also acquire possessions, own land, and rise to the tops of social hierarchies, especially where sow production and reproduction could be exploited. The third little pigs were sure that they were much safer from the Big Bad Wolf than their ancestral pigs, many of whose descendants continued to live in the forests or wild savannas where danger lurked. Life was good for small groups of pigs who had learned how to exploit others to their own benefit.

Birth was still communal and cooperative among sows in agricultural societies, and midwives in settled farming communities had many opportunities to learn from each other and to continue developing their skills—although during the witch hunts in Europe and North America (1500s–1700s), they did experience horrific persecution. Many thousands of midwives, other healers, the poor, and even children were tortured and executed until the craze finally passed.

Some of the fourth little pigs watched with resentment as intensive agriculture took over the most fertile land and armies fought to keep others out. Their desire to roam reflected the foraging legacy of wanderlust. They wove goat hair tents, and began herding animals through agricultural territory, exploiting high hills, low valleys, the wild steppes and plains, and developing humankind's fourth subsistence strategy—pastoralism—while very much enjoying their freedom. Because male pigs tended to own, care for, and manage the herds, and because they often had to fight for rights of passage through agricultural lands, pastoral warrior cultures developed that enhanced male pig power. Their domination of the animals they herded tended to be reflected in other aspects of social organization—including the near universality of patrilineal decent, patrilocal residence patterns, and sometimes segregation of the sexes. Life was good for the male pigs, but symbolic and social stratification by gender spelled trouble for females, especially where strict honor codes and the exchange of females as chattel challenged or entirely did away with female pig autonomy. Little is known about birth in early pastoral societies, though there are some references to birthing stools, suggesting that birth occurred in an upright position as it had for many thousands of years.

The fifth little pigs were sure they could improve on matters further. Farming could be industrialized, and by moving into cities and building large tenements made of bricks and cement that could sustain huge population densities, a workforce would be available to modify the fruits of agricultural labor into "value-added" products produced in large factories for sale under a capitalistic economic system. Yes, severe exploitation of piglets, enslaved groups, and recent immigrants would seem necessary to those in power, and infectious disease rates would rise, especially where sanitation and food quality were poor, but some small number of pigs could also amass huge stores of material wealth, especially where they owned the means of production.

With eventual improvements in sanitation, basic public health interventions, and an intentional decrease in family size as children became more expensive to raise, life expectancy rose, providing a long lifetime over which to satisfy the intense need to buy the products of industrialization. Life was good for a few of the fifth little pigs, but the masses were poor and exploited—an unfortunate yet presumed inevitable accompaniment to the rise of capitalism. Birth was also industrialized and standardized as it was moved from communities into hospitals where it could be controlled and regulated. Nature was being tamed, but thousands paid the price, laboring in industrial hospitals created to accommodate large numbers of births, where disease transmission was common and puerperal fever became one of the major causes of maternal pig death.

The sixth little technocratic pigs were so far removed from nature that they had lost all sense of its value and devoted themselves to inventing complex technologies, building gleaming cities of concrete and glass and paving over most things green. They and the many friends they had met through social media developed a technocratic society organized around a capitalistic ideology of progress through the development of high technology and the global flow of information. Beginning just a few decades ago, the forces of globalization, consumerism, and neocolonialism transformed even the most remote agriculturalists into dependents in an exploitative, global economy that produced vast inequities between high and low-resource nations. The sixth little pigs and a few of their elite investor friends benefited, while many others struggled to access even the most basic of resources. Soon environmentalist pigs began to notice that the nature that they had worked so hard to tame through technology was turning on them as industrialization heated the planet, melted the glaciers, and polluted the atmosphere and oceans.

And sure enough, the Big Bad Wolf did in fact show up in the form of the Climate Catastrophe, and via tsunamis and superstorms he huffed, and he puffed, and he blew down the few remaining houses of the first five little pigs, whose descendants all came running over to the houses of their distant, technocratic cousins, who rather than letting them in, separated parents and children and locked them in detention centers. Having slammed their doors just in time, the sixth little pigs found themselves safe within their McMansions far from the Big Bad Wolf, as well as from the masses who might critique their elitism. However, because love is stronger than hate, it was only a matter of time before the sixth little pigs too would come to their senses.

Eventually they came to see that the ways of living in earlier centuries had caused far less ecological damage than was occurring in industrial and late-modern technocratic societies. They did not want to give up their cars, computers, and smartphones, nor their settler colonialism, but they did wonder: perhaps there was a larger lesson to be learned from the story of the Big Bad Wolf? Perhaps the fear of nature it generated was preventing more pigs from wanting to respect and revere their natural environment and loosen their desire to control it?

Luckily, several of the little pigs' partners, already feminists, majored in the social sciences and some became midwives. Teaming up with grass roots community organizations, they traveled the world and spent time with social justice advocates in order to learn about where things had gotten off track. They came to realize that how we culturally manage birth is not so distinct from how we treat our planet and each other, and that indeed, childbirth is a lens through which to read the core beliefs and values of a society. While not all traditional birth practices were healthy or promoted justice, many of them were extremely beneficial and could be applied to help overturn the effects of inequality and institutional racism—including that which occurs through industrial and technocratic birth "management"—once, of course, such time-honored techniques had been scientifically (re)proven to work. Together they labored to re-capture ancient midwifery and other traditional knowledges. These knowledges ended up offering powerful correctives to the excesses of the technocracy, including those of technocratic obstetrics.

Evolutionary Medicine and the Discordance Hypothesis

Again, folktales often condense millennia of historical events into one story, as this one does. Humans have lived as hunter-gatherers from the time of our emergence as *Homo sapiens,* perhaps as long as 200,000–400,000 years ago (McDougall et al. 2005; Stringer 2016). The technocratic societies that many of us live and reproduce in today account for less than 1% of human history, and only 1%–2% of our biological makeup has evolved since the ape-human split between 5 and 7 million years ago, meaning that the vast majority of our genes are ancient in origin (Trevathan et al. 2008). While there have certainly been genetic changes since the development of agriculture around 10,000–12,000 years ago (Zuk 2013), the pace of our cultural evolution has generally been much faster than that of our biological evolution. As a result, our 35,000-year-old model bodies are not well-adapted to the technocratic and industrializing cultures many of us now live and birth in today (Armelagos et al. 2005; Eaton et al. 2002).

Evolutionary anthropology has shown us that our current diet, lifestyle, and reproductive patterns are quite different from those that produced the selective pressures under which humans and human childbirth evolved. This mismatch in genes and culture promotes, accelerates, and fosters many health issues, especially those associated with over-eating of highly processed foods that our bodies are ill-equipped to properly digest, under-exercising, and excessively or inappropriately intervening in childbirth (Cheyney 2010; Trevathan 2015; Rosenberg and Trevathan 2018). The notion that discontinuities between the conditions under which humans evolved and the conditions we live in today produce disease is called the *discordance hypothesis,* which forms the foundation for a subfield of Medical Anthropology called Evolutionary Medicine (Williams and Nesse 1991). Proponents of this approach attempt to propose evolutionarily informed solutions or treatments that are often premised on reducing these gaps (i.e., eating a "Paleolithic diet," getting our 10,000 steps per day, using midwives or doulas to support physiologic birth) (ibid.; Gluckman et al. 2016; Trevathan 2017; Rosenberg and Trevathan 2018).

Our approach in this chapter is *co-evolutionary,* meaning that we focus on our "dual-inheritance"—the complex intertwining of our biology and culture over time (Hewlett et al. 2002). We use "biocultural" and "co-evolutionary" throughout to emphasize the interactions between genes, culture, behavior, and unequal relationships of power (Goodman and Leatherman 1998) that combine to produce the cross-cultural birthing patterns we see today—patterns that we argue are far removed from what our evolved biology would predict and require. We also contend that finding ways to decrease the gap between how birth evolved and how the technocracy treats it today can help reduce maternal and neonatal death and suffering globally.

The Biocultural Evolution of Human Childbirth and Obligate Midwifery

Because non-human primates are adapted for quadrupedal locomotion, their pelves are generally wide enough in all diameters to allow for the uncomplicated descent of a relatively small fetal head, making for easier labors and births relative to human primates (Trevathan 2017; Rosenberg 1992) who generally have a much tighter fit. The difficulty of human birth relative to other primates is thought to stem from the so-called "obstetric dilemma" (Stoller 1995; DeSilva et al. 2017)—the conflicting evolutionary pressures on human pelvic morphology. On the one hand, the human pelvis must be wide enough side-to-side and narrow enough front-to-back to allow for efficient bipedalism (Lovejoy 1998). On the other, childbearers require a passageway that is wide, open, rounded, and spacious enough to accommodate the birth of relatively large-brained infants whose heads may be nearly the same size as, or larger than, the maternal pelvis (Figure 1.1).

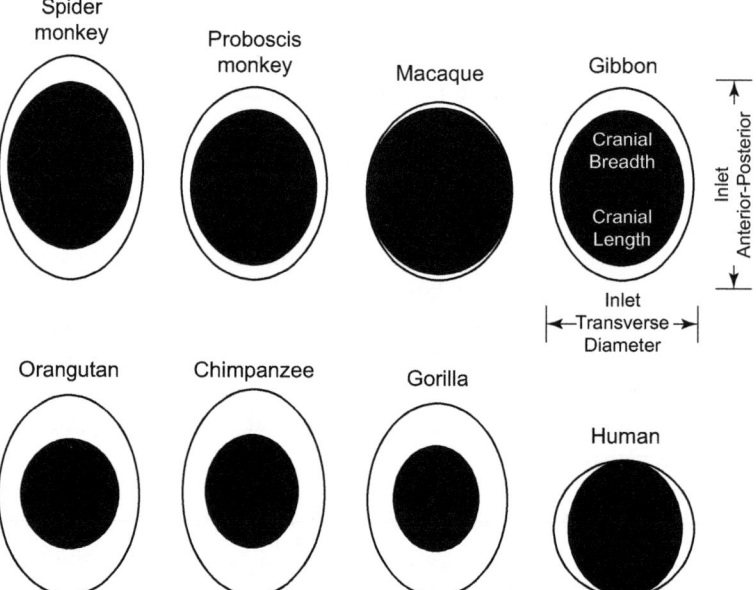

FIGURE 1.1   Relationship of the maternal pelvis size and shape (black outline) to the fetal head size and shape (black ovals). This figure illustrates why birth can take longer and feel so challenging to human mothers (from Trevathan 2010:93). Provided by Trevathan and used with permission.

These competing selective pressures[1] have resulted in an obstetric compromise: human babies must maneuver through a series of complex orientations—called the "cardinal movements" or "mechanisms of delivery"—as they travel through the changing diameters of the birth canal (Trevathan 2015, 2017; Trevathan and Rosenberg 2000) (Figure 1.2). As a result, researchers, with few exceptions (Walrath 2006), have tended to describe human birth as more painful and of longer duration relative to non-human primates, though for healthy mothers and babies, not necessarily more dangerous. Nonhuman primate babies can climb onto their mothers' backs and cling immediately after birth. But the larger brains of human infants made it necessary for them to be born earlier in their developmental cycle (a condition called "secondary altriciality"), ensuring that human babies would be relatively helpless at birth, requiring immediate nurturing. Together these factors encouraged the evolution of birth as a highly social process.

The Sociality of Birth and the Prevalence of Obligate Midwifery

The comparatively difficult nature of childbirth in our species has led researchers (Trevathan 1999; Rosenberg 1992, 2003) to reflect on how our uniquely human obstetric features might have shaped our birthing behaviors and cultural norms over time. For example, while non-human primates usually give birth alone and under the cover of night, human mothers almost always seek out assistance from female relatives, friends, and/or experienced birth attendants. Biological anthropologist Wenda Trevathan (1997, 1999) has reasoned that at some point in human history, the benefits of assisted birth would have outweighed the safety of solitary delivery— a condition she called "obligate midwifery." Trevathan did not argue that no person can ever safely give birth alone, but simply that having someone else present helped enough that over time this behavior was selected for. She found support for this argument in the cross-cultural observation that very few societies idealize unassisted birth. As Jordan noted in her classic *Birth in Four Cultures*: "The physiology of birth

---

1 More recent work on the obstetric dilemma has explored additional selective pressures that may have influenced the complexity of human birth mechanisms (see for example Betti and Manica 2018; Pavličev et al. 2020). Bipedalism may be primarily constrained by the inflexibility of the pubic symphysis (the fixed joint at the front of the pelvic girdle where the halves of the pubis meet) in humans. This joint opens much more widely during birth in most other mammals with large fetuses than it does in humans. Thus, rather than being constrained by bipedalism *per se*, the human birth canal may be constrained by trade-offs between (1) the disadvantages of a narrow pelvis for birth; and (2) its improved support for the abdominal viscera (the organs in the abdominal cavity) and for carrying the weight of a large fetus during the relatively long human gestation period. Gruss and Schmitt have argued that thermoregulation may also have shaped human pelvic morphology and resultant birth mechanics. They assert that "The advent of the modern birth canal...allowed early homo sapiens to deal obstetrically with increases in encephalization while maintaining a narrow body to meet thermoregulatory demands and enhance locomotor performance" (2015:1). Betti and Manica (2018) similarly acknowledge multiple additional evolutionary constraints on the female pelvis, and argue that human women are highly variable in their morphologies of the bony pelvis.

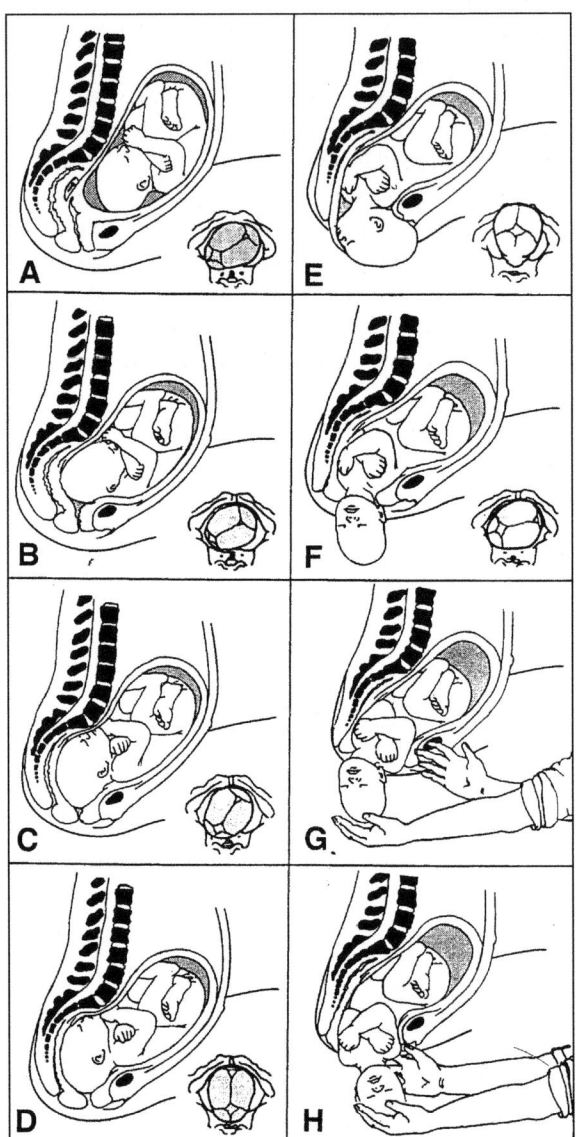

FIGURE 1.2   The "cardinal movements" or "mechanisms of delivery" that a human baby moves through during birth (provided by Wenda Trevathan and used with her permission). The fetus is entering the pelvis in Image A and emerging from the birth canal in Image H. This figure shows how the head moves through the pelvis; the fetal shoulders, which are widest side-to-side, must do the same thing.

and its interactional context (or the sociality of birth and its physiological context) constantly challenge all efforts to separate them" (1993:3). Thus, Jordan stressed the importance of a *biosocial* approach that unites the study of biological aspects of birth with the study of its usually social nature—we say "usually" here because in a very few cultures and subcultures, solitary birth is valued (see for examples Sargent 1989; Shanley 1994; Biesele 1997; Selin and Stone 2009; Miller 2021).

Nevertheless, in general, before birth moved into hospitals, across cultures it tended to be primarily a social event, with community members participating or helping alongside female relatives (see for example Wilson 2016; Tucker 2018). Trevathan (1997) has argued that this condition of "obligate midwifery"—the human tendency toward having a birth attendant—evolved in response to three important differences among the mechanisms of birth in humans relative to other primates: (1) Because human babies almost always emerge facing away from the mother—a position called "occiput anterior"—it is difficult for the mother to reach down, as non-human primates do, to catch the baby, and to clear an airway or remove the umbilical cord from around the infant's neck (Figure 1.3).

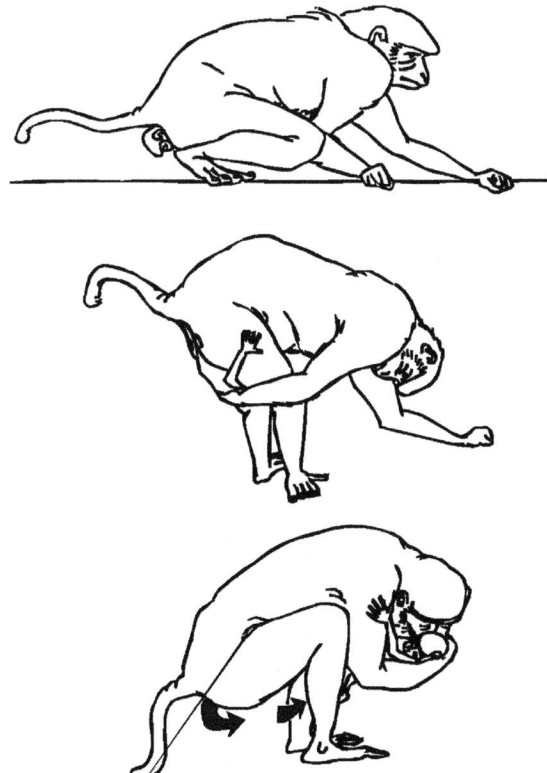

FIGURE 1.3 Solitary, occiput posterior delivery in a nonhuman primate with the mother's response (from Trevathan 2010:95, redrawn from Trevathan 1987). Provided by Trevathan and used with her permission.

(2) Modern humans give birth to *altricial*, or very developmentally immature, infants who require extensive care from the time of birth. The relative helplessness of the human infant may be an additional reason why extra hands at birth contribute to improved reproductive success, especially where mothers are exhausted by particularly long and difficult labors. (3) Trevathan (1997) noted that powerful emotions around labor and birth, including excitement, anxiety, fear, tension, joy, and uncertainty, may have provided the evolutionary impetus for women to seek out support. The emotions of childbirth that encourage birthing people to look for assistance and companionship may be seen as biocultural adaptations to the physiologic challenges that result from multiple, sometimes competing, selective pressures.

Taken together, the core components of human birth—the occiput anterior position of the baby, the altricial nature of human newborns, the powerful emotions surrounding birth, and the gregarious or social nature of humans—likely contributed to its transformation from a solitary event to a highly social enterprise (Figures 1.4 and 1.5), setting humans on a trajectory toward social and cultural interventions in birth (Trevathan 2017).

The Cultural Elaboration of Childbirth: Biomedical Hegemony and the Technocratic Model

The nuances of each culturally constructed birthing system—the dietary taboos, the ideal direction to face during birth, the rituals considered necessary for a successful birth, the first words whispered into the ears of newborn babies—are highly varied. However, a broad, historical view makes far more visible what the birthing systems of hunter-gatherers, horticulturalists, pastoralists, and early agriculturalists had or have in common. Up until the Industrial Age, just 260 years ago, the essential cultural practices associated with childbirth were relatively uniform. Birthing people around the world commonly moved freely during labor, changing positions frequently as a method for managing the pain associated with labor contractions and cervical dilation and to help the baby descend. They ate and drank as they pleased within the cultural confines of what was considered acceptable, nourishing, and safe for the mother and baby. They were attended by other women whom they knew well, in a place that was familiar to them—usually in their home or in the home of a female relative. They labored and birthed in upright or all-fours positions (thereby expanding the pelvis, capitalizing on gravity, and maximizing the efficiency of the abdominal muscles needed for pushing). They developed artifacts for upright birth like birthing stools and chairs, ropes thrown over beams to pull against, flexible hammocks, and poles for support. Midwives knelt down in front of upright mothers to receive their babies. Newborns were kept with their mothers skin-to-skin for warmth, and long-term exclusive breastfeeding, co-sleeping, slings, and other technologies kept baby and mother close during a year or more of *external gestation* (Montague 1971; McKenna 2003; Trevathan and McKenna 2003).

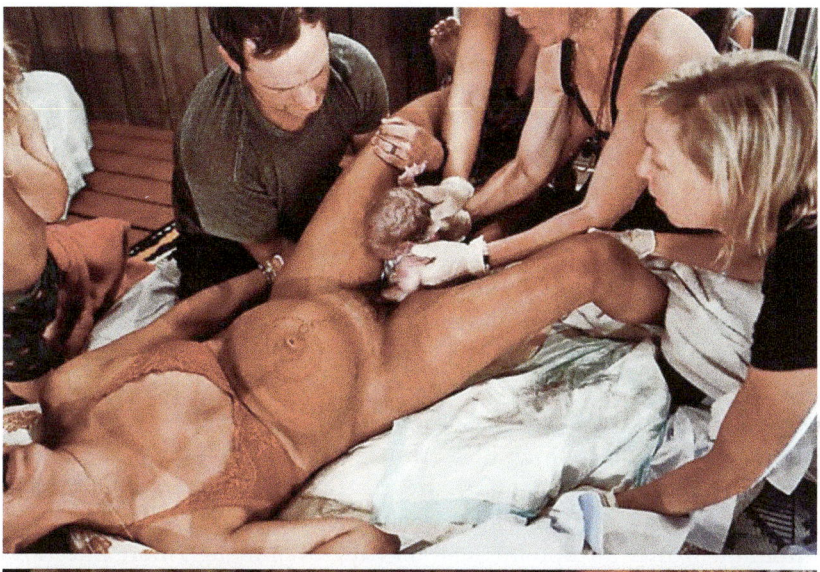

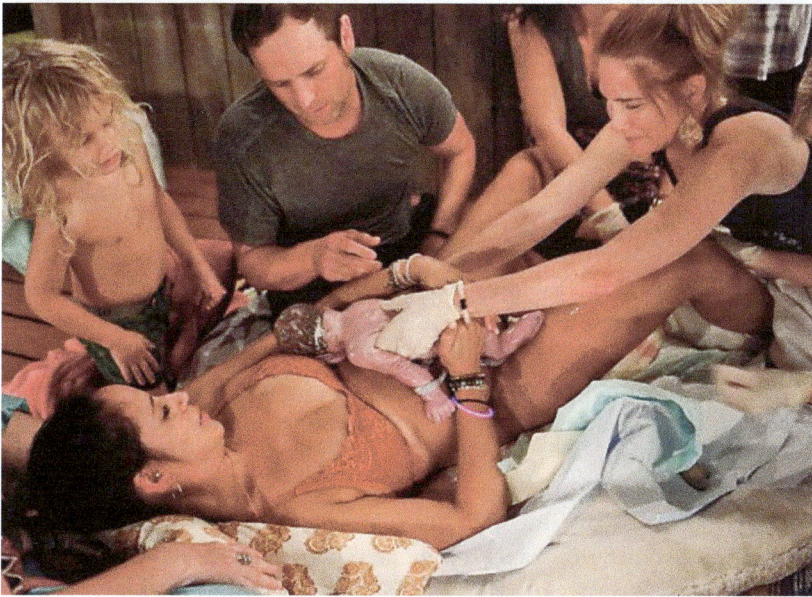

FIGURES 1.4 and 1.5 Missy (who is both an anthropologist and a practicing homebirth midwife) helps to untangle a baby from his cord so he can be lifted into his mother's arms. This mother had been upright and walking throughout her very fast labor (less than 2 hours) until she felt the urge to push, only lying down to help *slow* the descent of the baby to avoid the (usually shallow) perineal tearing that can happen in a fast birth. This was her fifth baby; she wanted to make sure she could birth gently, and she did. (Photos by Kala Noel, used with permission of the photographer and the parents.)

These basic cultural adaptations were normative in many cultures until the enormous social changes associated with industrialization moved birth from home to hospital and fundamentally changed it, while doing little to reduce mortality and morbidity (see Wertz and Wertz 1989; Wilson 1995; Cheyney and Davis-Floyd 2019). Several historians have argued that it was largely the industrialization of birth, and not birth itself, that contributed to the fear of birth that many describe today (ibid.; Ulrich 1990; see also Chapters 9 and 13). As in our folktale, before the widespread acceptance of germ theory, the unsanitary lying-in hospitals of industrialized nations produced massive epidemics of puerperal fever from the 18th to the very early 20th centuries (Leavitt 1986; Crawford 1990; Pollock 1990, 1997)—until the germ theory of disease developed by Louis Pasteur in 1881 finally became widely accepted and handwashing became standard practice.

From then on, precautions were taken in hospitals to prevent or decrease puerperal fever and other infections, with a primary focus on attempts at sterilizing, standardizing, and managing the birth process. Birthing mothers were painted from breasts to knees with iodine, forbidden to touch their own infants, and separated from them after birth, sometimes for days, even though more infections started (and still start) in nurseries than in babies kept with their mothers (Bertini et al. 2006; McDonald et al. 2007; Nguyen et al. 2007; James et al. 2008; Khan et al. 2015). Ritualized procedures like enemas and pubic shaving were instituted under the premise that they would prevent infections. Such "standards of care" were implemented in response to unfounded cultural beliefs about the "dirtiness" of the female body and are still common in far too many countries (Cuervo et al. 2000; Baservi and Lavender 2001; Reveiz et al. 2007). Current research has shown that the bacteria transferred from mother to baby during vaginal birth and breastfeeding—the microbiome—is critical to the prevention of multiple chronic diseases later in life (Iyer and Blumberg 2018; Montoya-Williams et al. 2018; Chapter 9). This information comes as no surprise to evolutionary biologists, who tend to respect the complex relationships that have resulted from millennia of natural selection. However, in technocracies, natural processes are commonly seen as needing technological improvement. The Big Bad Wolf, after all, must be tamed.

Over recent decades, the interventions that were introduced into the birthplace during industrialization have multiplied as more and more countries have embraced high-tech, invasive procedures. As a result, much of our knowledge of normal, unmedicated, physiologic birth has been lost (Davis-Floyd et al. 2018; Kennedy et al. 2018). Clinicians in many places have been de-skilled and may have little experience supporting physiologic birth in healthy, unmedicated birthing people.

Yet a midwifery revival has been taking place around the world over the last several decades; the ancient legacy of obligate midwifery survives and even thrives in many places today. As more midwives realize what is being lost, they are working to regain their positions as the keepers and researchers of knowledge about physiologic birth—speaking and practicing outside the dominant paradigm, holding open a conceptual space where technocratic birth may be challenged and viable premodern practices revived (Cheyney et al. 2014; Davis-Floyd et al. 2018; Kennedy et al. 2018; Daviss 2019; Daviss and Bisits 2021). Biomedical hegemony—the power-laden rule by cultural consent that constructs some models as authoritative (Jordan 1993, 1997) and others (like midwifery models of care; see Wang et al. 2012) as fringe, retrogressive, premodern, and thus "uncivilized"—means that today, birth in hospitals looks quite similar all over the world, yet quite different from the kind of births the first four little pigs would have experienced.

Dressed in hospital gowns and hooked up to intravenous lines that often carry synthetic oxytocin, prophylactic antibiotics, and narcotics for pain, many women labor and give birth on their backs or in semi-sitting positions that compress the pelvic outlet. The most notable differences in the contemporary medical treatment of birth have little to do with the specific customs of particular cultures, but much to do with the vast disparities between resource-rich and resource-poor countries. In many high-resource nations, women receive significantly more interventions, with pharmaceuticals and technologies applied at higher rates in more attractive and humane hospital settings. In many low-resource nations, women receive less expensive and outdated interventions like shaving, enemas, and episiotomies without the benefits of expensive interior decorating—or even of a birthing companion. In both high- and low-resource countries, cesarean birth rates are rising (see Chapters 9 and 14) without a concomitant improvement in maternal and fetal health outcomes (Althabe et al. 2006; Belizán et al. 2018), and iatrogenic morbidity (Villar et al. 2006, 2007; Liu et al. 2007) and maternal mortality disproportionately affect poor women and women of color (Krisberg 2019; Parks et al. 2019). Technology has tamed the Big Bad Wolf, damming, controlling, and homogenizing the raw, elemental river of birth, and often supplanting the knowledge of how to support its flow. In what follows, we will ask, what does the Big Bad Wolf still have to teach us?

Premodern Birthing Patterns and Why They Matter

In a society so consumed with technologies, it is perhaps not surprising that when we encounter a problem or a concern—like elevated maternal or neonatal ill-health or death—we ask: what technologies, interventions, or pharmaceuticals can be used to solve this problem? This phenomenon constitutes the *obstetric paradox*: Intervene in birth to keep it safe, thereby causing harm. As mentioned in the Introduction to this volume, here we extend the obstetric paradox to incorporate what anthropologist Peter Reynolds (1991:4) has called the "1-2 Punch" of the technocracy—what he also referred to as "mutilation and prosthesis"—wherein we intervene in nature via technology, cause new problems via that technology, and then attempt to solve those problems with more technology. Reynolds argues that *Punch 2 is the point*. We tend to think we have improved upon nature by prosthetizing it with technology, in what Robbie (Davis-Floyd 2003) calls *the myth of technological transcendence*—the notion that no matter how many problems we create with technology, we will solve them with more technology. But what if, sometimes, the answer is less, not more technology? Or technologies applied more selectively and in a manner that is more respectful and supportive of the evolved physiologic and psychosocial needs of childbearing people? What if an important part of the answer lies with the re-introduction of time-honored, premodern birthing practices?

As long-time midwifery researchers, and while there are certainly exceptions, we are both struck by the extent to which midwives have functioned as the keepers of time-honored birthing practices, combining them with more recent innovations when needed—a phenomenon that Robbie calls "postmodern midwifery" (Davis-Floyd et al. 2018). She defines the postmodern midwife (or obstetrician) as having the ability to use *informed relativism* to pick and choose what is likely to be most effective from varying knowledge systems (ibid.). The vast majority of the midwives we have met and worked with have never heard of evolutionary medicine nor of the discordance hypothesis described above. Yet because they tend to trust women's bodies, and to believe, based on their experience, that birth works well most of the time when women are healthy and adequately supported, they have, in effect, preserved a set of behaviors that are key to moving birth beyond the transnational, technological dualism of "too much too soon" (TMTS) or "too little too late" (TLTL) (Miller et al. 2016) to the right amount at the right time in the right way (RARTRW)—a way that honors the dignity and human rights of the childbearer. The preservation and reintroduction, where appropriate, of pre-modern birthing practices that better align with our evolved biologies may help to reduce the discordance between how humans evolved to give birth and how technocratic obstetrics "manages" it today (see Trevathan 2017; Rosenberg and Trevathan 2018).

Cross-cultural midwifery approaches, with their often-explicit rejection of some core components of the technocratic model, combined with their subversive, norm-challenging support of physiologic birth, provide an important point of comparison for critically examining the technocratic management of birth. The midwifery norms, for example, of encouraging food and fluid intake (Singata et al. 2013) and unrestrained movement in labor (Priddis et al. 2012; Lawrence et al. 2013), upright and hands-and-knees pushing positions (de Jonge et al. 2009; Gupta et al. 2017), and intensive emotional support during labor (Trevathan 2015, 2017; Bohren et al. 2017), along with active encouragement of skin-to-skin at birth (Moore et al. 2016), long-term, exclusive, on demand breastfeeding and co-sleeping (Gettler and McKenna 2011; Hauck et al. 2011; Das et al. 2014; McFadden et al. 2017) are all associated with significantly improved psychosocial and clinical outcomes for both parents and babies.

We propose that midwifery and other low-tech, high-touch models of care that attempt to preserve "natural" (read: those with a long history in human and non-human primates) birthing practices produce the positive outcomes documented in so many studies (see for example Sandall et al. 2016) because they reduce discordances between our evolved birthing biology and recent cultural norms via mechanisms that facilitate, rather than hamper, the physiologic and psychosocial needs of human mothers. A closer examination of three sets of premodern, reclaimed midwifery practices, re-viewed through the lens of evolutionary medicine, provides an evidence-informed template for the reform of contemporary technocratic models of birth.

Premodern Birthing Practices Set 1: Fluids and Food, Unrestrained Movement in Labor, and Physiologic Pushing Positions

The notion that women should lie in bed hindered by tubes and devices for fetal monitoring and intravenous fluid delivery is relatively recent and makes little sense from an evolutionary perspective (Trevathan 1999, 2017). A large body of clinical research documents the value of mobility and eating and drinking at will during labor, as well as the use of maternal positioning, such as squatting and hands-and-knees, that helps to speed and ease the complicated descent of the fetus through the pelvis (see Bodner-Adler et al. 2003; Gupta et al. 2017; Zhang et al. 2017; Berta et al. 2019). Food and fluids keep the mother hydrated and nourished, supplying the energy to labor and birth. Upright and hands-and-knees postures maximize the dimensions of the pelvis, while improving blood flow to the baby by preventing compression of the large vessels that run along the mother's spine. Women around the world who give birth in community settings, with midwives or holistic physicians, tend to labor and push in a variety of non-supine positions, in accordance with the physiologic urges that come with an unmedicated second stage (Dunham 2016; Trevathan 2017). However, high epidural rates in hospitals prevent many women in high-resource countries from utilizing the well-documented benefits of upright labor and pushing positions that optimize the curve of the human birth canal.

Technocratic models of labor and pushing rely instead on supine or semi-recumbent positions and high use of epidural analgesia—the latter of which has been shown to alter the course of labor, sometimes prolonging second stage (Amin-Somuah et al. 2011). While the timing of epidural analgesia initiation (i.e., before 6 cm dilation or after) has not been shown to consistently increase the risk of cesarean birth (Jones et al. 2012; Sng et al. 2014), the risk of instrumental (forceps or vacuum) vaginal delivery is increased when epidural-assisted births are compared to those without (Ami-Somuah et al. 2011). Discordances between evolved behavioral encouragements known to promote physiologic birth and non-physiologic TMTS interventions that can negatively influence the progress of labor and pushing may partially explain the high rates of operative vaginal and cesarean birth, as well as the associated maternal and neonatal morbidities that characterize modern, technocratic obstetrics (Althabe et al. 2006; Miller et al. 2016).

Premodern Birthing Practices Set 2: Obligate Midwifery and Continuous Labor Support vs. "Intimate Strangers"

The intimacy of time-intensive, continuous labor support provided by birth attendants who are a part of a woman's community or have come to know her well over the course of her pregnancy may play an additionally decisive role in how human birth unfolds. The calming presence of a familiar midwife, doula, or other companion is likely, for example, to help reduce levels of maternal stress hormones like cortisol that are known to inhibit the effects of oxytocin—the hormone that stimulates labor contractions (Jolly 1999; Buckley 2015). The complex evolutionary relationships between hormones produced during fear and/or pain responses and those that stimulate labor combine to produce the "white coat" effect. This effect is characterized by the lessening or complete cessation of labor contractions when childbearers feel afraid or anxious in response to perceptions of danger—sometimes from the presence of care providers who are strangers to the birthing family ("white coats")—compensated for in the hospital by the administration of synthetic oxytocin.

The release of adrenaline and cortisol in response to fear and stress, and the consequent slowing of labor, likely served an adaptive function in the distant past because such mechanisms prevent mammals—including humans—from birthing fragile infants under conditions of perceived danger. However, fear of pain, the hospital environment, specific procedures, or even just the feeling of self-consciousness that can come with laboring in front of "intimate strangers," and the contraction-dampening effects of stress hormones that can result are often not beneficial in a technocratic environment where birth must occur according to relatively rigid time schedules to be considered "normal."

In relation to the obligate midwifery that led to the evolutionary advantage toward increased survival described above, and with the underlying assumption that we still occupy Paleolithic bodies, then midwifery and other humanistic and holistic models of care that focus on trust (Anderson 2000; Dahlberg and Aune 2013), building relationships, and reducing maternal stress through intensive emotional and psychosocial support during labor partially explain the excellent outcomes associated with doula care and with midwife-attended birth in all settings (home, birth center, and hospital maternity units) (Olsen and Clausen 2012; Sosa et al. 2012; Stapleton et al. 2013; Cheyney et al. 2014; Zeilinski et al. 2015; Bohren et al. 2017; Alliman et al. 2019). Current technocratic approaches vastly underestimate the evolved psychosocial and physiologic needs of birthing people. These needs can (and often do) include being in a hospital for birth, when that is the setting that makes a woman feel safest. Thus, evolutionary birth is not an argument for community birth, though home and birth center protocols are far more supportive of the evolved physiology of birth (Dunham 2016) than those in hospitals. *Midwifery models of humanistic, compassionate, evidence-based care can be applied anywhere and by any practitioner.*

Premodern Birthing Practices Set 3: Low Intervention Birth–Long-Term Breastfeeding–Co-Sleeping Adaptive Complex

The intimacy and connectedness that facilitate human childbirth have also been extended and applied to early parenting behaviors and mother-baby co-evolutionary patterns among primates. Evolutionary biologist James McKenna (2020) has examined contemporary Euro-American childrearing practices like solitary sleep and scheduled feedings from the perspective of evolutionary medicine. His work challenges the common Western assumption that solitary crib sleep should be considered normative for human babies, concluding instead that there are great benefits to safe parent-infant co-sleeping and sensory proximity when combined with long-term, on-demand nursing (McKenna and Mosko 2001; McKenna and McDade 2005; WHO Recommendations on Infant Feeding 2020). "Co-sleeping" here refers to an array of sleeping arrangements, from bed-sharing to sleeping in "sensory proximity," wherein babies sleep close enough to adults to hear, smell, and feel their reassuring presence.

Close proximity in sleep facilitates the frequent nursing and skin-to-skin contact required for human babies who have evolved to consume and very quickly digest breastmilk. McKenna and Gettler (2016) assert that breastfeeding is so physiologically and behaviorally intertwined with and functionally dependent upon forms of co-sleeping that the term "breastsleeping" should be adopted to capture three critical factors that describe the evolved maternal-infant relationship in humans: (1) Immediate and sustained maternal contact throughout both day and night plays a critical role in helping to establish optimal breastfeeding (see also Das et al. 2014). (2) Normal infant sleep can only be understood by studying breastsleeping dyads "because of the ways maternal–infant contact affects the delivery of breastmilk, the milk's ingestion, the infant's concomitant and subsequent metabolism and other physiologic processes, maternal and infant sleep architecture, including arousal patterns, as well as breastfeeding frequency and prolongation" (McKenna and Gettler 2016:17). (3) Breastsleeping in mother–infant pairs is so vastly different behaviorally and physiologically from bottle-feeding that this relational context must be taken into consideration whenever the risks and benefits of sleep location are assessed.

The benefits of close sleep proximity, touch, and breastfeeding include the promotion of bonding, growth, neurological development, decreased stress response, and the regulation of breathing patterns in developmentally immature infants (Das et al. 2014; McKenna 2020; see Chapter 14 for a discussion of how

NICUs should be adapted to facilitate all these). Thus, long-term breastfeeding, parent-infant co-sleeping, and skin-to-skin (even when breastfeeding is not possible [Ludington-Hoe et al. 1991a, 1991b]) are all likely part of an adaptive complex that evolved to allow for intensive parental investment, optimal nutrition, improved immunity, social learning, and rapid postnatal brain growth. However, there are many challenges in contemporary technocratic society that make evolutionarily informed infant care practices difficult to implement, which include highly variable levels of parental leave and other supports for new families.

Birth and early parenting activists around the world have called us to think through the implications of the decline in continuous contact in early childrearing that characterized parenting practices until "plastic babysitter" technologies like monitors, swings, strollers, cribs, and car seats extensively replaced physical contact (Hrdy 1999; Small 1999, 2001; DeLoache and Gottlieb 2000). Midwives and holistic pediatricians who recognize the external gestation period (Montague 1971; McKenna 2003; Trevathan and McKenna 2003) argue that more high-touch (sometimes called "attachment") parenting practices often produce babies who are healthier (emotionally and physically) than bottle-fed, solitary-crib-sleeping, and stroller-carried infants. Humans are what evolutionary biologists call "cooperative breeders," meaning that we tend to raise our children in communities where family and friends share the work of caring for little ones (Hrdy 1999, 2017). These extra parental caregivers are called "allomothers," and cross-culturally, we see that humans tend to have many of them (Hrdy 2016). However, pressure to return to work outside the home soon after birth, unpaid maternity leave, and the breakdown of extended families who can provide allomother supports create enormous barriers for new parents who might otherwise choose to engage in attachment practices such as exclusive breastfeeding, co-sleeping, and "baby-wearing" facilitated by slings and wraps.

Because we see birthing behaviors as inextricably linked to mother-baby co-evolution and early parenting adaptations like exclusive, on-demand breastfeeding and sensory proximity of mother and baby during sleep, we propose an extension of McKenna's (2003) breastfeeding-co-sleeping adaptive complex to include low-intervention, physiologic birth as an approach that helps to decrease the discordance between human biology and technocratic birth. The alertness of unmedicated infants, combined with skin-to-skin contact post-birth, facilitates the cascade of hormonally regulated bonding that promotes exclusive and long-term breastfeeding (Trevathan and McKenna 2003; Huber and Sandall 2006).

Correctives from Evolutionary Medicine: Towards a Model of (R)Evolutionary Maternity Care

In this chapter, we have reviewed what we see as remarkable similarities in human birth mechanisms and cultural practices over time and argued that, pre-Industrial Revolution, these similarities were an outgrowth of our common evolutionary heritage as bipedal primates. Despite the multiple, culturally mediated differences in the ritual treatment of birth, our common evolutionary heritage and the evolved physiology of birth were relatively attuned in premodern societies. With industrialization, there emerged a fear-based need to control nature that, along with the hegemony of biomedicine, again produced relatively uniform cross-cultural birthing practices. Birth in the industrial and technocratic eras, while very similar cross-culturally, looks very different from what the first 4 little pigs in our folktale would have experienced. These transformations in the global management of birth exacerbate the *discordance* between the evolved physiologies of human childbirth and contemporary technocratic interventions during labor, birth, and the early postpartum periods. Through the lens of evolutionary medicine, we see several places where premodern birthing and childrearing patterns can be re-introduced in a way that honors the Upper Paleolithic bodies we occupy, while also helping us to move beyond TMTS or TLTL approaches to RARTRW care (see also Chapter 14).

Evolutionary approaches, while certainly not without limitations in that they carry their own set of contestable presuppositions, are valuable insofar as they provide yet another way of critically examining birth in cultures that supervalue technocratic approaches over more humanistic and holistic methods encompassed within midwifery and doula care. We encourage researchers, clinicians and parents (current, future, allo-, and other) to consider not only the immediate contexts of an individual pregnancy, but also the larger, evolutionary and social histories of our species that have shaped our biology and, to some extent, our culture and behaviors.

In addition, we advocate for a deeper and more explicit acknowledgment of the fact that recent human evolution has not unfolded within a power vacuum. The influences of colonization, industrialization, technocracy, racism, and gendered power inequities have generated massive inequalities among nations and among populations within countries (see Davis 2019a, 2019b). "Too much too soon" (TMTS) forms of biomedical obstetrics that have been exported around the world through colonialism and the maladaptive imitation of what appears to be "best" simply because it is "modern" cause harm, as do "too little too late" (TLTL) systems where resources are scarce and/or wherever laboring people are neglected, as TLTL care can also occur in high-resource countries—usually in socio-structurally stratified ways. Adjusting our critical lens to see birth within the larger and more holistic contexts of cross-cultural and evolutionary perspectives, we can develop approaches that combine the best of what technological innovations have to offer, while also embracing the wild beauty and instinctive power of the Big Bad Wolf in the birthplace (Figure 1.6). And so, we close by considering future reproductive possibilities through the literary device of a 7th little pig, drawing upon cyborgian theory (after Haraway 1991) to challenge the dualistic binary often drawn between nature and culture, the social and the technocratic, body and machine. Here is the next, futuristic part of our story.

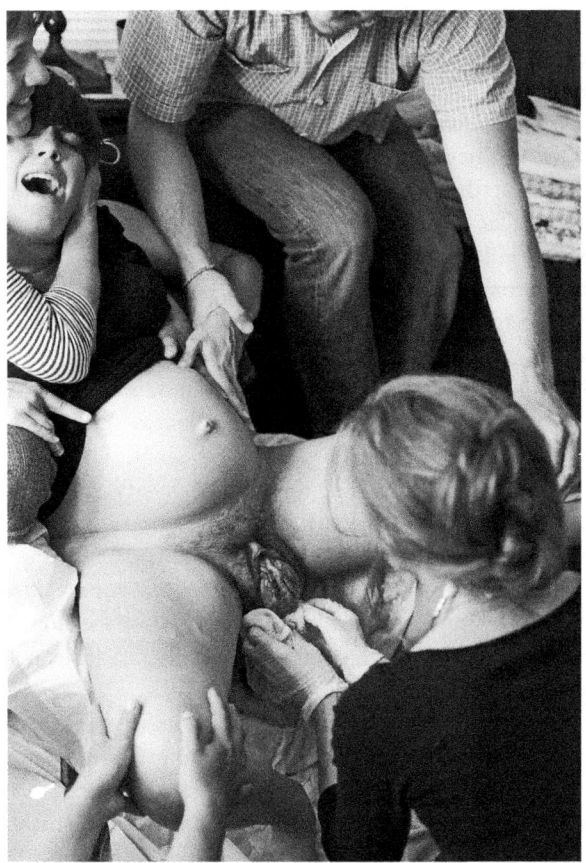

FIGURE 1.6 An untamed, physiologic, midwife-attended birth in Corvallis, Oregon, 2014. Photograph by Alicia Juniku, used with permission of the mother and the photographer.

The 7th Little Pig and Human-Technology Co-Evolution: Kiri's Story

The 6th little capitalist technocrat pig married a researcher interested in the human genome. Wanting to have children, yet struggling with infertility, they spent over $100,000 and used an in-vitro fertilization (IVF) method wherein one partner's eggs were mixed with donor sperm. Cells were then taken from the resulting embryos and tested for various genetic disorders and chromosome number using a method called pre-implantation genetic diagnosis. One healthy embryo was then implanted into the other partner, allowing both parents to contribute biologically to the offspring. Seven months later, Kiri (named after the iPhone's "Siri," of course) was born prematurely and spent eight weeks in the Neonatal

Intensive Care Unit (NICU), monitored constantly by sophisticated life-support machines. Kiri's parents placed a teddy bear in the isolette that played the sound of a human heartbeat—something the fetus had heard regularly in the womb (now replaced by the high-tech plastic incubator/artificial womb), and after birth would still have heard regularly had Kiri's parents been able to hold their baby

When they were finally able to take Kiri home, they found that Kiri could not sleep in their crib without the constant sound emanating from the teddy bear. Thus, Kiri began as a cyborg—a symbiotic fusion of human and machine—a process that started with a high-tech conception and birth and continued to unfold as Kiri grew. Kiri's primary attachments were to blankets and other objects, and especially to the teddy bear and later to a cellphone and an iPad, which by now were 3D and holographic so Kiri could actually enter into the stories they read via interactive goggles.

In high school, having limited access to affordable education (for that had not yet changed in the United States), Kiri—who had eventually decided on a gender identity and now preferred the pronouns "she, her, hers"—longed for a career in medicine, and so joined the military upon graduation, hoping to have her education funded this way. The military did help her complete her medical studies, and she became a well-respected researcher specializing in the human genome, just like one of her parents. Tragically, on a field research trip to Afghanistan, she was injured by an improvised explosive device (IED) and lost her leg. Kiri was sent home to obtain a prosthetic leg (Punch 1: mutilate a natural process with technology; Punch 2: prosthetically fix the damage with more technology.)

Over time, Kiri grew to love her high-tech leg and was amazed by how much she could do with it. Her connection to that leg led her to reflect on her cyborgian nature—she had always been dependent on machines, and now one was an integral part of her—along with the supersmart phone that rarely left her hands. Kiri started to think about this ongoing and ever-increasing fusion of human and machine, this cyborgian future being created. Her new interest made the military very happy, as they were able to assign her to their medical cyber-branch—a highly specialized team of researchers looking into the possibility of creating a meta-human—a human or group of humans with special abilities given to them via technologies that alter their genomes. After all, they reasoned, we are already co-creating ourselves with our technology, generating a new species, which they called *techno-sapiens*. Kiri herself became one of their experiments, having technologies implanted into her arm and ear so she could always be connected.

After trying for several years to conceive, Kiri discovered she too was infertile secondary to uterine cancer (which was on the rise due to all the chemical toxins accumulating in the environment). Unwilling to give up on the possibility of giving birth, she received a uterine transplant and again, Punch 2 worked. The transplanted uterus contained a tiny computer chip that allowed researchers to monitor how Kiri's body was accepting the new organ. After several attempts at becoming pregnant with her new uterus, the doctors discovered that Kiri's partner's sperm count was far below normal—something the experts attributed in part to his constant smartphone use and his habit of carrying this device in his front pants pockets. And yet, Kiri still wanted a child, so, again using IVF, she became pregnant with her own cyborgian child, whom she and her partner sex-selected for XX chromosomes. Research on the human genome had not yet reached the point where hair and eye color, nor intelligence, could be selected for, but Kiri wondered what choices her child and her grandchildren would be able to make.

Kiri did not like being pregnant—feeling large and unwieldy, having morning sickness, and being unable to bend over to strap her shoes—so she was fascinated by, and spent time researching, the possibility of growing babies in artificial wombs. But one day during her yoga class, while in deep meditation, Kiri heard the voice of her baby warn that they were in the wrong position and needed help. Kiri was amazed. She loved technology, but was also quite intuitive, and as such, was willing to trust her experience as real. She immediately changed her mind not only about artificial wombs, but also about where and with whom to give birth. Kiri found a local midwife who checked the baby's position and discovered that the baby was in fact presenting breech. After trying some re-positioning exercises that were unsuccessful, the midwife performed an external version, while Kiri silently spoke to the baby, urging movement with the pressure of the midwife's hands. She felt some fear from the baby, but kept whispering to trust, and soon the baby turned into the vertex position.

About two weeks later, Kiri the cyborg, who had only recently come to trust the evolved organic biology of her body and the process of birth, embraced the Big Bad Wolf and the raw power it represented, and had an intense, beautiful, and wildly out-of-control birth with a midwife, her partner, and a doula by her side (along with various colleagues from her research lab who were desperate to see an unmedicated, physiologic birth). She chanted and sang, rocked her body in an ancient dance, and yelled out gutturally from deep inside her soul as her baby made its way into the world. Kiri discovered the power of her own birth song, and felt triumphant beyond words as she pushed out little Quinn Riley while standing up facing and embracing her partner. Quinn was perfectly healthy, yet with one anomaly. Via the placenta's attachment to the uterine wall, the microscopic computer chip used to monitor the transplanted uterus had traveled through the umbilical cord and become encased in Quinn's brain, opening up new possibilities for studying brain growth and for furthering human-technology co-evolution—which we leave our readers to imagine...

As Kiri held Quinn in her arms, she realized she had been privileged to experience the best of both worlds over her lifetime—access to sophisticated medical technology when it served her and trust in the power of her own body when needed. She saw the need to "right-size" maternity care globally and so became an activist and researcher, committing her career to finding ways to move beyond the TMTS/TLTL dualism to offer RARTRW care—the right amount at the right time in the right way—that is, in a way that explicitly respects the dignity and autonomy of all childbearing people everywhere. Kiri loved the present and looked forward to the future, yet wanted to remember and honor parts of the past.

Conclusion: Birthing Techno-Sapiens

Our future will write the rest of this story, so for now we leave it up to your imagination. Given the rapid technological advances in this digitally interconnected world, it seems clear that we have taken human evolution into our own hands and are co-evolving ourselves with our technologies, re-creating ourselves as techno-sapiens. The 7th little pigs and their progeny will likely live on Planet Earth as cybernetic organisms—a fusion of human and machine. In fact, millions of us are already cyborgs—we have artificial knees, hips, hearts, prosthetic legs, arms, hands. Google and other tech companies are working to design machines that can provide sight to the blind and have already provided hearing to some who are deaf. NASA engineers Robbie interviewed (Davis-Floyd 2000) insisted that there are *no limits* to where we can go with technology. What will this mean for humankind? For how we give birth? Will the pendulum swing back towards a more moderated integration of human and machine, of nature and culture, of technological intervention and trust in the wisdom of our bodies shaped by millions of years of evolution? We have no doubt that the next generation of reproductive anthropologists will have plenty to think and write about.

When it comes to birth, will we continue on our present path, until most babies are born by cesarean (see Chapter 9)—or possibly incubated in artificial wombs (Chapter 8)? Or will the scientific evidence eventually preponderate? Will we go "back to the future" by humanizing our birthing systems to fully support the normal physiology of birth and allow all people the full spectrum of choice in birth setting and provider type? (See National Academies of Science, Engineering, and Medicine 2020.) That *full spectrum of choice* is what we ceaselessly advocate for: from home to birth center to hospital, from midwives to obstetricians, from entirely organic births to scheduled cesarean births. All parents should have the right to fully informed choice, and to compassionate, respectful treatment during parturition *and* during life.

Together, can we create a world in which those are the norms? We ask our readers to look back at our long biocultural and evolutionary paths, to consider where we are along them now, and to give some thought to where we will go next. These are issues that many young people, who may have long lives ahead of them—possibly to 100 years or more—will have to navigate as we make choices that perpetuate, resist, or moderate the techno-sapiens, cyborgian future of our planet and all the creatures that live upon it.

Acknowledgments

This chapter has been greatly expanded, revised, and updated from "Birth and the Big Bad Wolf: An Evolutionary Perspective," by Melissa Cheyney and Robbie Davis-Floyd, in *Childbirth across Cultures: Ideas and Practices of Pregnancy, Childbirth, and the Postpartum,* edited by Helaine Selin and Pamela K. Stone, Springer 2009, pp. 1–22. We thank Springer Publishing for permission to borrow the sections of it that we use here. This chapter also appeared as a two-part article in the *International Journal of Childbirth,* which allowed us to flesh out our ideas, update our information, and refine our thinking considerably on these subjects. We thank IJC for allowing us to combine it back into one and publish it in this volume.

References

Alliman J, Stapleton SR, Wright J, Bauer K, Slider K, Jolles D. 2019. Strong Start in Birth Centers: Socio-Demographic Characteristics, Care Processes, and Outcomes for Mothers and Newborns. *Birth* 46(2):234–243.

Althabe F, Sosa C, Belizán JM, Gibbons L, Jacquerioz F, Bergel E. 2006. Cesarean Section Rates and Maternal and Neonatal Mortality in Low-, Medium-, and High-Income Countries: An Ecological Study. *Birth* 33(4):270–277.

Anderson T. 2000. Feeling Safe Enough to Let Go: The Relationship between a Woman and Her Midwife During the Second Stage of Labour. In: *The Midwife–Mother Relationship,* ed. Kirkham M. London: Palgrave Macmillan, 92–119.

Anim-Somuah M, Smyth RM, Jones L. 2011. Epidural Versus Non-Epidural or No Analgesia in Labour. *Cochrane Database of Systematic Reviews* 12(12):CD000331. doi:10.1002/14651858.CD000331.pub3.

Armelagos G, Brown P, Turner B. 2005. Evolutionary, Historical and Political Economic Perspectives on Health and Disease. *Social Science and Medicine* 61(4):755–765.

Baservi V, Lavender T. 2001. Routine Perineal Shaving on Admission in Labour. *Cochrane Database of Systematic Reviews* 1:CD001236.

Belizán JM et al. 2018. An Approach to Identify a Minimum and Rational Proportion of Caesarean Sections in Resource-Poor Settings: A Global Network Study. *The Lancet Global Health* 6(8):e894–e901.

Berta M, Lindgren H, Christensson K, Mekonnen S, Adefris M. 2019. Effect of Maternal Birth Positions on Duration of Second Stage of Labor: Systematic Review and Meta-Analysis. *BMC Pregnancy and Childbirth* 19(1):466. doi:10.1186/s12884-019-2620-0.

Bertini GP, Nicolett F, Scopetti P, Manoocher DC, Orefici G, Orefici G. 2006. Staphylococcus Aureus Epidemic in a Neonatal Nursery: A Strategy of Infection Control. *European Journal of Pediatrics* 165(8):530–535.

Betti L, Manica A. 2018(1889). Human Variation in the Shape of the Birth Canal Is Significant and Geographically Structured. *Proceedings of the Royal Society of London, Series B* 285. www.ncbi.nlm.nih.gov/pubmed/20181807.

Biesele M. 1997. An Ideal of Unassisted Birth: Hunting, Healing, and Transformation among the Kalahari Ju/'hoansi. In: *Childbirth and Authoritative Knowledge: Cross Cultural Perspectives*, eds. Davis-Floyd R, Sargent C. Berkeley: University of California Press, 474–499.

Bodner-Alder B, Bodner KO, Kimberger P, Lozanov P, Husslein P, Mayerhofer K. 2003. Women's Position During Labour: Influence on Maternal and Neonatal Outcomes. *Wiener Klinische Wochenschrift* 115(19–20):720–723. doi:10.1007/BF03040889.

Bohren MA, Hofmeyr GJ, Sakala C, Fukuzawa RK, Cuthbert A. 2017. Continuous Support for Women during Childbirth. *Cochrane Database of Systematic Reviews* 7:CD003766. doi:10.1002/ 14651858.CD003766.pub6.

Buckley SJ. 2015. *Hormonal Physiology of Childbearing: Evidence and Implications for Women, Babies, and Maternity Care*. Washington, DC: Childbirth Connection Programs, National Partnership for Women & Families.

Cheyney M. 2010. *Born at Home: Cultural and Political Dimensions of Maternity Care in the United States*. Florence, KY: Wadsworth.

Cheyney M, Bovbjerg M, Everson C, Gordon W, Hannibal D, Vedam S. 2014. Outcomes of Care for 16,924 Planned Home Births in the United States: The Midwives Alliance of North America Statistics Project, 2004 to 2009. *Journal of Midwifery and Women's Health* 59(1):17–27. doi:10.1111/jmwh.12172.

Cheyney M, Davis-Floyd R. 2019. Birth as Culturally Marked and Shaped. In: *Birth in Eight Cultures*, eds. Davis-Floyd R, Cheyney M L. Grove, IL: Waveland Press, 1–16.

Crawford P. 1990. The Construction and Experience of Maternity in Seventeenth-Century England. In: *Women as Mothers in Pre-Industrial England*, ed. Fildes V. London: Routledge, 3–38.

Cuervo LG, Rodriguez MN, Delgado MB. 2000. Enemas during Labor. *Cochrane Database of Systematic Reviews*: CD000330.

Dahlberg U, Aune I. 2013. The Woman's Birth Experience—The Effect of Interpersonal Relationships and Continuity of Care. *Midwifery* 29(4):407–415. doi:10.1016/j.midw.2012.09.00.

Das RR, Sankar MJ, Agarwal R, Paul VK. 2014. Is "Bed Sharing" Beneficial and Safe during Infancy? A Systematic Review. *International Journal of Pediatrics* 2014:1–16. doi:10.1155/2014/4685.

Davis DA. 2019a. Obstetric Racism: The Racial Politics of Pregnancy, Labor, and Birthing. *Medical Anthropology* 38(7):560–573. doi:10.1080/01459740.2018.1549389.

Davis DA. 2019b. *Reproductive Injustice: Racism, Pregnancy, and Premature Birth*. New York: New York University Press.

Davis-Floyd R. 2000. Commercializing Outer Space: The SATWG Stories. In: *Late Editions VII, Para-Sites*, ed. Marcus G. Chicago: University of Chicago Press, 149–163.

Davis-Floyd R. 2003 [1992]. *Birth as an American Rite of Passage*, 2nd ed. 2003. Berkeley: University of California Press.

Davis-Floyd R, Matsuoka E, Horan H, Ruder B, Everson CL. 2018. Daughter of Time: The Postmodern Midwife. In: *Ways of Knowing about Birth: Mothers, Midwives, Medicine, and Birth Activism* by Davis-Floyd R. Long Grove, IL: Waveland Press, 221–264.

Davis-Floyd R, Laughlin CD. 2016. *The Power of Ritual*. Brisbane: Daily Grail Press.

Daviss BA. 2019. *Rethinking the Physiology of Vaginal Breech Birth: Evidence-Based Guide to Upright Delivery*. Ottawa, Ontario: Informed Descent Publishing. www.understandi ngbirthbetter.com.

Daviss BA, Bisits A. 2021. Bringing Back Breech. In: *Birthing Models on the Human Rights Frontier: Speaking Truth to Power*, eds. Daviss BA, Davis-Floyd R. New York: Routledge. Chapter 7, in press.

de Jonge A, Rijnders ME, van Diem MT, Scheepers PL, Lagro-Janssen AL. 2009. Are There Inequalities in Choice of Birthing Position?: Sociodemographic and Labour Factors Associated with the Supine Position During the Second Stage of Labour. *Midwifery* 25(4):439–448. doi:10.1016/j.midw.2007.07.013.

DeLoache J, Gottlieb A. 2000. *A World of Babies: Imagined Childcare Guides for Seven Societies*. Cambridge: Cambridge University Press.

DeSilva JM, Laudicina NM, Rosenberg KR, Trevathan W. 2017. Neonatal Shoulder Width Suggests a Semirotational, Oblique Birth Mechanism in Australopithecus Afarensis. *The Anatomical Record* 300(5):890–899.

Dunham B. 2016. Home Birth Midwifery in the United States: Evolutionary Origins and Modern Challenges. *Human Nature* 27(4):471–488. doi:10.1007/s12110-016-9266-7.

Eaton SB, Eaton III SB, Cordain L. 2002. Evolution, Diet, and Health. In: *Human Diet: Its Origin and Evolution*, eds. Ungar PS, Teaford MF, Westport CT: Bergin and Garvey, 7–17.

Gettler LT, McKenna JJ. 2011. Evolutionary Perspectives on Mother–Infant Sleep Proximity and Breastfeeding in a Laboratory Setting. *American Journal of Physical Anthropology* 144(3):454–462. doi:10.1002/ajpa.21426.

Gluckman P, Beedle A, Buklijas T, Low F, Hanson M. 2016. *Principles of Evolutionary Medicine*. Oxford: Oxford University Press.

Goodman A, Leatherman T. 1998. Traversing the Chasm between Biology and Culture: An Introduction. In: *Building a New Biocultural Synthesis: Political-Economic Perspectives on Human Biology*, eds. Goodman A, Leatherman T. Ann Arbor: University of Michigan Press, 3–42.

Gruss LT, Schmitt D. 2015. The Evolution of the Human Pelvis: Changing Adaptations to Bipedalism, Obstetrics and Thermoregulation. *Philosophical Transactions of the Royal Society of London Series B Biological Sciences* 370(1663):20140063. doi:10.1098/rstb.2014.0063.

Gupta JK, Sood A, Hofmeyr GJ, Vogel JP. 2017. Position in the Second Stage of Labour for Women without Epidural Anaesthesia. *Cochrane Database of Systematic Reviews* 5:CD002006. doi:10.1002/14651858.CD002006.pub4.

Haraway D. 1991. *Simians, Cyborgs and Women. The Reinvention of Nature*. London: Free Association Books.

Hauck FR, Thompson JM, Tanabe KO, Moon RY, Vennemann MM. 2011. Breastfeeding and Reduced Risk of Sudden Infant Death Syndrome: A Meta-Analysis. *Pediatrics* 128(1):103–110. doi:10.1542/peds.2010-3000.

Hewlett BS, De Silvestri A, Guglielmino CR. 2002. Semes and Genes in Africa. *Current Anthropology* 42(2):313–321.

Hrdy SB. 1999. *Mother Nature: Maternal Instincts and How They Shape the Human Species*. New York: Ballantine Books.

Hrdy SB. 2016. Variable Postpartum Responsiveness among Humans and Other primates with "Cooperative Breeding": A Comparative and Evolutionary Perspective. *Hormones and Behavior* 77:272–283. doi:10.1016/j.yhbeh.2015.10.016

Hrdy SB. 2017. Comes the Child before Man: How Cooperative Breeding and Prolonged Postweaning Dependence Shaped Human Potential. In: *Hunter-Gatherer Childhoods:*

Evolutionary, Developmental, and Cultural Perspectives, eds Hewlett BS, Lamb M. London: Routledge, 65–91.

Huber U, Sandall J. 2006. Continuity of Carer, Trust and Breastfeeding. *MIDIRS Midwifery Digest* 16(4):445–449.

Iyer SS, Blumberg RS. 2018. Influence of the Gut Microbiome on Immune Development During Early Life. In: *Physiology of the Gastrointestinal Tract,* 6th ed. London: Academic Press, 767–774.

James L et al. 2008. Methicillin-Resistant Staphylococcus Aureus Infections among Healthy Full-Term Newborns. *Archives of Disease in Childhood: Fetal and Neonatal Edition* 93(1):F40–F44.

Jolly A. 1999. *Lucy's Legacy: Sex and Intelligence in Human Evolution.* Cambridge, MA: Harvard University Press.

Jones L et al. 2012. Pain Management for Women in Labour: An Overview of Systematic Reviews. *Cochrane Database of Systematic Reviews* 3:CD009234. doi:10.1002/14651858. CD009234.pub2.

Jordan B. 1993. *Birth in Four Cultures: A Crosscultural Investigation of Birth in Yucatan, Holland, Sweden, and the United States.* Long Grove, IL: Waveland Press.

Jordan B. 1997. Authoritative Knowledge and Its Construction. In: *Childbirth and Authoritative Knowledge: Cross-Cultural Perspectives,* eds. Davis-Floyd R, Sargent C. Berkeley: University of California Press, 55–79.

Kennedy HP et al. 2018. Asking Different Questions: A Call to Action for Research to Improve the Quality of Care for Every Woman, Every Child. *Birth: Issues in Perinatal Care* 45(3):222–231. https://onlinelibrary.wiley.com/doi/full/10.1111/birt.12361.

Lawrence A, Lewis L, Hofmeyr GJ, Styles C. 2013. Maternal Positions and Mobility During First Stage Labour. *Cochrane Database of Systematic Reviews* 8:CD003934. doi:10.1002/14651858.CD003934.pub3.

Leavitt JW. 1986. Under the Shadow of Maternity: American Women's Responses to Death and Debility Fears in Nineteenth-Century Childbirth. *Feminist Studies* 12(1):129–154.

Liu S, Liston RM, Joseph KS, Heaman M, Sauve R, Kramer MS. 2007. Maternal Mortality and Severe Morbidity Associated with Low-Risk Planned Cesarean Delivery Versus Planned Vaginal Delivery at Term. *Canadian Medical Association Journal* 176(4):455–460.

Lovejoy OC. 1998. The Evolution of Human Walking. *Scientific American.* 259(5):118, 122–123, 125.

Ludington-Hoe S, Hadeed A, Anderson G. 1991a. Physiologic Responses to Skin-to-Skin Contact in Hospitalized Premature Infants. *Journal of Perinatology: Official Journal of the California Perinatal Association* 111(1):19–24.

Ludington-Hoe S, Hadeed A, Anderson G. 1991b. *Randomized Trials of Cardiorespiratory, Thermal and State Effects of Kangaroo Care for Preterm Infants.* Paper presented at the biennial meetings of the Society for Research in Child Development. Seattle, Washington.

Martin E. 1987. *The Woman in the Body.* Boston: Beacon Press.

McDonald JR et al. 2007. Methicillin-Resistant Staphylococcus Aureus Outbreak in an Intensive Care Nursery: Potential for Interinstitutional Spread. *Pediatric Infectious Disease Journal* 26(8):678–683.

McDougall I, Brown F, Fleagle J. 2005. Stratigraphic Placement and Age of Modern Humans from Kibish, Ethiopia. *Nature* 433(7027):733–736.

McFadden A et al. 2017. Support for Healthy Breastfeeding Mothers with Healthy Term Babies. *Cochrane Database of Systematic Reviews* 2:CD001141. doi:10.1002/14651858. CD001141.pub5.

McKenna J. 2003. Sudden Infant Death Syndrome in Cross-Cultural Perspective: Is Infant-Parent Sleeping Protective? In: *The Manner Born: Birth Rites in Cross-Cultural Perspective*, ed. Dundes L. Walnut Creek CA: Altamira Press, 63–178.

McKenna J. 2020. *Safe Infant Sleep: Expert Answers to Your Cosleeping Questions*. Washington, DC: Platypus Media.

McKenna J, Gettler LT. 2016. There Is No Such Thing as Infant Sleep, There Is No Such Thing as Breastfeeding, There Is Only Breastsleeping. *Acta Paediatrica* 105(1):17–21. doi:10.1111/apa.13161.

McKenna J, McDade T. 2005. Why Babies Should Never Sleep Alone: A Review of the Cosleeping Controversy in Relationship to SIDS, Bedsharing and Breastfeeding. *Paediatric Respiratory Reviews* 6(2):134–152. doi:10.1016/j.prrv.2005.03.006.

McKenna J, Mosko S. 2001. Mother-Infant Co-Sleeping: Toward a New Scientific Beginning. In: *Sudden Infant Death Syndrome: Problems, Progress and Possibilities*, eds. Byerd R, Krous H. New York: Arnold, 258–272.

Miller J. 2021. Solitary and Kin-Assisted Rarámuri Birth: Ideals and Realities. In: *Birthing Models on the Human Rights Frontier: Speaking Truth to Power*, eds. Daviss BA, Davis-Floyd R. London: Routledge, Chapter 16, in press.

Miller S. et al. 2016. Beyond Too Little, Too Late and Too Much, Too Soon: A Pathway Towards Evidence-Based, Respectful Maternity Care Worldwide. *Lancet* 388(10056):2176–2192. doi:10.1016/S0140-6736(16)31472-6. Pub Med PMID: 27642019.

Montague A. 1971. *Touching: The Human Significance of Skin*. New York: Harper and Row Publishers.

Montoya-Williams D, Lemas DJ, Spiryda L, Patel K, Neu J, Carson TL, Carson TL. 2018. The Neonatal Microbiome and Its Partial Role in Mediating the Association between Birth by Cesarean Section and Adverse Pediatric Outcomes. *Neonatology* 114(2):103–111.

Moore ER, Bergman N, Anderson GC, Medley N. 2016. Early Skin-to-Skin Contact for Mothers and Their Healthy Newborn Infants. *Cochrane Database of Systematic Reviews* 11:CD003519. doi:10.1002/14651858.CD003519.pub4.

National Academies of Sciences, Engineering, and Medicine. 2020. *Birth Settings in America: Outcomes, Quality, Access, and Choice*. Washington, DC: The National Academies Press. doi:10.17226/25636.

Nguyen DM, Bancroft E, Mascola L, Guerara R, Yasuda L. 2007. Risk Factors for Neonatal Methicillin-Resistant Staphylococcus Aureus Infection in a Well-Infant Nursery. *Infection Control and Hospital Epidemiology* 28(4):406–411.

Olsen O, Clausen JA. 2012. Planned Hospital Birth Versus Planned Home Birth. *Cochrane Database of Systematic Reviews* 9:CD000352.pub2. doi:10.1002/14651858.

Ortner S. 1974. Is Female to Male as Nature Is to Culture? In: *Woman, Culture, and Society*, eds. Rosaldo MZ, Lamphere L. Stanford: Stanford University Press, 120–135.

Pavlicev M, Romero R, Mitteroecker P. 2020. Evolution of the Human Pelvis and Obstructed Labor: New Explanations of an Old Obstetrical Dilemma. *American Journal of Obstetrics and Gynecology* 222(1):3–16. doi:10.1016/j.ajog.2019.06.043.

Pollock LA. 1990. Embarking on a Rough Passage: The Experience of Pregnancy in Early-Modern Society. In: *Women as Mothers in Pre-Industrial England*, ed. Fildes V. London: Routledge, 39–67.

Pollock LA. 1997. Childbearing and Female Bonding in Early Modern England. *Social History* 22(3):287–306.

Priddis H, Dahlen H, Schmied V. 2012. What Are the Facilitators, Inhibitors, and Implications of Birth Positioning? A Review of the Literature. *Women and Birth: Journal of the Australian College of Midwives* 25(3):100–106.

Reveiz L, Gaitan HG, Cuervo LG. 2007. Enemas During Labour. *Cochrane Database of Systematic Reviews* 4:CD000330.

Reynolds P. 1991. *Stealing Fire: The Atomic Bomb as Symbolic Body*. Palo Alto, CA: Iconic Anthropology Press.

Rosenberg K. 1992. The Evolution of Modern Human Childbirth. *American Journal of Physical Anthropology* 35(S15):89–124.

Rosenberg K. 2003. "Comments. Response to D. Walrath, Rethinking Pelvic Typologies and the Human Birth Mechanism *Current Anthropology* 44(1):5–31.

Rosenberg K, Trevathan W. 2018. Evolutionary Perspectives on Cesarean Section. *Evolution, Medicine, and Public Health* 1(1):67–81. doi:10.1093/emph/eoy006.

Sandall J, Soltani H, Gates S, Shennan A, Devane D. 2016. Midwife-Led Continuity Models Versus Other Models of Care for Childbearing Women. *Cochrane Database of Systematic Reviews* 4:CD004667.pub5. doi:10.1002/14651858.

Sargent C. 1989. *Maternity, Medicine, and Power: Reproductive Decisions in Urban Benin*. Berkeley: University of California Press.

Selin H, Stone PK, eds. 2009. *Childbirth across Cultures: Ideas and Practices of Pregnancy, Childbirth, and the Postpartum*. Springer.

Shanley L. 1994. *Unassisted Childbirth*. Westport, CT: Bergin and Garvey.

Singata M, Tranmer J, Gyte GM. 2013. Restricting Oral Fluid and Food Intake during Labour. *Cochrane Database of Systematic Reviews* 8:CD003930.pub3. doi:10.1002/14651858.

Small MF. 1999. *Our Babies, Ourselves: How Biology and Culture Shape the Way We Parent*. New York: Anchor Books.

Small MF. 2001. *Kids: How Biology and Culture Shape the Way We Can Raise Young Children*. New York: Anchor Books.

Sng BL, Leong WL, Zeng Y, Siddiqui FJ, Assam PN, Lim Y … Sia AT. 2014. Early Versus Late Initiation of Epidural Analgesia for Labour. *Cochrane Database of Systematic Reviews* 10:CD007238.pub2. doi:10.1002/14651858.

Sosa G, Crozier K, Robinson J. 2012. What Is Meant by One-to-One Support in Labour: Analysing the Concept. *Midwifery* 28(4):451–457. doi:10.1016/j.midw.2011.07.001.

Stapleton SR, Osborne C, Illuzzi J. 2013. Outcomes of Care in Birth Centers: Demonstration of a Durable Model." *Journal of Midwifery and Women's Health* 58(1):3–14. doi:10.1111/jmwh.1200.

Stoller M. 1995. The Obstetric Pelvis and Mechanism of Labor in Nonhuman Primates. *American Journal of Physical Anthropology* 20:204.

Stringer C. 2016. The Origin and Evolution of Homo Sapiens. *Philosophical Transactions of the Royal Society of London Series B Biological Sciences* 371(1698). www.ncbi.nlm.nih.gov/pubmed/20150237.

Trevathan W. 1997. An Evolutionary Perspective on Authoritative Knowledge About Birth. In: *Childbirth and Authoritative Knowledge*, eds. Davis-Floyd R, Sargent C. Berkeley: University of California Press, 80–90.

Trevathan W. 1999. "Evolutionary Obstetrics." In: *Evolutionary Medicine*, eds. Trevathan W, Smith EO, McKenna J. New York: Oxford University Press, 183–208.

Trevathan W. 2010. *Ancient Bodies, Modern Lives: How Evolution Has Shaped Women's Health*. New York: Oxford University Press.

Trevathan W. 2015. Primate Pelvic Anatomy and Implications for Birth. *Philosophical Transactions of the Royal Society Series B: Biological Sciences* 370(1663). doi:10.1098/rstb.2014.0065. www.ncbi.nlm.nih.gov/pubmed/20140065.

Trevathan W. 2017 [1987]. *Human Birth: An Evolutionary Perspective*, 3rd ed. New York: Routledge.

Trevathan W, McKenna J. 2003 [1994]. Evolutionary Environments of Human Birth and Infancy: Insights to Apply to Contemporary Life. *Children's Environments* 11:88–104.

Trevathan W, Rosenberg K. 2000. The Shoulders Follow the Head: Postcranial Constraints on Human Childbirth. *Journal of Human Evolution* 39(6):583–586.

Trevathan W, Smith EO, McKenna J. 2008. *Evolutionary Medicine and Health: New Perspectives*. New York: Oxford University Press.

Ulrich LT. 1990. *A Midwife's Tale*. New York: Vintage Books.

Villar J et al. 2006. Caesarean Delivery Rates and Pregnancy Outcomes: The 2005 WHO Global Survey on Maternal and Perinatal Health in Latin America. *Lancet* 367(9525):1819–1829.

Villar J et al. 2007. Maternal and Neonatal Individual Risks and Benefits Associated with Caesarean Delivery: Multicentre Prospective Study. *British Medical Journal* 335(1025):1–11.

Walrath D. 2006. Gender, Genes, and the Evolution of Human Birth. In: *Feminist Anthropology: Past Present and Future*, eds. Geller P, Stockett M. Philadelphia: University of Pennsylvania Press, 55–69.

Wang Z, Sun W, Zhou H. 2012. Midwife-Led Care Model for Reducing Caesarean Rate: A Novel Concept for Worldwide Birth Units Where Standard Obstetric Care Still Dominates. *Journal of Medical Hypotheses and Ideas* 6(1):28– 31. doi:10.1016/j.jmhi.2012.03.013.

Wertz RW, Wertz DC. 1989 [1977]. *Lying-In: A History of Childbirth in America*, 2nd edition. New York: Free Press.

WHO Recommendations on Infant Feeding. 2020. www.who.int/nutrition/topics/infantfeeding_recommendation/en/.

Williams G, Nesse R. 1991. The Dawn of Darwinian Medicine. *Quarterly Review of Biology* 66(1):1–22.

Wilson A. 1995. *The Making of Man-Midwifery: Childbirth in England 1660–1770*. Cambridge, MA: Harvard University Press.

Wilson A. 2016. *Ritual and Conflict: The Social Relations of Childbirth in Early Modern England*. London: Routledge.

Zhang H et al. 2017. A Randomised Controlled Trial in Comparing Maternal and Neonatal Outcomes between Hands-and-Knees Delivery Position and Supine Position in China. *Midwifery* 50:117–124. doi:10.1016/j.midw.2017.03.022.

Zielinski R, Ackerson K, Low LK. 2015. Planned Home Birth: Benefits, Risks, and Opportunities. *Journal of Midwifery and Women's Health* 7:361. doi:10.2147/IJWH.S55561.

Zuk M. 2013. *Paleofantasy: What Evolution Really Tells Us about Sex, Diet, and How We Live*. New York: WW Norton & Company.

2

EGG FREEZING ACTIVISTS:

Extending Reproductive Futures to Cancer Patients, Single and Minority Women, and Transgender Men

Marcia C. Inhorn

Introduction: The Global Rise of Egg Freezing

In 1978, Louise Brown, the world's first "test-tube baby," was born in England, allowing her working-class parents, Lesley and John Brown, to overcome 9 years of heart-breaking involuntary childlessness. Forty years later, more than 8 million in vitro fertilization (IVF) babies have been born (ESHRE 2018), comprising a whole generation of IVF-conceived "techno-sapiens."

But IVF has also led to other births, including a multitude of IVF-related assisted reproductive technologies (ARTs) designed to overcome intractable reproductive barriers. As Sarah Franklin (2013) has argued, IVF has been a "platform" technology for other innovations, including preimplantation genetic diagnosis (PGD) (Franklin and Roberts 2006), human embryonic stem cell (hESC) research on unused IVF embryos (Franklin 2013), and even the future possibility of human reproductive cloning (Franklin 2007).

The most recently conceived repro-technology is "oocyte cryopreservation," or egg freezing. First tried in the early 1980s—with the first reported frozen egg baby born in 1986—egg freezing remained technologically challenging because of lethal ice crystal formation and concerns about chromosomal damage to the human egg (Lockwood 2011). While cryopreservation of human sperm and embryos had been mastered by the 1980s, the successful freezing of human eggs remained elusive. Not until the early 2000s was a new method of flash-freezing called "vitrification" introduced (Mertes and Pennings 2012). Vitrification is a process by which oocytes are treated with cryoprotective substances and then submerged into liquid nitrogen. The cells cool so rapidly to −320 degrees Fahrenheit that they become "vitrified," or glass-like in structure. Unlike older slow freezing methods, vitrification takes minutes rather than hours. Most importantly, with vitrification, the egg survival rate post-rewarming increases from 70% to 90%, with good evidence that fertilization and pregnancy rates are similar between fresh and frozen (and then rewarmed) eggs (Cobo et al. 2016). Furthermore, in terms of reproductive outcomes, no increases in chromosomal abnormalities, birth defects, or developmental deficits have been found in children born from frozen eggs (IFFS 2019). Thus, vitrification has proved to be a "game changer" in the world of oocyte cryopreservation, simplifying the procedure and increasing its efficiency (Inhorn et al. 2021).

A clear-cut need for egg freezing through vitrification was first seen in the world of clinical oncology. Women at risk of losing their reproductive ability via chemotherapy could now freeze their eggs, potentially preserving their ability to conceive genetically related offspring (Inhorn et al. 2018a, 2018b). Given the success of vitrification in clinical trials with cancer patients, healthy women concerned about their own age-related fertility decline began to volunteer for these studies. By 2012, both the American Society for Reproductive Medicine (ASRM) and the European Society for Human Reproduction and Embryology (EHSRE) lifted the "experimental" label, allowing the clinical use of both *medical egg freezing* (MEF) for cancer patients (as well as for women with other fertility-threatening conditions) (Inhorn et al. 2017, 2018a, 2018b), and *elective egg freezing* (EEF)[1] for healthy women hoping to preserve their remaining reproductive potential (Inhorn et al. 2018c, 2018d, 2019).

Calling egg freezing "one of the most significant recent advancements in assisted reproduction technology," the International Federation for Fertility Societies issued a 2019 global report depicting the global spread of egg freezing. Of 82 countries surveyed, 68 (83%) reported that MEF was being performed in their countries, while 56 (68%) also reported the performance of EEF. Eighteen of 42 (43%) countries reported that both MEF and EEF were being frequently performed in their IVF clinics (IFFS 2019).

Yet the 2019 IFFS survey did not report on the extent of *transgender egg freezing* (TEF)[2]—potentially one of the most revolutionary aspects of this new cryopreservation technology. With the growing social acceptance of gender assignment technologies, individuals assigned female at birth can now preserve their eggs before initiating testosterone therapy in their gender transitions (Birenbaum-Carmeli et al. 2020). An international survey of fertility preservation providers in 9 countries (Tishelman et al. 2019) showed that TEF is on the rise around the world, thereby extending reproduction to transgender men and preserving their potential for future fatherhood.

In the United States, all forms of egg freezing have increased in usage since the ASRM lifted the experimental label. Today, most American IVF clinics

---

1 Although the terminology to describe egg freezing is quite variable in the literature, I have forwarded these terms and acronyms, "medical egg freezing" (MEF) and "elective egg freezing" (EEF), to most accurately represent women's own preferences.
2 "TEF" is my own term and acronym, intended to align with medical egg freezing (MEF) and elective egg freezing (EEF).

now offer MEF and EEF routinely (the extent of TEF remains unknown), and multiple EEF commercial clinics and egg banks have opened in major urban areas across the US (see Chapter 3). The response to egg freezing on the part of US women has been quite significant. Within the first year of clinical acceptance (2013), approximately 5,000 egg MEF and EEF cycles were undertaken in the US. Five years later (2018), that number had more than doubled, to 11,000 cycles, according to the Society for Assisted Reproductive Technology (SART). Over the past decade, it is estimated that 36,000 US women have frozen their eggs.

Despite the rise of MEF and EEF—and to a lesser extent TEF—in the US, there are still many barriers for those who would access this technology. Most importantly, egg freezing is an expensive technology (see Chapter 3), not covered by most health insurance plans (Inhorn et al. 2018a, 2018b). Cost concerns are especially daunting for young cancer patients, who rarely have the financial resources to undertake a cycle of MEF, especially under extreme time pressure prior to chemotherapy. Young women and their families must raise sufficient funds on a rapid timescale, usually within days of a cancer diagnosis.

Given these problems of access, egg freezing has been the site of much "behind-the-scenes" activism, primarily on the part of "early adopters," who saw the need for this technology in their own lives, and then worked to make egg freezing more known, available, and affordable to others. Indeed, egg freezing technology has co-evolved with human interaction, specifically through the work of *egg freezing activists,* as I call them here. These individuals were not necessarily part of reproductive activist circles, and thus initiated egg freezing activism mostly on their own. Their major focus was on changing policies among employers, insurers, and professional organizations to make egg freezing more visible, affordable, and beneficial to others. Some of these activists described their approach to change as "vocal" and insistent, while others adopted quieter, yet "proactive" measures.

In this chapter, we will meet 4 of these egg freezing activists: Corinne, a cancer survivor who formed a successful MEF non-profit; Julie, a single professional in Silicon Valley who fought hard for EEF to be funded by a major tech firm; Kamila, an employee of a global reproductive rights organization, who advocated for EEF coverage, as well as access for women of color; and Andrew, a young transgender man, who worked with his university employer to initiate TEF services and insurance coverage. (All names of individuals and organizations in this chapter are pseudonyms.) As we will see, all of these egg freezing activists succeeded as change agents—creating reproductive futures for *cancer patients, single and minority women,* and *transgender men.*

The Ethnographic Study

These stories were collected as part of an ethnographic study of oocyte cryopreservation in the United States. Between June 2014 and August 2016, I undertook in-depth ethnographic interviews with 150 individuals who had undertaken at least one cycle of egg freezing. These included 33 MEF patients, the majority with cancer diagnoses; 114 EEF users, most of them single women who underwent EEF in their late 30s (or early 40s) because they lacked a reproductive partner; 2 women who underwent EEF because their husbands were infertile; and 1 transgender man who undertook TEF in his mid-20s. These individuals were recruited through four IVF clinics (2 academic, 2 private), 3 of which were located in major cities along the East Coast and one in the San Francisco Bay/ Silicon Valley region. Participants often led our discussions, narrating their egg freezing stories and their decision-making processes in detail.

The participants in this study were diverse. About two-thirds were white, and about one-third were non-white, including 30% of the MEF patients and 31% of the EEF recipients. Black, Latinx, Asian American, mixed race, and women of Middle Eastern heritage were represented in this study. Especially among the MEF patients from working-class backgrounds, affording MEF was a significant struggle. In fact, across the MEF and EEF groups, the major recommendation of study participants was to make egg freezing more accessible by bringing the cost down and/or increasing its insurance coverage. This also provided a major focus for egg freezing activism, as we shall see.

In the 4 stories that follow, Corinne, Julie, Kamila, and Andrew explain how they came to adopt activist stances and what they hoped to achieve by them. Such activism is part of the untold history of egg freezing and its birth in American society.

Egg Freezing Activists

Corinne—MEF for Young Cancer Patients

At the turn of the new millennium, when egg freezing was still considered experimental and vitrification not yet perfected, Corinne discovered, at the tender age of 22, that she had a rare form of tongue cancer. She was told by her physician that chemotherapy would put her at high risk for permanent sterility, the thought of which made her panic. But, in an unlikely turn of events, Corinne found her way to egg freezing:

> To kind of paint the picture at this point, I had just recovered from surgery, where they had removed one third of my tongue. So I was, like, lying in bed, on pain meds, it was hard to talk. And, literally, I was watching the movie "You've Got Mail." Well, in the movie, one of the women drops the kids off with a babysitter and says, "I'm going to have my eggs harvested." And I really ran downstairs to my mom, like, "Mom! Egg freezing is possible! I want to freeze my eggs! Then I can do chemo!" And it was really silly, obviously, that it was in this movie. But I thought, if it's in the movie, it exists.

Recovering from her tongue surgery, Corinne began calling different research centers around the country to ask about egg freezing:

> Essentially, it was so unusual—so experimental—that everyone told me it wasn't possible. You can bank sperm or freeze embryos, everyone said. You know, you can have donor sperm, freeze embryos, etc. But that's not what I wanted. The donor sperm kind of scared me at that age…I kept calling the same centers over and over, because they had different receptionists who would say different things. And so on my fifth or sixth call to [a California university] someone answered the phone, honestly, by mistake. It was either a nurse or a doctor, [who] said, "Oh my gosh! We have a new egg freezing clinical trial for cancer patients! We would love to see you. Come in tomorrow!" And 11 days later, my eggs were frozen. And then I started chemo on time and everything was fine. But yeah, it was definitely, there was no information out there. I was basing it on a Hollywood movie, and what different receptionists were telling me at different times during the day.

Corinne's elation made going through her second round of chemotherapy much easier:

> I was so excited about my egg freezing experience! You know, I was in this whole journey, where I sort of resigned my eggs and my body over to medicine. Those were my favorite appointments, those were my favorite injections, where all this stuff was happening to me. And I think part of why this was my favorite was because I was actually planning for the future. It was some tangible hope. So, in the chemo room…you're kind of in there with a bunch of people, including with some people who were my age, my peers. [Fertility preservation was] what I really wanted to talk about. So, the first day I was talking about it, and would ask people what they had done. You know, "Have you banked your sperm?" No one else knew that infertility was a risk, let alone that there were these options, often in the same hospital. And so I'm essentially telling them they might be becoming sterile right now, with the needle in their arm, and they didn't know that before. And so that hit me really hard, and…I felt two things. One, I felt the obligation of truth. Like, I need to do something to give back. And a little bit of survivor's guilt. And I felt like I had this secret, because I knew that everyone was being sterilized, and I knew that there were these amazing options out there, and it was sort of beyond me why no one was linking the two. And so that led me to do some research and see, "Is anyone talking about this? Is this just a bad experience in my hospital, with my physician, or is this a problem in the treatment of young cancer patients?" And I determined it was just like a void in the treatment of young cancer patients.

After recovering from her second round of cancer treatments, Corinne decided to start a small non-profit organization to fill in this void:

> Essentially it had two goals. One was to make sure that every cancer patient is informed of their risk. Research at the time suggested less than 10% of cancer patients were being informed of the fertility risk. And so my goal was that at the end of the day, you shouldn't be sterilized without your knowledge and information. Everyone should know this. And so (1) we wanted to change that, and then (2) we wanted to increase access—access being defined by knowing where the resources are in your area, and actual financial access. And so essentially, we were able to achieve Number 1. It's now an ASCO [American Society of Clinical Oncology] guideline, which is the main body of oncologists, that every patient must be informed. So it's now malpractice if the doctor doesn't inform…Of course, in operation it's not perfect. But we were able to change a standard of care, and then with regards to insurance and access, we got a lot of financial assistance from them, and then worked with a lot of insurance companies to get them to change their benefits…I pushed the "insurance for fertility" agenda, and now egg freezing—fertility preservation—is covered by a number of insurers, for cancer patients only, because of my work. We didn't get every [insurance] company out there…But for the most part our goals are achieved.

Corinne added, "It's exciting. I didn't know back then that I was at Ground Zero of something huge."

Julie—EEF Activism for Single Women in Tech

Julie, also a California native, found herself still single at the age of 35, with no partner in sight, even though she worked as an IT director in the heavily male-dominated Silicon Valley tech industry. This was in the era before all of the Silicon Valley tech giants—Apple, Facebook, Google, and Intel—were offering egg freezing as part of their "fertility benefits" for company employees. Julie worked for one of those companies when she decided to freeze her eggs:

> I know there's a lot of information out there now about how [the company] covers egg freezing. They did not three years ago when I did it. I would actually like to think that my very vocal feedback to our internal benefits group around it maybe played some sort of a role in them eventually moving to this…I was incredibly vocal going through that entire time…I felt like the insurance company really didn't know how to deal with a situation like mine. I mean, even the questions they were asking about infertility and having a partner…You could tell it was just something that was completely foreign to them and they didn't know how to respond.

Like most Fortune 500 companies, Julie's tech firm only offered fertility benefits—namely, full insurance coverage for infertility diagnosis and treatment,
including IVF—to married couples. Single women like Julie facing age-related
fertility concerns were not eligible for fertility coverage. In the many conversations Julie had with the company's HR department and insurers, she began to
feel a sense of discrimination as a single woman hoping to preserve her remaining reproductive potential. She also thought about how LGBTQAI+ employees
might be treated in this situation:

> I really felt like they didn't even know how to ask the questions. I mean,
> everything was about "your partner"...Even three years ago, going through
> this, it was all about your male partner. Now I do have a male partner, but
> I was even thinking on the flip side, you know, if I had a female partner
> at that point in time, how would they have approached that? And it was
> funny: Not only on the insurance side, but even when I was going through
> the classes to learn how to inject myself and all of that. I was the only single
> person in there. And I even remember one of the women saying to me,
> "Well, you know, don't worry; my husband didn't come with me to the
> first class, either." And I said: "Well, I'm actually not married. I don't have
> a partner. I'm actually going through this because I'm going to be freezing
> my eggs." It's already an emotional time and an emotional issue. And, like I
> said, for a lot of people it can feel like, "What's wrong with me?" You kind
> of feel like...you should be able to reproduce. And just all of their ques-
> tions! "How often are you having sex?" Really? Is this really necessary?
> "How many doctors have you seen?" Just the way that they ask the ques-
> tions and phrase the questions to go through this. It's incredibly invasive at
> a time when you are already feeling emotional, overwhelmed. It's a very
> sensitive topic, and there's just no sensitivity in how this is handled.

Still, Julie persisted in her vocal advocacy of egg freezing, eventually convincing
her tech firm to subsidize egg freezing for single women employees. In retro-
spect, she was both bewildered and bemused by the negative media attention this
decision garnered in American society:

> It's funny to me, even now. Obviously, there's been a lot more coverage of
> it recently, and especially with both Apple and Facebook announcing that
> they cover it as a benefit for their own employees...It's funny for me to see
> how things get blown out of proportion. All these stories came out that
> said that Apple and Facebook are paying female employees to freeze their
> eggs. And that then, in turn, "Well, they're paying you because they don't
> want you to have kids, because they don't want you to walk away from the
> workforce." And it just made me laugh so hard, because I said, "They're
> not paying to freeze your eggs! They're saying that they're going to cover
> it if you decide to do that." They're not offering any financial incentive.

In terms of her own finances, Julie was required to pay $16,000 out of her own pocket for her single cycle of egg freezing. But once the company benefits were in place, Julie's $750 annual egg storage fees were covered. For Julie, however, the best "company benefit" was meeting another employee who would soon become her husband. Following two unsuccessful IVF cycles together, they turned to Julie's frozen eggs—rewarming 36 of them, fertilizing 24 of them, transferring 2 to Julie's womb, and freezing 22 embryos. In the middle of my interview with Julie, she received a phone call from the clinic. Recent blood test results showed that Julie was pregnant—probably with frozen-egg-conceived twins.

Kamila—EEF as a Reproductive Choice, Including for Black Women

Kamila was a New York-based communications specialist, who had spent most of her mid-30s working for an international reproductive rights organization. Kamila was in a relationship, but not sure that she wanted to have children with this man, or even become a mother. Still, she decided to pursue egg freezing at the age of 38:

> I just know that I want the choice. Right? Like, I want the option to decide that if I'm in a relationship and I decide that we want to start a family, have children, that I have that ability. But, also, if I decide that I don't, that's okay, too.

Kamila checked with her medical insurance, only to discover that egg freezing was one of the only reproductive technologies *not* covered by the reproductive rights organization for whom she worked:

> You know, we had great healthcare coverage! But what it didn't cover was the egg freezing process…And my health insurance would have covered the process if I was doing IVF and if I could have shown a pattern of having a fertility issue—showing that I tried to get pregnant for six months and was unsuccessful. I was like, "No. That's not exactly what I'm doing here"…I think Google and some of the other…very progressive organizations were offering that as a lifestyle bonus to their employees. And so my thing was, "Come on! This is [a reproductive rights organization]! So if everything else is covered, then you guys definitely need to get behind this as well."
> I was the one who was like, "Listen, if I'm on the road all the time, this is the part of my lifestyle, then my insurance should cover it to the same extent that [they cover IVF]." One of the great things about [the organization] is they cover unlimited IVF for their employees…And so my response to our HR department was, "If you guys are covering all of these great procedures and we are [a reproductive rights organization], then you

should support my decision." So now [they] will cover egg freezing! They had to do some negotiating with the insurance companies and were able to get it covered. So I'm pretty proud of that. To have unlimited coverage for egg freezing is just above and beyond—pretty amazing!

In addition to the changes Kamila was able to enact in her reproductive rights organization, she was also keen on making egg freezing more visible in the Black community. So she began documenting her process on Instagram and Facebook—recording videos of herself and "talking about how I was feeling and all of those things." As the co-founder of a Black women's mentoring organization, it was very important to Kamila that she share her egg freezing story, because, as she said, "the voice of the African-American woman is missing":

> I think that there's just an increased shaming of women that is above and beyond anything that you can imagine. And I really don't think that it's anything to be ashamed of…So many women would say, "I did it, but I just didn't share my story." I think that the sense of keeping it to ourselves is because there is an inherent shame attached to it, especially in the African-American community. I think the shame for women is that you're expected to be married, to have a family, and to have kids by a certain age, and with no problems attached to it. I think that in the African-American community, religion, especially Christianity, plays a huge role there. And so the idea that you are trying to control something that is outside of God's plan, I think, is a big thing… The shame is overwhelming. And I think the shame is related to just women making decisions on their own and for their own health…And if you take that and put it in communities of color, and then you put it in the South (laughing)! I mean, you just, you know. You're pushing a brick wall there.

Kamila continued, sharing her thoughts on the importance of reproductive choice and bodily autonomy for African-American women:

> I think reproductive healthcare in and of itself is an issue among all women, but has a very sensitive vibe in the African-American community, from the historical ability to control our own bodies and our own reproductive healthcare. So, for me, it was very important to do the procedure, but to also share it with someone who may…need that voice to know that it's okay, and that it's our choice. Like, it's really our choice and our decision to make, and what it means to have, you know, bodily autonomy. I control what I do. So I wanted to share that message.

Interestingly enough, after Kamila completed her egg freezing cycle, the young women in her office "went crazy! You know, wanting to know more information on how they could do it." So, I actually got the policy reversed," Kamila explained, "and I want to be proud of myself for standing up and saying, 'This is something I wanted to do, so I did it.'"

Andrew—TEF "Proactivism" for Transgender Men

Kamila, Julie, and Corinne were educated professional women confident in their abilities to push for change and reproductive choice. Andrew was a young, relatively uneducated, working-class transgender man, only 25 at the time of our interview. A recent graduate from a culinary technical school, he was working as an assistant chef in a university dining hall. Always a tomboy, Andrew became motivated to transition from female to male after following Caitlyn Jenner's well-publicized gender affirmation. At that point, Andrew started to mobilize, reading everything he could get his hands on and describing himself as "proactive."

Andrew's entrée into the physical process of gender transition began with a visit to a new primary care physician, who referred him to others who could help him on his way. After making numerous telephone calls and inquiries, Andrew soon discovered that he was the first person at the university where he worked to request TEF, which was definitely not covered by his university's health insurance plan. From that point on, Andrew spent many hours with university benefits personnel to justify insurance coverage. Without it, Andrew explained, TEF was entirely out of reach.

Nervously, Andrew waited for a decision, which had to be approved by a board of medical experts. Fortunately, the decision handed down was a positive one, based on the rationale that the use of testosterone in the gender transition is equivalent to the use of chemotherapy in young cancer patients. Both have sterilizing effects.

Andrew, who was told by his therapist that he was "the first transgender case to get accepted," was elated by the decision:

> I'm very, very grateful…All of the doctors I've seen just showed me so much that I can trust them. I feel like I have great support [from] them. So this is very new to them and new to me as well… so we're kind of going through this together for the first time. I am so lucky [that] it's just been a smooth ride.

At the time of his interview, Andrew had just undergone his first TEF cycle. Without the insurance coverage, it would have cost him a total of $8,100. Yet his only expenses were a $90 co-pay and a $600 annual storage fee. At this point, Andrew was also hoping that 3 additional egg freezing cycles would be approved—comparable to the 4 IVF cycles approved for married couples under the state's insurance mandate:

> I will do all four if I can. I just feel like this is kind of, you know, my one shot right now to have children, and I feel really strongly about this. And

it is something that is very important to me, before I start pursuing, you know, the transition…And I'm also thinking about donating or selling a couple cycles of my eggs…if I'm allowed four cycles. It's something I want to consider. Because I feel like I'm very grateful for the position I'm in and having all the help I have and financial aid, just, you know, has been a blessing. I want to give back as well.

As a practicing Catholic who had been confirmed, accepted all of the sacraments, attended church each Sunday, and believed in God, Andrew had a strong sense of moral responsibility. He hoped to use his own transition and egg freezing experiences to improve the situation for other transgender men living in the US:

Like I said, this was a very important thing for me, being able to have my own children, and I didn't want to harm that in any way…I may not be carrying them, but I'm saving and preserving my eggs…for the future… There's so many unique things about me that I just question all the time, and I told [the doctor that] I'm definitely willing to do any kind of research. Yeah, I just feel like very powerful. I feel like my eggs will be powerful. I feel like I will have numerous amounts of them…I feel like I definitely was made who I am for a reason.

Conclusion

In closing this chapter on egg freezing activism, it seems important to hark back to the title of this volume—*Birthing Techno-Sapiens: Human-Technology Co-Evolution and the Future of Reproduction*. I argue that egg freezing constitutes an apt example. As seen in this chapter, egg freezing through oocyte vitrification: (1) was birthed from IVF; (2) was its most recent birth, considered the newest in the world of assisted reproduction; (3) was made possible by early adopters, some of whom served as human subjects under experimental conditions; (4) was forwarded through human-technology co-evolution, beginning with cancer patients, then single women facing age-related fertility decline, then transgender men; (5) was the site of significant egg freezing activism among individuals who benefited from this technology; and (6) was a way for all of these humans to potentially extend their reproductive futures.

As this chapter has also shown, egg freezing activists in America have worked hard to achieve significant reproductive gains, including: (1) creating an egg freezing non-profit for cancer patients; (2) extending egg freezing insurance coverage to women in the tech industry; (3) advocating for egg freezing as a single woman's reproductive right; (4) making egg freezing more transparent, imaginable, and accessible for minority women; and (5) mandating egg freezing insurance coverage for transgender men. Only through in-depth ethnography with egg freezing activists and others like them can we begin to tell the story of egg freezing—a true exemplar of human-technological co-evolution in the 21st-century United States.

Acknowledgments

I thank Robbie Davis-Floyd for inviting me to contribute to this important volume. I am also grateful to my study colleagues Daphna Birenbaum-Carmeli, Joseph Doyle, Norbert Gleicher, Pasquale Patrizio, and Lynn M. Westphal, as well as my research assistants Rose Keimig, Mira Vale, and Ruoxi Yu. Other invaluable assistance came from Jennifer DeChello, Jeannine Estrada, Sandee Murray, and Tasha Newsome. This study was generously funded by a grant from the US National Science Foundation, Cultural Anthropology, and Science and Technology Studies Programs (BCS-1356136).

References

Birenbaum-Carmeli D, MC Inhorn, P Patrizio. 2020. "Transgender Men's Fertility Preservation: Experiences, Social Support, and the Quest for Genetic Parenthood." *Culture, Health and Sexuality.* doi:10.1080/13691058.2020.

Cobo A, JA Garcia-Velasco, A Coello, J Domingo, A Pellicer, J Remohí. 2016. "Oocyte Vitrification as an Efficient Option for Elective Fertility Preservation." *Fertility and Sterility* 105(3): 755–764.

ESHRE. "More Than 8 Million Babies Born from IVF since the World's First in 1978." www.eshre.eu/ESHRE2018/Media/ESHRE-2018-Press-releases/De-Geyter.

Franklin SB. 2007. *Dolly Mixtures: The Remaking of Genealogy.* Durham, NC: Duke University Press.

Franklin SB. 2013. *Biological Relatives: IVF, Stem Cells and the Future of Kinship.* Durham, NC: Duke University Press.

Franklin SB, C Roberts. 2006. *Born and Made: An Ethnography of Preimplantation Genetic Diagnosis.* Princeton, NJ: Princeton University Press.

Inhorn MC, D Birenbaum-Carmeli, P Patrizio. 2017. "Medical Egg Freezing and Cancer Patients' Hopes: Fertility Preservation at the Intersection of Life and Death." *Social Science and Medicine* 195: 25–33.

Inhorn MC, D Birenbaum-Carmeli, LM Westphal, J Doyle, N Gleicher, D Meirow, H Raanani, M Dirnfeld, P Patrizio. 2018a. "Medical Egg Freezing: The Importance of a Patient-Centered Approach to Fertility Preservation." *Journal of Assisted Reproduction and Genetics* 35(1): 49–59.

Inhorn MC, D Birenbaum-Carmeli, LM Westphal, J Doyle, N Gleicher, D Meirow, H Raanani, M Dirnfeld, P Patrizio. 2018b. "Medical Egg Freezing: How Cost and Lack of Insurance Coverage Impact Women and Their Families." *Reproductive Biomedicine and Society Online* 5: 82–92.

Inhorn MC, D Birenbaum-Carmeli, J Birger, LM Westphal, J Doyle, N Gleicher, D Meirow, M Dirnfeld, D Seidman, A Kahane, P Patrizio. 2018c. "Elective Egg Freezing and Its Underlying Socio-Demography: A Binational Analysis with Global Implications." *Reproductive Biology and Endocrinology: RB&E* 16(1): 70.

Inhorn MC, D Birenbaum-Carmeli, LM Westphal, J Doyle, N Gleicher, D Meirow, M Dirnfeld, D Seidman, A Kahane, P Patrizio. 2018d. "Ten Pathways to Elective Egg Freezing: A Binational Analysis." *Journal of Assisted Reproduction and Genetics* 35(11): 2003–2011.

Inhorn MC, D Birenbaum-Carmeli, LM Westphal, J Doyle, N Gleicher, D Meirow, M Dirnfeld, D Seidman, A Kahane, P Patrizio. 2019. "Patient-Centered Elective Egg

Freezing: A Binational Qualitative Study of Best Practices for Women's Quality of Care." *Journal of Assisted Reproduction and Genetics* 36(6): 1081–1090.

Inhorn MC, D Birenbaum-Carmeli, P Patrizio. 2021. "Elective Egg Freezing." In: *Female and Male Fertility Preservation*, eds. M Grynberg, P Patrizio. New York: Springer, in press.

International Federation of Fertility Societies (IFFS). 2019. "International Federation of Fertility Societies' Surveillance (IFFS) 2019: Global Trends in Reproductive Policy and Practice, 8th Edition." *Global Reproductive Health* 4(1): e29.

Lockwood GM. 2011. "Social Egg Freezing: The Prospect of Reproductive 'Immortality' or a Dangerous Delusion?. " *Reproductive Biomedicine Online* 23(3): 334–340.

Mertes H, G Pennings. 2012. "Elective Oocyte Cryopreservation: Who Should Pay?" *Human Reproduction* 27(1): 9–13.

Tishelman AC, ME Sutter, C Chen, A Sampson, L Nahata, VD Kolbuck, GP Quinn. 2019. "Health Care Provider Perceptions of Fertility Preservation Barriers and Challenges with Transgender Patients and Families: Qualitative Responses to an International Survey." *Journal of Assisted Reproduction and Genetics* 36(3): 579–588.

3

THE SPECULATIVE TURN IN IVF:

Egg Freezing, Reproductive Futures, and the Financialization of Fertility

Lucy van de Wiel

Introduction: The Speculative Turn in Contemporary IVF

Contemporary IVF is undergoing a speculative turn, which is characterized by an increasing number of tests and treatments that are future-oriented, risk-focused, and speculative in nature. Beyond a treatment for current experiences of infertility, IVF is increasingly oriented towards the pre-emptive and proactive treatment of future infertility. This proactive approach is reflected in the growing popularity of cryopreservation technologies—particularly oocyte cryopreservation (OC), or egg freezing—both in existing fertility clinics and in new specialized start-ups. In the US, fertility companies provide and heavily market egg freezing as a widely indicated means of counteracting age-related fertility decline. Thereby changing the indication for fertility treatment, predictive technologies for fertility testing have also become an integral part of a new ethos of proactive fertility management. Major IVF clinics offer fertility check-ups—so-called "fertility MOTs"[1]—and a growing number of start-ups specialize in data-driven testing innovations, which use reproductive health data and predictive analytics to offer personalized estimations of future reproductive chances. Investments in these preservation and prediction technologies reflect how a speculative orientation to future fertility is increasingly central to contemporary IVF practices.

In part, this speculative turn follows the emergence of new oocyte vitrification technologies that significantly improve the prospects for female fertility preservation (Kuwayama et al. 2005). Especially after the American Society

---

1 MOT is an acronym used in the UK to refer to a general medical examination, derived from the mandatory annual Ministry of Transport (MOT) car inspection.

for Reproductive Medicine's (ASRM) 2012 declaration that egg freezing was no longer considered "experimental"—and in spite of the Society's less widely quoted reservations about OC's use to circumvent age-related infertility—egg freezing has rapidly gained in popularity and is now on offer in 97% of US IVF clinics (ASRM 2012; CDC 2018:22). Uniquely, egg freezing is both an infertility treatment for the fertile and a fertility treatment for the infertile. Younger, fertile women are freezing their eggs in preparation for future infertility, while frozen eggs enable the possibility of conception after the onset of age-related infertility. Through this double movement, categories of fertility, infertility, and what we may call "post-fertility" are mobilized in new ways. This chapter addresses how processes of financialization are paving the way for a future remaking of fertility in which a new norm of "proactive fertility management" also implicates a widely indicated reliance on biotechnological interventions.

The speculative turn in assisted reproduction is also characterized by speculative investments in these technologies by investors, entrepreneurs, employers, and patients alike. Although the relations between reproduction, cellular life, and capital have been extensively theorized through concepts of biocapital, biovalue, and bioeconomies (Helmreich 2008), the shifting power dynamics in the fertility sector resulting from large equity investments, increasing consolidation, and the institutionalization of financial instruments for IVF payment have received relatively little attention. Processes of financialization are crucial for understanding the rising popularity of egg freezing, as they play a key role in establishing the infrastructures through which OC may be accessed and in reorganizing reproductive health care more broadly.

In this chapter, I analyze the financialization of fertility by first developing a conceptual framework based on the literature on biocapital and cellular life. Focusing on fertility, I subsequently describe the role of equity investments in the emergence of egg freezing start-ups and the concomitant expansion and consolidation of fertility services. I then discuss how financial products such as subscription plans and insurance for egg freezing establish a dynamic between investment and indebtedness through which ongoing fertility is enacted and constituted. In so doing, I argue that both the material conditions and the underlying logics of financialization function as enabling conditions and interpretative frames for a reinvented, speculative, and precarious notion of fertility and its futurities.

The financial investments and broader commercial and clinical infrastructures constructed around the promise of fertility preservation of course do not determine specific experiences of egg freezing, but they do play a key role in constructing the material realities that organize OC practices, thereby mainstreaming egg freezing across larger groups of potential clients, integrating egg freezing into future treatment plans, and rationalizing OC through new treatment logics that are changing the meaning of fertility in the 21st century.

Financialization, Fertility, and Cryopreservation

Dominant discourses of egg freezing—particularly in the US context—align neatly with neoliberal rationalities by appealing to ideas about "self-responsibilization" for the ongoingness of fertility and maximization of one's future reproductive potential (Brown 2015). A growing body of scholarship has addressed egg freezing in relation to neoliberalization. It has highlighted the responsibilization of individual women for reproductive aging, as popular risk-focused discourses on fertility are characterized by an "implicit injunction to stay informed [and] to live the future in the present body" (Van de Wiel 2015:123). Carroll and Krolokke (2018) analyze egg freezing as an enactment of "responsible" reproductive citizenship that "anticipates coupledom" and genetic relatedness. Rottenberg likewise reads egg freezing as symptomatic of a middle-class neoliberal governmentality based on smart self-investments for enhanced returns in the future, while Emily Jackson highlights the possibility of blame and retrospective regret as the flipside of this responsibilization of one's future fertility (Rottenberg 2016; Jackson 2017).

Herein, I analyze how the widely observed neoliberal rationality of OC is situated in the context of contemporary regimes of financialized capitalism. From its very inception, fertility treatment has been closely aligned with capital accumulation and privatized health care. In the UK, where the first IVF baby was born and the first IVF clinic was founded in 1980 by the clinicians responsible for Louise Brown's conception (Steptoe and Edwards 1978), the emergence of this new medical sector coincided with Margaret Thatcher's rise to power. Marilyn Strathern has described the "enterprising up" of IVF in this context, and Sarah Franklin has analyzed IVF in relation to the "enterprise culture" of Thatcherism (Strathern 1990; Franklin 1997). Gay Becker (2001:39) documented the embeddedness of IVF experiences in the ethos of the American Dream (see also Franklin 2013:240). The neoliberal responsibilization of future fertility with OC emerges in the wake of these histories of IVF.

Yet egg freezing is also quintessentially a reproductive technology of the contemporary moment, in which a shift towards financialization in the fertility sector—particularly the largely for-profit US sector—meets a speculative turn in IVF enabled by (cryo)preservation and prediction technologies. Financialization here includes "changes in management ideology that increasingly orient firms to financial markets (i.e. 'shareholder value')," "the growing influence of financial products, [and] the extension of debts in underserved communities" (Krippner et al. 2017, n.p.). To understand the phenomenon of egg freezing, then, we need to not only focus on clinicians and patients, but also on the firms and financiers that shape this part of the reproductive bioeconomy. This requires addressing not only the sale of commodities (e.g., goods and services), but also the financial value ascribed to egg freezing through capital investments in fertility companies themselves (Birch 2017:472). What is at stake in this focus on financialization in the fertility sector is not so much the fact of commercialization, but rather the

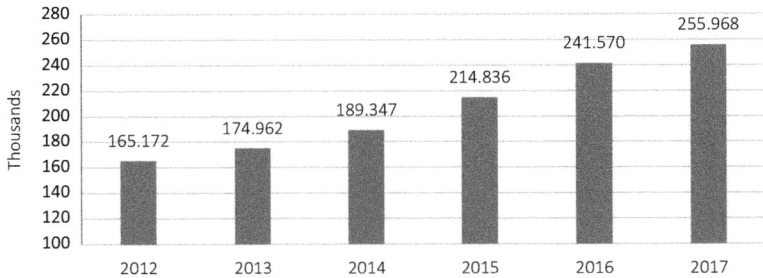

FIGURE 3.1   IVF cycles in US (SART [Society for Assisted Reproductive Technology] 2019). (Graph produced by author.)

shift in power relations and the reconceptualization of female fertility in the face of the changing financial dynamics that govern the industry and *its* viability.

This chapter, then, draws attention to the growing importance of fertility—to be distinguished from reproduction—within the accumulation strategies of the US IVF sector, focusing particularly on the interrelated accumulation of reproductive time and the accumulation of fertility capital through OC. It explores the relations between cryopreservation and financialization in the new forms of indebtedness, financing, and investment that are co-emerging with contemporary egg freezing practices.

Equity for Cryo-Eggs

The increasing popularity of egg freezing is situated in a global fertility sector that has experienced a decade of consistent growth and was—until the COVID-19 crisis—projected to continue expanding at an annual growth rate of almost 10% (GVR 2020).[2] In keeping with this trend, the total number of IVF cycles in the US has steadily grown every consecutive year (see Figures 3.1 and 3.2). Although egg freezing only accounts for a small percentage of US IVF cycles—less than 4% are performed for oocyte banking even though the procedure is on offer in 97% of clinics—this technology has received widespread attention in popular media and academic scholarship (CDC 2018; SART 2019). In spite of these small—albeit rapidly growing—numbers of women freezing their eggs, the promise of cryopreserving female fertility has also attracted investors' interest. Since 2016, millions of dollars of private equity and venture capital have been invested in egg freezing businesses, which materialize the promise of egg freezing as a growth technology that may be targeted at a wide group of younger,

---

2 Estimations of the IVF market size vary wildly and methods for determining these figures are not transparent. These market reports do, however, offer an indication of the broader trends in the IVF sector.

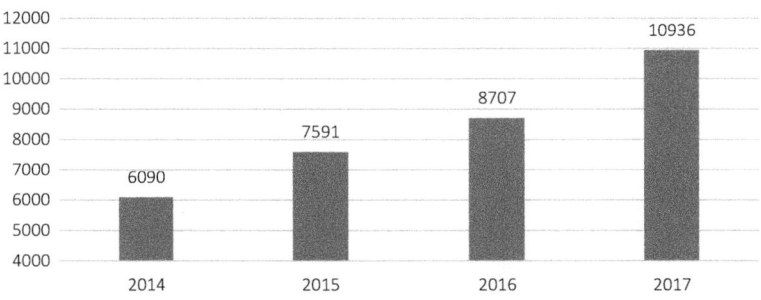

FIGURE 3.2 Egg freezing cycles in US (SART 2019). (Graph produced by author.)

fertile women, who may or may not want to have children in the future—a far greater segment of the population than those currently accessing IVF.

Buoyed by private equity and venture capital investments, egg freezing–focused start-ups are emerging rapidly and are changing the landscape of US IVF. Prelude Fertility, for example, is one major new player focused on egg freezing, founded in 2016 with the aid of a $200 million equity investment. Extend Fertility has operated for a decade through its network of IVF clinics and, in 2016, opened the world's first egg-freezing-only clinic in New York. This business is backed by private equity from North Peak Capital and received a further $15M in 2019 from Regal Healthcare Capital Partners. Kindbody was founded in 2018 with $6.3M seed funding and describes itself as "the future of women's health, fertility and wellness." It brings egg freezing to the streets of urban centers with yellow "fertility vans," or "boutique mobile locations," which offer information on egg freezing and on-site fertility testing (Kindbody 2019). Ova Egg Freezing is another new start-up founded in 2017; it is a member of the Donor Egg Bank USA Network, which was in turn acquired by Generate Life—a major cryopreservation company that combines sperm, egg, and cord blood banking after a massive merger and acquisition deal worth an estimated $1 billion by San Francisco-based private equity firm GI Partners (Ditkowsky 2018).

Beyond clinical services, some of the major new egg freezing start-ups offer financial products. For example, Progyny sells fertility insurance, including coverage for egg freezing, to employers. Such fertility benefits caused an international media hype when Apple and Facebook began offering egg freezing coverage to their employees in 2014; since then, a growing number of Fortune 500 companies have followed suit. Progyny secured almost $100 million in equity to grow its corporate fertility benefit business, a process aided by a strategic alliance with Mercer, the world's largest HR company (Lee 2016; Crunchbase 2019b). In 2019, Progyny entered the NASDAQ stock market and raised almost $150 million (Javeed 2019). Carrot Fertility secured $39.2M in funding to provide fertility benefits to employers. Future Family received $114M in venture capital and debt financing to offer loans and subscription plans for egg freezing and other fertility treatments (Crunchbase 2019a). Symptomatic of the financialization of fertility, the funding attracted for these companies highlights the significance of financial products in the mainstreaming of US egg freezing.

Collectively, these new egg freezing companies have a widespread reach; they create nation-wide networks of fertility clinics, manage influential online platforms, and their innovations receive widespread media and academic commentary. Rather than simply providing the means for their emergence, the significant investment capital poured into egg freezing companies propels a much broader transformation in assisted reproduction. Birch and Tyfield describe the biotechnology sector as underpinned by a "regime in which financial asset values are more important than revenues from the sale of biotechnology commodities" (2013:322). In other words, the key is not primarily the amount of revenue the company generates, but the (speculative) value of the company itself, based on its potential for future growth. These financial investments thus simultaneously enable the current emergence of new egg freezing enterprises, signal the valuation of the promissory value of OC, and materialize the speculation of the future growth of this practice.

The private equity investments in egg freezing companies, then, point not simply to the capital market's interest in the profit that may be generated from (more) women freezing their eggs. Rather, it reflects a more ambitious vision that positions cryopreservation at the heart of a step-change from reproduction to fertility in contemporary IVF. As Stuart Hogarth (2017) has argued, the ongoing growth of US private equity has led to a new model of business development, which relies on securing equity investment by presenting a vision for creating value that is by necessity futural and speculative in nature—and which aligns with the investment culture organizing relevant capital markets. For example, Hogarth argues that the investment culture of Silicon Valley is organized by the ideal of "disruptive innovation" characterized by "a compelling vision of socially beneficial market transformation communicated by a passionate CEO, a belief in the transformative power of information technology," and "the ambition for global growth and market dominance" (2017:256–258). By zooming in on the case of Prelude Fertility, we can consider the discursive, financial, and infrastructural dimensions of equity-backed egg freezing companies and the "disruptive" visions of speculative fertility that propel them.

Prelude and Speculative Fertility

The largest recent OC investment was $200 million committed to Prelude Fertility, an ambitious fertility company founded in 2016 that primarily focuses on egg freezing. Its CEO, Martin Varsavsky, is a serial entrepreneur specialized in real estate and cloud computing; Prelude Fertility is his 7th enterprise, and his first time branching out to the fertility sector. Varsavsky partnered with Lee Equity to acquire RBA IVF clinics and My Egg Bank, one of the largest US egg banks, to form Prelude Fertility (Dorbian 2016). With enough funding to acquire numerous other, existing IVF clinics, Prelude became the second largest US fertility company in its first year, thereby reflecting the "disruptive" effects of private equity in the organization of US IVF (Dresner Partners 2018).

Exemplifying Hogarth's characteristic of a "charismatic" CEO with a vision (2017:258), Varsavsky's plan revolves around oocyte cryopreservation as a means to mainstream infertility treatment. Marketing Prelude as a "fertility company" rather than an *in*fertility clinic, Varsavsky presents the so-called "Prelude Method"—a treatment package that combines cryopreservation, IVF, and embryo genetic screening, as "a complementary strategy to starting a family by having sex":

> As opposed to people who solely rely on sex to make babies, people who rely on both sex and Prelude have a much greater chance of achieving their parental goals of having healthy babies when they are ready. Prelude uses the technology available to infertile people, on fertile people. At Prelude we believe that something as important as having [...] a healthy baby should not be left to chance. (Varsavsky 2016, n.p.)

Blurring distinctions between those who do and don't need fertility treatment, the Prelude Method exemplifies post-fertility and echoes Sunder Rajan's description of a parallel phenomenon in post-genomics: "a reconfiguration of subject categories away from normality and pathology and toward variability and risk, thereby placing *every* individual within a probability calculus as a potential target for therapeutic intervention" (2006:167). Similarly, the Prelude Method expands the target population of IVF to fertile people and also expands the IVF cycle to include embryo screening technologies, thereby providing two axes of growth. Moreover, unlike the potential birth of a baby after an IVF cycle, egg freezing does not have an equally clear endpoint for marking reproductive success. The potential for repeat cycles to accumulate more cryo-eggs presents another rationale for growth.

This approach to ensuring that people can "have a healthy baby when they are ready" by extending fertility to a later point in life is matched with a model of proactive, technologized fertility risk management earlier in life. The notion that young women should be "proactive" in managing their fertility in the face of the progressive loss of their embodied eggs is at the core of several egg freezing companies' missions. Prelude describes itself as "a comprehensive fertility company with a focus on providing proactive fertility care," as reflected in its slogan: "It's time to take charge of your fertility" (Prelude Fertility 2017a). Likewise, Extend Fertility presents itself as "the first service in the country to focus exclusively on women who want to proactively preserve their fertility options" and Progyny as the "leading digital healthcare company combining data and science to provide the first end-to-end, proactive fertility solution for employers" (Bartasi 2016, n.p.; Extend Fertility 2017, n.p.). The emphasis on proactive fertility care suggests a contradistinction with the existing—by implication *reactive*—model of IVF, in which people access treatment when they experience infertility or other barriers to reproduction (see Chapter 2). Instead, *proactive* fertility care requires active, technologized management earlier in life to "preserve options" and maintain the possibility of having (biogenetically related) children later on.

In "promissory capitalism," promises and expectations become capitalized through private equity and venture capital investments. Speculative investment in the eggs' freezability aligns with the promissory value of the future return for patients, companies, and investors alike. As *promise* becomes the "one fundamental of post-Fordist production," which functions as a means to "anticipate and escape the possible 'limit' to its growth long before it has even actualized," cryopreservation enables the temporal manipulation of cellular life to meet the speculative, futural orientation of a "finance-dominated regime of accumulation" (Cooper 2008:23–24). A variation of the "double reproductive value" of stem cells (Franklin 2006), the freezable eggs here hold a double speculative value through the cryo-enabled promise of both a future financial return and a future return of fertility.

Varsavsky's vision for the potential future growth of his fertility company— and the concomitant financial value for investors—is thus coupled with a reconceptualization of fertility that facilitates this future growth. Overcoming the "limits to production" inherent in a "reactive" model of IVF that relies only on the treatment of infertile people, the possibility of pre-emptively treating future infertility through cryopreservation broadens the target group, while the risk-avoidant Prelude Method allows for an expansion of each IVF cycle with additional genetic screening technologies.

It is this vision of a widely indicated, extendable fertility that held the promise of future growth for Lee Equity, Prelude's investors. Meeting the "ambition for market dominance" characteristic of disruptive innovation (Hogarth 2017), Prelude used their equity investment to acquire a nationwide network of 31 IVF clinics across the US. While the US fertility industry is highly fragmented—75% of clinics account for less than 0.24% of total cycles—egg freezing companies are establishing nationwide networks for fertility preservation. Whether through acquisitions (Prelude), strategic alliances with clinics (Progyny), or combining brick-and-mortar with mobile clinics (Kindbody), each of these companies has a broad geographical reach. These equity investments in speculative fertility thus re-organize US IVF by enabling network formations that position egg freezing companies as parent or umbrella organizations.

In order to reach a new group of potential patients, consolidated OC companies can also centralize marketing budgets to reframe IVF as a tool for comprehensive, proactive fertility management. A case in point, Prelude's expanding network of clinics allows for the concentration of marketing efforts—exactly what the investors had in mind. Lee Equity was interested in the growth potential of IVF, given the rising age of first-time mothers and the legalization of same-sex marriage. Yet they also recognized fertility awareness as a means to broaden demand for IVF. Collins Ward, a partner at Lee Equity, says that the "biggest surprise" he encountered in the fertility industry is the "low awareness of fertility services." So the investment in Prelude was coupled with the "significant costs" of a big marketing push intended to, in Ward's words, "speak to younger patients and younger Americans who live in social and digital media." It is this drive to "increase awareness" that bears the promise of "a sizable upside in years to come" by proactively appealing to a new group of potential patients, who are themselves encouraged to be proactive about fertility (quoted in Robbins 2017, n.p.). Now comprising a nation-wide network, Prelude's mission "to educate a generation of women of childbearing age about their fertility" and its "commitment to improving fertility awareness, and providing a proactive approach to family building" has a widespread reach (Prelude Fertility 2017b).

Prelude's online platform reframes fertility in line with the company's vision of mainstreaming proactive fertility management. It shows beautiful yet relatable young adults against a splash of stylish colors. Confident smiles are enframed with statements such as:

> "Find that right person." "Focus on your career." "Finish your education." "The age of your eggs (not you) is the number one cause of infertility." (Prelude Fertility 2017a)

Prelude's website contrasts with the visuals of babies that dominate the majority of IVF websites (Hawkins 2013). Although other reproductive technologies are also on offer, the homepage prominently features egg freezing with a carousel of quotes, such as:

> Stop the hands of the biological clock with Prelude.
> It used to be that women had few options, but not anymore.

In keeping with these statements, Prelude's slogan of "Options Preserved" echoes a vision that, as Strathern (1990) reminded us, has been there since the conception of IVF, when the idea that the "child ought to exist by choice" was embedded in the wider matrix of the prevalent "enterprise culture": "NRTs are presented as opening up reproductive options, the vision of a biology under control, of families free to find their own form (pp. 3–4).

Yet here the focus lies less on the option of having a child and more on the continuation of fertility—as a precondition for achieving relationship, career, and reproductive goals. In the absence of (the desire for) a child, fertility instead refers to a state of having options and the particular relation to futurity that implies.

Beyond marketing, the fertility companies' online platforms are also key instruments in managing widespread networks. These platforms connect participating network members and take on functions previously covered by the clinic. Ongoing medical and emotional support is offered through concierge services and wellness apps (Progyny, Future Family), which provide a centralized discursive framing of the "entire fertility journey." Kindbody takes this one step further through its patient portal, which provides the foundation for "building a centralized data platform, allowing for standardized decision-making, and building predictive protocols to define and scale best practices" (Kindbody 2018b). The equity-based egg freezing companies thus affect IVF's broader infrastructure through acquisitions and network formation, the centralization of marketing, and patient support through online platforms and the adoption of cloud-based services that enable standardization across the network.

Financing Fertility

As egg freezing infrastructures are thus expanding through financial investments, the resulting high stakes in increasing the number of women who freeze their eggs coincides with a shift towards encouraging younger potential patients to "freeze now" to take advantage of their "peak fertility." This appeal to younger people, who typically have less access to the significant sums needed for egg freezing, is matched with financing options offered to broaden access to OC treatment, which represent yet another dimension of the financialization of fertility. Prelude, Extend Fertility, and Future Family present subscription plans for egg freezing with fixed payments of $99–$300/month, while Progyny and Carrot Fertility offer egg freezing insurance to employers. This section discusses the major financial instruments adopted in the mainstreaming of egg freezing and considers how they set up a dynamic of indebtedness and investment as part of contemporary cryopreservation practices.

Reflecting the trend towards promoting earlier freezing, Kindbody spreads the word about egg freezing and fertility decline with its promotional fertility vans, in which passersby can receive free fertility education and fertility tests. In the pastel-colored yellow van, printed statements in photo frames convey the rationale behind earlier freezing:

> You will never be as fertile as you are today.

Coupled with the "facts" that "we are born with all the eggs we will ever have" and that "the quantity and quality of eggs declines with age," these statements convey a temporal logic in which fertility is continually slipping away—a slippage that may be halted with OC: "freezing eggs is like freezing time" (Kindbody 2018a). In keeping with this logic, OVA Egg Freezing (2017) states:

> Your fertility is never going to be as young as it is today—so why wait?

This emphasis on the ongoingness of fertility decline—and the suggested urgency of freezing eggs as early as possible—coincides with the push to market egg freezing to younger women. Prelude Fertility's president Susan Herzberg, for example, states that egg freezing "used to resonate primarily with women in their late 30s," but Prelude is "now targeting women in their 20s and early 30s" (Ferla 2018). The senior OVA nurse specialist and "Bachelor" reality TV winner Whitney Bischoff likewise asserts that "we really want to [reach] the younger crowd because that's the best time to do it" (2015).[3]

Because younger women especially are less likely to be able to afford OC—costs average around $10,000/cycle—these marketing efforts are often paired with payment plans. Within a treatment rationale that promotes earlier freezing, it is better to freeze young eggs now and pay later, rather than save up and freeze older eggs. In this way, the capital investments in the promise of the expansion of egg freezing as a mainstream practice are complemented with additional revenue produced through financial instruments such as fertility loans and subscription plans. Consequently, broadening the target group for egg freezing can increase revenue by creating new norms and needs for both clinical and financial services.

The distribution of consumer credit through clinics is widespread throughout the fertility industry. The average cost for an IVF cycle in the US is currently around $23,474 and is a major barrier to accessing treatment (FertilityIQ 2020). Almost 50% of US fertility clinics mention credit on their websites, often through third-party fertility lenders, such as CapexMD and Prosper (Hawkins 2009:863; Jacoby 2009:148). Reflecting a national context characterized by a fee-for-service health care and higher treatment fees, 70% of women using fertility treatment in the US accrued debt. Almost half of these women incurred over $10,000 in debt and younger women (25–34) borrowed significantly more than their seniors (Market Cube 2015). Firms in the industry estimate that fertility-related loans totaled about $4 billion in 2011 (Silver-Greenberg 2012).

Although the debt financing of IVF can expand access, legal scholars have raised concerns about potential conflicts of interest arising from arrangements between clinics and lenders, given the power and trust relation between doctors and patients and the potential financial incentives for prescribing both particular treatments and the means to finance them (Jacoby 2009; Hawkins 2009). So while fertility loans may be valuable to patients struggling to afford treatment, such loans may also change the dynamics between financial and reproductive decision making for patients and professionals alike. Nonetheless, as Melissa Jacoby (2009:170,175) asserts, fertility companies that wish to expand "must move beyond the elite to those of more modest means. Specialty consumer credit

---

3 Commenting on US egg freezing more broadly, the ASRM Ethics Committee notes that it is "concerned about [...] the line between education of young women and inappropriately aggressive marketing to them." (ASRM 2018). In their analysis of the quality of information about social egg freezing on the websites of 147 US clinics, Avraham and colleagues (2014) found that the majority of websites did not follow the ASRM guidelines on OC and related advertising.

could be a key ingredient to this expansion, particularly when partnered with other financial products."

Similarly, the egg freezing companies' encouragement of earlier freezing may also entail an invitation into a debt relation between the patient and the fertility (financing) company. The creation of dedicated fertility lending companies attests to the fact that the debt financing of egg freezing functions as a revenue source in its own right. Companies such as Extend Fertility work with external lenders for their subscription plans, which charge between 7% and 22% interest rates and 1%–6% origination fees, depending on one's credit score. In this way, the financial risk taken by clinics to recruit younger people with fewer financial means is transferred to lenders, who subsequently pass this risk on to clients through varying rates and fees—in line with Lazzarato's observation that financialized capitalism demands "that one take upon oneself the costs and risks externalized by [...] corporations" (2012:51). In this process, value is created through a circular shifting of financial and reproductive risk: as patients shift the risk of future infertility to the clinic, clinics transfer the risk of non-payment to lenders, who, in turn, move this risk to patients through differential rates and fees (Figure 4.3). In this dynamic exchange of reproductive and financial risk, fertility lending thus aligns companies' capital accumulation with patients' fertility accumulation through OC. By promoting both a proactive treatment rationale and fertility financing, this *debt financing model of egg freezing* creates value through a double temporal movement of anticipation and deferral; it combines treating future infertility in the present and paying for present treatment in the future.

Lastly, besides fertility financing, fertility insurance is another financial product that is rapidly growing in popularity as a result of capital investments in cryopreservation. Having secured almost $100M in venture capital, market leader Progyny has a widespread reach with its online platforms, over 600 affiliated clinics, and coverage of over 2.1 million people (CNBC 2018; Progyny 2020). Its fertility benefit streamlines egg freezing into an elaborate IVF package presented as "the first end-to-end proactive fertility solution for both large, self-insured employers [and] today's informed consumer looking to manage their reproductive health" (Progyny 2016). Progyny presents its proactive fertility program to employers as a means to improve return on investment—both by limiting costs for absenteeism and multiple pregnancies associated with "reactive" IVF, and by fostering a "family friendly" and innovative image (Abdou 2016). Progyny thus integrates proactive fertility management into the workplace by positioning OC as a tool for employees to self-invest in future fertility and a tool for employers to increase return on investment. Significantly, by aligning the financial investment rationales for employers and the reproductive investment rationales for their patient-employees, Progyny institutionalizes a speculative approach to fertility, which positions egg freezing as the entry point into a long-term, highly technologized, proactive fertility management plan for a growing number of women.

Conclusion: Financializing Fertility

This chapter focuses on the remarkable emergence of egg freezing in the last decade and explores the ways in which processes of financialization play a central role in the organization of contemporary US IVF and the widespread mainstreaming of OC in particular. Situated in a broader context of financialized capitalism, the growing popularity of egg freezing is propelled by large capital investments in cryopreservation in recent years. The growth potential of egg freezing and the promissory nature of proactive fertility preservation align directly with the logic of promissory capitalism underlying equity investment markets. (Hogarth 2017:266). It is therefore not surprising that the niche of oocyte cryopreservation has been particularly successful in attracting finance capital and, consequently, egg freezing is now at the heart of a consolidating trend of the US fertility industry that is both reorganizing the sector and changing the discursive construction of fertility through these growing enterprises.

As became clear in the case of Prelude Fertility, equity-backed expansion, acquisition, and consolidation strategies can subsume traditional IVF practices under the umbrella of growing egg freezing enterprises. Even when clinics are not directly acquired, the new egg freezing companies have a widespread reach through marketing efforts directed at broader target groups and financial products that cover treatment costs by bundling egg freezing with other treatments. By bringing together payment, concierge support, and fertility information, centralized online platforms moreover become key framing instruments for organizing and promoting egg freezing treatment across nation-wide networks; the concomitant normalization of fertility preservation represents yet one more move towards what is described in this volume as a *techno-sapiens* future.

The major egg freezing companies also offer financial products such as subscription and insurance plans. Subscription plans are presented as a means to democratize access to treatment, yet, in so doing, they set up a dynamic of investment and indebtedness in the process of preserving fertility. Characteristic of financialization, this brings debt relations to the heart of assisted reproduction and sets up additional sources of OC-related revenue through financial instruments, while enabling more spending on treatment cycles. Both subscription and insurance plans streamline egg freezing into a wider set of treatments, thereby adopting OC as a stepping-stone into a longer-term trajectory of proactive technologized fertility management.

By means of the expansive growth and reach of fertility companies—through mergers and acquisitions, network formation, online marketing, and financial products—egg freezing is thus changing the landscape of IVF. Fertility can now be frozen in time and separated from the bodies that used to embody it. The financialization of fertility, in this context, references the significant financial investments in a future in which ever more women freeze their eggs, the role of private equity and venture capital in establishing the clinical and commercial infrastructures through which egg freezing becomes accessible, the alignment of the financialized logics of the capital market and those underlying dominant treatment rationales, and the role of financial products in shaping both the stories and the streamlining of fertility preservation. Together, these developments are indicative of a shift from reproduction to fertility in IVF, in which treatment need not necessarily be aimed at having a child in the face of infertility, but rather at the proactive management of a more speculative fertility throughout the life course. As a result, the introduction and financial backing of egg freezing presents not simply another reproductive option, but has instigated a step-change in IVF and is changing what it means to be "fertile" in the 21st century.

Acknowledgments

This chapter is an abridged and revised version of Van de Wiel (2020). I thank *New Genetics and Society* for their permission to reprint the parts of the original article that appear in this chapter.

References

Abdou, Jenna. 2016. *How Progyny Is Modernizing Family Planning with CEO Gina Bartasi.* 33 Voices. www.youtube.com/watch?v=y5YjDlfBlBs#t=462.808435.

ASRM, Ethics Committee of the American Society for Reproductive Medicine. 2018. "Planned Oocyte Cryopreservation for Women Seeking to Preserve Future Reproductive Potential: An Ethics Committee Opinion." *Fertility and Sterility* 110(6):1022–1028. doi:10.1016/j.fertnstert.2018.08.027.

ASRM Office of Public Affairs. 2012. "ASRM Lifts 'Experimental' Label from Technique." *American Society for Reproductive Medicine*, October 22. http://elireshefmd .com/fertility-experts-issue-new-report-on-egg-freezing-asrm-lifts-experimental -label-from-technique/.

Avraham, Sarit, Ronit Machtinger, Tal Cahan, Amit Sokolov, Catherine Racowsky, Daniel S Seidman. 2014. "What Is the Quality of Information on Social Oocyte Cryopreservation Provided by Websites of Society for Assisted Reproductive Technology Member Fertility Clinics?" *Fertility and Sterility* 101(1):222–226. doi:10.1016/j.fertnstert.2013.09.008.

Bartasi, Gina. 2016. "Gina Bartasi, Chief Executive Officer at Progyny, Inc." *LinkedIn*, December. www.linkedin.com/in/gina-bartasi/.

Becker, Gay. 2001. *The Elusive Embryo: How Women and Men Approach New Reproductive Technologies.* Berkeley: University of California Press.

Birch, Kean. 2017. "Rethinking Value in the Bio-Economy." *Science, Technology, and Human Values* 42(3):460–490. doi:10.1177/0162243916661633.

Birch, Kean, David Tyfield. 2013. "Theorizing the Bioeconomy Biovalue, Biocapital, Bioeconomics or… What?" *Science, Technology and Human Values* 38(3):299–327. doi:10.1177/0162243912442398.

Bischoff, Whitney. 2015. "'Bachelor' Winner Whitney Bischoff: Why Freezing My Eggs at 27 Was One of the Best Decisions of My Life." *Splinter*, July 2. https://sp linternews.com/bachelor-winner-whitney-bischoff-why-freezing-my-eggs-179384 9303.

Brown, Wendy. 2015. *Undoing the Demos: Neoliberalism's Stealth Revolution.* New York: Zone Books-MIT.

Carroll, Katherine, Charlotte Kr"løkke. 2018. "Freezing for Love: Enacting 'Responsible' Reproductive Citizenship Through Egg Freezing." *Culture, Health and Sexuality* 20(9):992–1005. doi:10.1080/13691058.2017.1404643.

CDC. 2018. *Assisted Reproductive Technology: Fertility Clinic Success Rates Report 2016.* Atlanta: Centers for Disease Control and Prevention. ftp://ftp.cdc.gov/pub/Publicat ions/art/ART-2016-Clinic-Report-Full.pdf.

CNBC. 2018. *Progyny 2018 Disruptor 50.* May 22. www.cnbc.com/2018/05/22/progyn y-2018-disruptor-50.html.

Cooper, Melinda E. 2008. *Life as Surplus: Biotechnology and Capitalism in the Neoliberal Era.* Seattle: University of Washington Press.

Crunchbase. 2019a. "Future Family." *Crunchbase.* www.crunchbase.com/organization/ future-family.

Crunchbase. 2019b. "List of Progyny's 10 Funding Rounds Totaling $99.5M." *Crunchbase.* www.crunchbase.com/search/funding_rounds/field/organizations/funding_total/ progyny.

Ditkowsky, Lisa. 2018. "White Paper: The Fertility Field Mergers & Acquisitions (M&A): Frothy or the Next Frontier?" *Pllush Capital Management*, August 17. www.pllush.com/ blog/fertility-ivf-donor-eggs-shady-grove-fertility-centers-illinois-private-equ.

Dorbian, Iris. 2016. "Lee Equity Partners Co-Launches New Fertility Company Prelude." *PE Hub (Blog)*, October 17. www.pehub.com/2016/10/lee-equity-partners -co-launches-new-fertility-company-prelude/.

Dresner Partners. 2018. "Staying Ahead of the Curve: Healthcare—Women's Health Sector." *Dresner Partners*, June. www.dresnerpartners.com/ace-files/Fertility_June_2 018.pdf.

Extend Fertility. 2017. *Extend Fertility: A Premier Egg Freezing Service Extend Fertility.* https://extendfertility.com/.

Fertility, IQ. 2020. "The Cost of IVF by City." *FertilityIQ.* www.fertilityiq.com/topics/ ivf/the-cost-of-ivf-by-city.

Franklin, Sarah. 1997. *Embodied Progress: A Cultural Account of Assisted Conception.* London: Routledge.

Franklin, Sarah. 2006. "Embryonic Economies: The Double Reproductive Value of Stem Cells." *BioSocieties* 1(1):71–90.

Franklin, Sarah. 2013. *Biological Relatives: IVF, Stem Cells, and the Future of Kinship.* Durham: Duke University Press.

GVR. 2020. "IVF Market Size Worth $37.7 Billion by 2027 | CAGR: 9.5%." *Grand VIEW Research*, February. www.grandviewresearch.com/press-release/global-ivf -market.

Hawkins, Jim. 2009. "Doctors as Bankers: Evidence from Fertility Markets." *Tulane Law Review* 84(July):841–898.

Hawkins, Jim. 2013. "Selling ART: An Empirical Assessment of Advertising on Fertility Clinics' Websites." *Indiana Law Journal* 88(4):1147–1179.

Helmreich, Stefan. 2008. "Species of Biocapital." *Science As Culture* 17(4):463–478. doi:10.1080/09505430802519256.

Hogarth, Stuart. 2017. "Valley of the Unicorns: Consumer Genomics, Venture Capital and Digital Disruption." *New Genetics and Society* 36(3):250–272. doi:10.1080/14636778.2017.1352469.

Jackson, Emily. 2017. "The Ambiguities of 'Social' Egg Freezing and the Challenges of Informed Consent." *BioSocieties*, April: 1–20. doi:10.1057/s41292-017-0044-5.

Jacoby, Melissa B. 2009. "The Debt Financing of Parenthood." *Law and Contemporary Problems* 72(3):147–175.

Javeed, Mohammad Shayan. 2019. "Fertility Services Company Progyny Raises $149.5M in Nasdaq IPO." *S&P Global*, October 29. www.spglobal.com/marketintelligence/en /news-insights/trending/0QtsiLp6WXe0p47T2Sa0rA2.

Kindbody. 2018a. "Egg Freezing Facts." *Kindbody*. https://kindbody.com/egg-freezing-f acts/.

Kindbody. 2018b. "Kindbody Purchases Cloud-Based Software From IVFqc." *PR Newswire*, August 4. www.prnewswire.com/news-releases/kindbody-purchases-clo ud-based-software-from-ivfqc-300696756.html.

Kindbody. 2019. "Kindbody—The Future of Women's Health, Fertility and Wellness." *Kindbody*. https://kindbody.com/.

Krippner, Greta, Benjamin Lemoine, Quentin Ravelli. 2017. "The Politics of Financialization." *Revue de la Régulation* 22(22). doi:10.4000/regulation.12637. https ://journals.openedition.org/regulation/12637.

Kuwayama, Masashige, Gábor Vajta, Osamu Kato, Stanley P Leibo. 2005. "Highly Efficient Vitrification Method for Cryopreservation of Human Oocytes." *Reproductive Biomedicine Online* 11(3):300–308.

La Ferla, Ruth. 2018. "These Companies Really, Really, Really Want to Freeze Your Eggs." *The New York Times*, September 6, sec. Style. www.nytimes.com/2018/08/29 /style/egg-freezing-fertility-millennials.html.

Lazzarato, Maurizio. 2012. *The Making of the Indebted Man: An Essay on the Neoliberal Condition.* Los Angeles, CA: Semiotexte. https://monoskop.org/images/6/62/La zzarato_Maurizio_The_Making_of_the_Indebted_Man_An_Essay_on_the_Neol iberal_Condition_2012.pdf.

Lee, Bruce M. 2016. "Mercer Forms Strategic Alliance with Progyny." *Mercer*, January 7. www.mercer.com/newsroom/mercer-progyny-alliance.html.

Market Cube. 2015. "Fertility Treatments in the United States: Sentiment, Costs and Financial Impact." *Prosper Blog*, May 20. https://blog.prosper.com/2015/05/20/fert ility-treatments-in-the-united-states-sentiment-costs-and-financial-impact/.

OVA. 2017. "New to Egg Freezing? The Top 10 Questions You Should Ask." *OVA Blog (Blog)*, January 1. www.ovaeggfreezing.com/2017/01/01/new-to-egg-freezing-the -top-10-questions-you-should-ask/.

Prelude Fertility. 2017a. *Prelude Fertility.* Prelude Fertility, Inc. www.preludefertility.com/.

Prelude Fertility. 2017b. "Prelude Fertility Expands Network with Pacific Fertility Center in San Francisco." *PR Newswire*, September 25. www.prnewswire.com/news -releases/prelude-fertility-expands-network-with-pacific-fertility-center-in-san-f rancisco-300524534.html.

Progyny. 2016. "Progyny to Present at 34th Annual J.P. Morgan Healthcare Conference." *PRWeb*, January 8. www.prweb.com/releases/2016/01/prweb13155994.htm.

Progyny. 2020. *Annual Report 2019.* New York: Progyny. investors.progyny.com/static-f iles/f46e36c9-a659-4f03-b7d6-4be56066bace.

Robbins. 2017. "Investors See Big Money in Infertility. And They're Transforming the Industry." *STAT*, December 4. www.statnews.com/2017/12/04/infertility-industry -investment/.

Rottenberg, Catherine. 2016. "Neoliberal Feminism and the Future of Human Capital." *Signs: Journal of Women in Culture and Society* 42(2):329–348. doi:10.1086/688182.

SART. 2019. *National Summary Report.* Society for Assisted Reproductive Technology. www.sartcorsonline.com/rptCSR_PublicMultYear.aspx.

Silver-Greenberg, Jessica. 2012. "In Vitro: A Fertile Niche for Lenders." *Wall Street Journal*, February 24. www.wsj.com/articles/SB100014240529702039608045772 41270123249832.

Steptoe, PC, RG Edwards. 1978. "Birth after the Reimplantation of a Human Embryo." *Lancet* 312(8085):366.

Strathern, Marilyn. 1990. "Enterprising Kinship: Consumer Choice and the New Reproductive Technologies." *Cambridge Anthropology* 14(1):1–12.

Sunder Rajan, Kaushik. 2006. *Biocapital: The Constitution of Postgenomic Life.* Durham, NC: Duke University Press.

Van de Wiel, Lucy. 2015. "Freezing in Anticipation: Eggs for Later." *Women's Studies International Forum* 53(November–December):119–128. doi:10.1016/j. wsif.2014.10.019.

Van de Wiel, Lucy. 2020. "The Speculative Turn in IVF: Egg Freezing and the Financialization of Fertility." *New Genetics and Society* 39(3):306–326. doi:10.1080/14 636778.2019.1709430.

Varsavsky, Martin. 2016. "But Daddy, How Are Babies Made?" *Martin Varsavky (Blog),* October 7. http://english.martinvarsavsky.net/paternity/but-daddy-how-are-babies-made.html#comments.

4

SOCIOLOGY AS TECHNOLOGY:

A Toolkit for Studying In Vitro Gametogenesis

Noémie Merleau-Ponty

Introduction: Attempting In Vitro Gametogenesis

A "gamete" is a mature sexual reproductive cell—a sperm or egg—that unites with another cell to form a new organism. The terms "in vitro gametogenesis (IVG)," "stem cell derived gametes," and "artificial or synthetic gametes" refer to the use of embryonic or adult cells to make spermatozoa and eggs. A "germ cell" is the sexual reproductive cell before it matures into a gamete. Academic IVG research in various countries uses undifferentiated cells known as stem cells from either embryos or somatic cells to focus on "germline" (the lineage of cells culminating in the germ cells) development. In vitro human germline development faces two constraints: (1) Because they form early in fetal development, *in vivo* germ cells are inaccessible to researchers. In vitro cultures of embryos end after 14 days, precisely when germ cells begin to develop and germ cell formation in donated aborted fetuses is nearly complete. (2) No robust experimental platform for the study of human germ cell formation exists.

In 2011, following fertilization of artificial gametes, mouse pups were born in a Japanese laboratory (Hayashi et al. 2011). In 2015, Naoko Irie, a Japanese researcher in the laboratory of Azim Surani at the Gurdon Institute in Cambridge, UK, published an important article about human germ cell biology in the influential journal *Cell* (Irie et al. 2015). Irie showed that the SOX17 gene is specific to humans, who turn out to be quite different from mice (which were until recently the primary model of study). Unsurprisingly, the article attracted worldwide attention, even outside of the academic community, because of the reproductive potential of creating human artificial gametes and perhaps even curing a number of infertilities.

From 2017–2019, I worked with biologists at the Gurdon Institute in Cambridge UK, conducting interviews with biologists and attending biological and bioethical talks on gamete development. I spent 5 months in Professor Azim Surani's laboratory, working with Dr. Naoko Irie and observing experiments by other researchers in the lab. I also participated in team activities such as lab meetings and meals. My mentor for the project was Professor Sarah Franklin, whose research on in vitro fertilization nurtures contemporary studies of reproductive technologies and fertility.

"After IVF" (Franklin 2013), the findings of studies of primordial germ cells fuel applicative projections and a broad range of reproductive hopes, including same-sex reproduction (having a baby with a same-sex partner), solo reproduction, multi-reproduction, post-chemotherapy reproduction, post-sterilization reproduction, and post-menopausal reproduction, to name only a few.

Nothing is publicly known about Naoko Irie's routine work. After I forwarded a TED talk video to her about in vitro gametogenesis that cited her article, she told me, "They should see how it's done in the lab." She is not a fan of American-style, over-enthusiastic speculation about future innovations, and she reminded me once again about the painfully dull experimental routine that involves years of successive failures before it eventually may allow the publication of a single article. The arduous process of "crafting" biology is a standard feature of the culture of everyday research (Meskus 2018), although it simultaneously energizes the imaginaries of rapid technological breakthroughs. What does this broad gulf between the dogged pace of research and the rapid spread of imaginaries teach us about making reproductive technologies and creating techno-sapiens?

Unlike a linear view of the translation of scientific work into technological applications, the practice of biotechnological research and online representations coexist and are thought of by biologists *as not working together*. Colleagues warn about misrepresentations of their research in the media or in bioethical publications—a layer of complexity often expressed as the dialectics between "scientific hype and reproductive hope." This gap is one of the significant challenges of translating stem cell research into biomedical practices (Gardner et al. 2015). Still, discourses about IVG are "good to think with," because they weave the notion that "biology is a technology" of sex and social reproduction into various social media (Franklin 2013).

My work emphasizes the importance of nurturing alternative narratives that might otherwise be silenced by dominant expectations. Far from offering linear, easy-going translations based on scientific authority, biologists express doubts, questions, difficulties, and wonder, some of which are described in this chapter. In a laboratory in which academic labor constructs in vitro gametogenesis, my presence was enacted as an interdisciplinary experiment. I attempted to culture stems cells alternatively with Irie to create one of these alternative narratives. I brought some tools from my own petri dish, or culture medium, where at the time I held a position as a research associate in the Reproductive Sociology Research Group based in the Sociology Department at the University of Cambridge.

Toward the end of this chapter, I propose "sociology as technology" as an alternative to linear translational thinking. This conceptual tool, built through my ethnographic practice with the biologists whom I had come to study, is also a response to the gap between slowness and rapidity, as well as an invitation to think in novel ways about the future of technology-making.

Relating Kin or Forgetting Progenitors?

After 8 years of research in a Japanese laboratory, as noted above, mice pups were born following the fertilization of artificial gametes induced from stem cells (Hayashi et al. 2011). This technique is also being used with human cells in laboratories around the world, and primordial human germ cells have been successfully produced in a British laboratory (Irie et al. 2015). The technical challenges to creating an "in vitro system" based on human cells led one biologist to observe that "the question of future potentials, it's quite a long way off." Still, given the emphasis on "translating" the biosciences into technologies, scientific publications using mice nourished the imagination of artificial gametes for humans.

With the exception of Japan, where IVG is banned from producing human embryos for research, no other countries have implemented regulations for this research field (Ishii, Pera, and Greely 2013). In a translational atmosphere in which the media assume that applications of basic science are imminent (López and Lunau 2012), despite the many challenges to actually making IVG work, biologists and bioethicists nevertheless continue to write, albeit cautiously, about the social implications and value of this research. Two intersecting topics emerge from their thinking: (1) IVG as a technology for curing infertility by using biology to make artificial gametes and relating kin; (2) IVG as a model for the study of gamete development as "cell memory loss," or the erasure of certain biological traces of the progenitor's past life embedded in their cells.

IVG as Making Artificial Gametes: Relating Kin

The possibility of making artificial gametes is linked to the well-known cultural value on genetic substance as constructing kinship (Schneider 1980; Carsten 2011; Porqueres i Gené 2015; Merleau-Ponty 2017). Body parts, particularly gametes, carry relational capacities. They not only make new bodies through biological mechanisms, but also identify people and relate them to each other as kin. They thus reproduce not only biology, but also social relations, embodied as "blood." In 2015, a group of biologists in the Netherlands published a review of IVG that interpreted the development of this technique as a reproductive technology:

> Although they are currently still at an experimental stage [...] deciding to introduce artificial gametes in clinical practice...requires a point of view that goes beyond biologic parameters. First, artificial gametes could

change the field of MAR [Medically Assisted Reproduction] dramatically by discarding the entire concept of infertility, and potentially allowing new groups of patients (e.g. heterosexual couples without functional gametes, post-menopausal women and gay couples) to have genetically related children. Second, we are unable to acquire informed consent from the children that will be conceived. (Hendriks et al. 2015)

Additionally, because chemotherapy often affects fertility, cancer survivors are frequently seen as potential beneficiaries of IVG (see Chapter 3). Concerns with these applications include not only the lack of consent from potential future children, but also the prospect of the mass production, screening, and selection of embryos (Palacios-González et al. 2014; Cohen et al. 2017), which are futuristically imagined in Chapter 5.

IVG also extends the value of genetics to sustain kinship relations beyond naturalistic and heteronormative reproduction to the possibility of the "democratization of reproduction." It could thus theoretically become possible for every human—regardless of their fertility status or sexuality—to conceive genetically related children (Testa and Harris 2005:165). In that spirit, writing for the Nuffield Council of Bioethics (UK), ethicist Anna Smajdor observed that:

> Artificial gametes (AGs) might enable anyone to produce gametes regardless of whether they ever had 'natural' gametes, and irrespective of their age, sex, relationship status, or sexuality. The prospect of creating sperm from women's cells and eggs from men's cells might also democratize reproduction in enabling same sex couples to have children that are the offspring of both partners, something which has never before been feasible. Thus AGs offer the possibility of genetic reproduction to people who are not typically regarded as being infertile. (Smajdor 2015)

There are two principal representations of artificial gametes with regard to reproduction and kinship: (1) a classical interpretation of reproductive technology as an enabler of genetically based parenthood; and (2) a tool for questioning the heteronormativity of these reproductive patterns. However, when the focus is not on future applications of IVG but on how it is currently used in scientific articles, it becomes apparent that IVG is not perceived as a reproductive technology for making artificial gametes but as a system for studying gametes' biological development and, more specifically, for advancing understanding of a single critical event: epigenetic reprogramming.

Forgetting Progenitor Memory: IVG as a Model for Studying Primordial Germ Cells and Epigenetic Reprogramming

"Epigenetics" is a common biological term that describes the molecular phenomena surrounding genes and the ways in which they are expressed and/or modified by environmental influences or other mechanisms. Epigenetic marks help determine how genes are made (un)available for transcription in RNA and proteins in cells. Some social science publications emphasize the fact that "epigenetics" introduce environmental factors into reproduction, blurring the boundaries between biology, health, and politics (Lamoreaux 2016; Meloni 2016; Lappé et al. 2019). In primordial germ cell formation, biologists point to the fact that some information from progenitors' cells must be "erased" or "forgotten" for a new organism to initiate a life cycle afresh.

During an interview, a Gurdon Institute (Cambridge, UK) biologist claimed:

> The big event [in gametogenesis] is epigenetic reorganization including DNA demethylation, which is extremely rare to see in the other cell types. So, this is the way to reset all the information for the next generation. (Interview 2, 2018)

"DNA demethylation" is the erasure of epigenetic marks located on DNA. These marks are known to induce the expressions of genes (by turning them on or off). Epigenetic reprogramming in gamete development was first described in mice (Hackett et al. 2013; Seisenberger et al. 2012). It is said to allow "primordial germ cells" to gain "totipotency"—the potential to develop into various specialized tissues in response to external or internal stimuli—within the fetus. Whereas every other cell type specializes during gestation, gametes alone retain the capacity to build every cell type (on condition that they mature and encounter another gamete in order to co-fertilize). Epigenetic reprogramming of cell information is thus represented as a critical event in the constant remaking of life through never-ending generations of new cells and individual organisms.

Epigenetic reprogramming is associated with the idea that "cellular memory" is "erased" (von Meyenn and Reik 2015). In the same vein, a stem cell biologist whom I interviewed argued that gamete development and epigenetic reprogramming are "a bit like a computer disk. [You] wipe out everything [and put] new information on." This approach may contradict the interpretation of IVG as a model for creating artificial gametes and relating people through reproduction and kinship. One approach values genetic substance as a kinship maker, initiating a discussion about democratizing reproduction by offering universal access to fertility. The alternative approach introduces ideas of cell memory loss and forgetting genitor—i.e., "parental"—embodiment. Yet surprisingly, these two approaches to reproduction—enabling and relating kinship and forgetting kin relatedness—are not contradictory. Amander Clark's laboratory, for example, promotes its research as both studying epigenetic reprogramming and attempting to offer solutions for patients rendered infertile by cancer treatments who wish to biologically reproduce (see Chapter 2). The differences between these two ways of writing about IVG and gamete development also suggest a gap in translating basic science into viable reproductive technologies.

Benchwork in Translational Times

Biological translation is often described as "bench to bed" (from the laboratory to the clinic). Because it suggests that the process is short and smooth, this frequent expression can be misleading. Indeed, as previously noted, scientists often stress the laborious nature of benchwork. In the summer of 2019, Professor Azim Surani invited me to present my research on IVG to his team at the Gurdon Institute in Cambridge (UK). I described my past work on in vitro fertilization, briefly summarized and analyzed the "relate and forget" dialectic described above, and mentioned my plans to spend time in their lab. A stunned silence followed the presentation. Azim Surani had assured me that lab meetings were generally lively, but no one reacted. Probably to alleviate this awkward moment, he briefly remarked that media representations and benchwork were two very different things. The notion of artificial gametes was obviously out of place when referring to what biologists actually do in the laboratory with germ cells. I tried to avoid revealing my distress by taking notes about these remarks, firmly believing that I was experiencing a powerful ethnographic event.

A few months later, I discussed this initial encounter in an interview with a doctoral candidate in the same lab. While I was describing one of my principal findings—that it would be a long time before artificial gametes would be functional—we also reminisced about my audience's stunned faces. My interlocutor replied:

> Artificial gametes: What? Are you serious? Let's just think about the fact that this cell lineage dedicated to reproduction is specified in the early weeks of fetal development, and then stops for 12 to 15 years, until puberty eventually starts the process of making fully functional gametes. Would biologists be able to remake the very first steps? What about those years of dormancy and what about all the mechanisms involved during puberty?

In her characteristically direct way, she added: "We need to be very careful. [...] For example, when a journalist is interviewing Azim and then he over-inflates everything, that's such a pity. [...] Because it's a big lie, it's not true that we are creating artificial [human] gametes, this is not true." Naoko Irie specifically asked me to emphasize this statement after seeing a draft of this chapter, arguing that this "is critical when one talks about IVG, which may also take 13 years to get gametes in vitro." So, what is it that the laboratory is currently creating if not artificial human gametes?

Simply put, the team's core contribution to germ cell development is *biological knowledge*—more specifically, an understanding of the molecular pathways involved in the specification of reproductive cells. In fact, medically assisted reproduction is not even cited in discussions of biomedical translational horizons and possibilities, while developmental knowledge and heritable diseases feature prominently. It is not so much *reproductive* medicine per se that is emphasized, but *regenerative* medicine that encapsulates the place of the lab's research within the far broader spectrum of stem cell research. Azim Surani (2015) stated for *The Conversation*:

> Imagine combining the procedures in one patient, for example a woman with a disease-causing mutation who does not wish to pass this mutation to her child. Starting with a cell taken from her skin, this is reprogrammed to a primordial germ cell, in which the DNA is then edited to remove the mutated gene. The primordial germ cell is developed into an egg and used to create an embryo for IVF, to be screened and transplanted back into her womb. The child and its subsequent descendants would be free of the mutated gene.

This scientist's approach focuses on biological regeneration as a source of applicative imagination. This approach, however, is closely connected to existing "selective reproductive technologies" such as prenatal and pre-implantation diagnoses (Gammeltoft and Wahlberg 2014). Recent debates about germline editing have also inspired social scientists to investigate what potential users think of such technologies. These studies have shown that regeneration is less of a concern than the recognition of disability rights, which are potentially challenged by the implication that living with mutated genes is inherently negative (Boardman and Hale 2018; Boardman 2020; see also Chapter 7). At the bench, meanwhile, considerations of the future significance of such technologies for patients with mutated genes seem to be absent. Instead, the interest of the laboratory is whether biological mechanisms associated with disease and health can be unraveled and potentially modified.

Biology is a discipline, both as a human endeavor to create new knowledge and as a set of behaviors guided by values like "effort," "diligence," and the kinds of repetitive and hyper-structured labor that involve long periods of time and frequent failures. Indeed, ethnographic fieldwork in these labs reveals not only the kinds of biology actually undertaken in them, but also the sociological context in which they are undertaken. The short history of the stem cell field is built around numerous unknowns that researchers explore, using experimentation and exchange within a highly competitive environment (Eriksson and Webster 2008). Human germ cell biology is especially "disciplined" because no prior knowledge exists on which to base new research. Naoko once told me that doing this work is like "walking in the dark." Not only is there no previous literature, but before 28 days of human development—when abortion clinics, pending patient permission, donate fetuses—in vivo comparison is impossible. Indeed, as Naoko added, "it's a new way of doing biology and you have to be extremely resilient." Beyond testing different culture conditions, there are no guidelines, no protocols, and no grounds for comparison—just pure research. At the beginning, it took Naoko 4 years to recapitulate the first event of human germ cell development. In summarizing this blend of psychology, technology, and science making, Naoko illustrates how basic science is a process of discovery and application that is far from linear:

This project requires [you] to be optimistic and to be sure that you will get something. It is very risky because if you get nothing, you get nothing. After trying so many things, you build some kind of instinct. [...] If you doubt your technique you cannot be sure of anything. If your tool is not right, you bring a lot of anxiety. It takes time and effort to build your tools. Even published papers—you are not entirely sure. I can wonder and go back to the first step again. But, at some point, you have to rely on something. Other groups will publish another way: is it the real way? With mouse models, it is less difficult because you can test in vivo. With human models you cannot. It also depends on how you set the goals and if you know what you want to see.

She portrays her project as a back and forth process involving failure, doubt, rethinking, and persistence in an uncertain environment. This quote also suggests that an important aspect of basic research requires letting go of one's assertiveness and accepting the unknown for what it teaches us: the humility and the patience to be able to repeatedly start all over again. As Naoko summarizes the process, "You cannot control everything. Not all of it is in your hands."

Not all researchers are as cautious as the two discussed above. I met one postdoctoral researcher from Japan who was less reserved about predicting the successful development of artificial gametes: "I don't think it's so far away," he said. While remaining cautious about the biology involved, he stressed the ethics of scientific practice, what Charis Thompson (2013) would call "good science." He told me that it took "just five years" between the first paper on mice gamete development and the development of functional mice gametes.

However, one important difference between mice and humans remains the in vivo timing. Mice gametes develop in vivo in 20 days, but human gametes follow a different developmental calendar. First, oocytes in human female infants are fully developed by the time they are born and remain dormant until puberty when, in males, spermatozoa start to be produced. According to my interlocutor, another major difference between mouse and human models that presents an even greater challenge is that mice can be "used" and "sacrificed," "but you cannot do that with women." This researcher made it clear that his research field is helpful because it contributes to our understanding of how human gametes develop, but that it should not be used to conceive an actual human baby. Similar ethical concerns about the biological risks of IVG-conceived offspring have appeared in the journal *Science* (Lippman and Newman 2005).

Ethnographic work can often reveal unexpected narratives. Building on the bioethical idea of "the democratization of reproduction" (Smajdor 2015)—i.e., universal access to biological reproduction—I would like to discuss *the democratization of biotechnology conception*, which would entail two objectives: (1) the interdisciplinary creation of tools that (2) could be used to include a wider range of perspectives in the conception of biotechnologies. For these endeavors, I firmly believe that ethnographic, feminist-oriented social science is especially well-suited because of its bottom-up, qualitative approach and its inclusive, intersectional political agenda. I argue that *sociology can be practiced as a technology for the democratization of biotechnology*, and from my personal perspective, it should be. (Let's debate!)

Sociology as Technology: A Toolkit for Democratizing Biotechnology

"Flow Cytometry" is a biotechnique to identify the physical and chemical characteristics of cells. It is a decisive step in a biological experiment because results can be "seen" in the form of specific diagrams that indicate the presence or absence of the characteristics being sought through culture conditions. On August 21, 2019, I sat with Naoko looking at the charts on the screen in front of us. In contrast with cell culturing, this aspect of biological work lends itself to informal conversation because once the tube is placed under the needle, it is simply a matter of time before the chart appears on the screen. This is Naoko's "favorite time" because she is able to see the answers to her question. In the short term, she says, she would like to see "a double positive" in her cells (whatever that means!). In the long run, though, she wonders about making artificial gametes and her role in society. Is her work controversial? "You can be helpful while I am struggling with this technical stuff every day," she concludes.

In what capacity can I be helpful? As an ethnographer trained as a social anthropologist and a former member of the Reproductive Sociology Research Group? This is the frame of my skill set, which centers around specific ethnographic tools such as relationality, talking, interviewing, hanging around, listening, observing, taking photos, reading, writing, and presenting. This skill set enabled me to identify and describe the gap between futuristic projections of the applicability of IVG and the actual routine work and views of some of the biologists working on this technology.

My work with the Reproductive Sociology Research Group took a somewhat audacious turn when, with the mentorship of Sarah Franklin and my co-worker Karen Jent (2018), I began to think about *sociology as a technology*—a term that came to me after a meeting with two stem cell biologists with whom Franklin and I were collaborating. Sarah and I were discussing how seminar sessions offered spaces in which sociologists could intervene in a way that rewired biologists' knowledge of their sociality, in turn perhaps empowering women to participate more fully in typically male-dominated Q&A sessions. "Yes," I added, "as you described how biology is a technology, what we are doing is sociology as technology." We smiled at each other—giving birth to a new social science concept is always a special moment—and I stared at Sarah in shock until she said, "You'd better write this down!"

In my view, the practice of sociology as a technology relies on an interdisciplinary approach that entails not only being in the laboratory (and thereby enabled to develop an alternative narrative), but also integrating sociological tools into the lab's daily functioning. I reminded everyone that I am a social scientist and that my work in their lab entails intervening in their routines in a potentially disruptive but entirely empathetic and attentive way. My job was to enact a different way of being part of a basic science laboratory by using my ethnographic tools to explore gaps between basic science and applications or media translations of the scientific work. By questioning how the reproductive futures of artificial gametes and benchwork could be seen as separated by these gaps, I was able to make the gaps work for my ethnographic praxis.

It is possible that the gaps I identified do not work as well for biological scientists, many of whom tend to perceive such distinctions as irrelevant. Artificial gametes and scenarios generated by the media have very little to do with these scientists' daily struggles. From a feminist perspective, this is an unsurprising dimension of translational practices, especially if we think of Marisol de la Cadena book's *Earth Beings* (2015), in which she translates into English her conversations with Mariano and Nazario Turpo—*Runakuna* or Quechua people (see Chapter 10). She thinks of anthropological work as a practice of translation. She writes: "I translated what they said into what I could understand, and this understanding was full of the gaps of what I did not get" (Cadena 2015:3).

Other voices have joined Cadena's profound, humble, participatory, interdisciplinary, and democratic move towards a more inclusive form of diversity. Sociological tools have proven helpful in reproducing historical perspectives for a democratic future. For example, the journal *Nature* featured Sarah Franklin's (2019:630) commentary about ethics and eugenics to mark the 150th anniversary of the publication of Darwin's 1859 *On the Origin of Species*. The conclusions of her remarks constituted a democratic call for inclusive, socially committed science-making:

> It turns out that what we have in common is less a single biological essence—or the ability to alter it—than a shared responsibility for human and non-human futures. The implication of this new model is that the most ethical science is the most sociable one, and thus that scientific excellence depends on greater inclusivity. We are better together—we must all be ethicists now.

My answer to Naoko's invitation to "help" is nurtured by my learning experience as a team member at Cambridge. I could not help Naoko on my own, but I could ask her questions and interrogate the texts that I have cited. And, as I have sought to do in this chapter, I can participate in Franklin's call to make scientific excellence sociable and more inclusive of a variety of perspectives, including those stemming from the social sciences.

This chapter has explored a number of issues ranging from the ethics of testing the functionality of synthetic gametes and of embryo selection to the scientific difficulties of accessing IVG. The chapter has also highlighted tensions between regenerative approaches to IVG, which potentially could remove mutated genes from germlines, and its prospective reproductive applications in terms of disability rights (see Chapter 17).

Yet numerous other relevant issues remain unaddressed herein. Colleagues working on related topics are exploring issues such as the role of power in the merging of knowledge production, venture capitalism, and entrepreneurial science, while also raising fundamental questions about social and reproductive justice (Wiel 2020; Kirskey, in press; see also Chapter 3). As Marit Melhuus (2007) aptly points out regarding the legal and ethical debates surrounding IVF in Norway, "procreative imaginations" provide sites from which to consider the high-stakes interplay between wonder, values, and power dynamics in the face of technologies that are accompanied by controversies and inequalities.

Because I mostly envision this chapter as a means of inspiring debate—a tool for enabling discussion, which is both the product and the medium of sociological technology—I propose that the debate be kept open by the addition of a few more questions: Who would use IVG if it were actually available, and for what purposes? Would they use it simply to increase biological knowledge and understandings of hereditary diseases, or to actually cure these diseases and create artificial gametes for those who can afford them? (These imagined possibilities are futuristically described as realities in Chapter 5). And what does an inclusive, intersectional democratic technology-making process look like? How do "we" get there? That is my take on a *sapiens* who is also *techno*. If we frame our questions with care and investigate them using interdisciplinary tools, there is hope that we will uncover some answers, naturally.

Acknowledgments

This chapter was supported by Wellcome Grant "Changing (In)Fertilities" number 209829/Z/17/Z as well as CNRS IRIS UMR8156-U997. A special thank you to Robbie Davis-Floyd and Naoko Irie for their insightful comments as well as to John Angell for language editing.

References

Boardman F. 2020. "Human Genome Editing and the Identity Politics of Genetic Disability." *Journal of Community Genetics* 11(2):125–127. https://doi.org/10.1007/s12687-019-00437-4.

Boardman F, R Hale. 2018. "How Do Genetically Disabled Adults View Selective Reproduction? Impairment, Identity, and Genetic Screening." *Molecular Genetics & Genomic Medicine* 6(6):941–956. https://doi.org/10.1002/mgg3.463.

Carsten J. 2011. "Substance and Relationality: Blood in Contexts." *Annual Review of Anthropology* 40(1):19–35. https://doi.org/10.1146/annurev.anthro.012809.105000.

Cohen IG, GQ Daley, EY Adashi. 2017. "Disruptive Reproductive Technologies." *Science Translational Medicine* 9(372). https://doi.org/10.1126/scitranslmed.aag2959.

de la Cadena M. 2015. *Earth Beings: Ecologies of Practice across Andean Worlds.* Durham, NC: Duke University Press. https://doi.org/10.1215/9780822375265.

Eriksson L, A Webster. 2008. "Standardizing the Unknown: Practicable Pluripotency as Doable Futures." *Science As Culture* 17(1):57–69. https://doi.org/10.1080/095054 30701872814.

Franklin S. 2013. *Biological Relatives: IVF, Stem Cells, and the Future of Kinship.* Durham, NC: Duke University Press.

Franklin S. 2019. "Ethical Research — The Long and Bumpy Road from Shirked to Shared." *Nature* 574(7780):627–630. https://doi.org/10.1038/d41586-019-03270 -4.

Gammeltoft TM, A Wahlberg. 2014. "Selective Reproductive Technologies." *Annual Review of Anthropology* 43(1):201–216. https://doi.org/10.1146/annurev-anthro-1023 13-030424.

Gardner J, A Faulkner, A Mahalatchimy, A Webster. 2015. "Are There Specific Translational Challenges in Regenerative Medicine? Lessons from Other Fields." *Regenerative Medicine* 10(7):885–895. https://doi.org/10.2217/rme.15.50.

Hackett JA, R Sengupta, JJ Zylicz, K Murakami, C Lee, TA Down, MA Surani. 2013. "Germline DNA Demethylation Dynamics and Imprint Erasure through 5-Hydroxymethylcytosine." *Science* 339(6118):448–452. https://doi.org/10.1126/science.1229277.

Hayashi K, H Ohta, K Kurimoto, S Aramaki, M Saitou. 2011. "Reconstitution of the Mouse Germ Cell Specification Pathway in Culture by Pluripotent Stem Cells." *Cell* 146(4):519–532. https://doi.org/10.1016/j.cell.2011.06.052.

Hendriks S, EAF Dancet, AMM van Pelt, G Hamer, S Repping. 2015. "Artificial Gametes: A Systematic Review of Biological Progress Towards Clinical Application." *Human Reproduction Update* 21(3):285–296. https://doi.org/10.1093/humupd/dmv001.

Irie N, L Weinberger, WWC Tang, T Kobayashi, S Viukov, YS Manor, S Dietmann, JH Hanna, MA Surani. 2015. "SOX17 Is a Critical Specifier of Human Primordial Germ Cell Fate." *Cell* 160(1–2):253–268. https://doi.org/10.1016/j.cell.2014.12.013.

Ishii T, RAR Pera, HT Greely. 2013. "Ethical and Legal Issues Arising in Research on Inducing Human Germ Cells from Pluripotent Stem Cells." *Cell Stem Cell* 13(2):145–148. https://doi.org/10.1016/j.stem.2013.07.005.

Jent KI. 2018. *Making Stem Cell Niches: An Ethnography of Regenerative Medicine in Scotland and the United States.* Thesis. University of Cambridge. https://doi.org/10.17863/CAM.26468.

Kirksey E. in press. *The Mutant Project. Inside the Global Race to Genetically Modify Humans.* New York: St. Martins Press.

Lamoreaux J. 2016. "What If the Environment Is a Person? Lineages of Epigenetic Science in a Toxic China." *Cultural Anthropology* 31(2):188–214. https://doi.org/10.14506/ca31.2.03.

Lappé M, RJ Hein, H Landecker. 2019. "Environmental Politics of Reproduction." *Annual Review of Anthropology* 48(1):133–150. https://doi.org/10.1146/annurev-ant hro-102218-011346.

Lippman A, SA Newman. 2005. "The Ethics of Deriving Gametes from ES Cells." *Science* 307(5709):515–517. https://doi.org/10.1126/science.307.5709.515c.

López JJ, J Lunau. 2012. "ELSIfication in Canada: Legal Modes of Reasoning." *Science As Culture* 21(1):77–99. https://doi.org/10.1080/09505431.2011.576240.

Melhuus M. 2007. "Procreative Imaginations: When Experts Disagree on the Meanings of Kinship." In: *Holding Worlds Together. Ethnographies of Knowing and Belonging,* eds. ME Lien, M Melhuus, 37–56. Oxford: Berghahn Books.

Meloni M. 2016. *Political Biology: Science and Social Values in Human Heredity from Eugenics to Epigenetics.* Basingstoke: Palgrave Macmillan.

Merleau-Ponty N. 2017. "In Vitro Fertilization in French and Indian Laboratories: A Somatotechnique?" Translated by John Angell. *Ethnologie Francaise* 167(3):509–518.

Meskus M. 2018. *Craft in Biomedical Research: The IPS Cell Technology and the Future of Stem Cell Science*. Palgrave Macmillan US. https://doi.org/10.1057/978-1-137-46910-6.

Palacios-González C, J Harris, G Testa. 2014. "Multiplex Parenting: IVG and the Generations to Come." *Journal of Medical Ethics* 40(11):752–758. https://doi.org/10.1136/medethics-2013-101810.

Porqueres, Gené, Enric. 2015. *Individu, Personne et Parenté en Europe*. Paris: Éditions de la Maison des Sciences de L'homme.

Schneider DM. 1980. *American Kinship: A Cultural Account*. Chicago, IL: University of Chicago Press.

Seisenberger S, S Andrews, F Krueger, J Arand, J Walter, F Santos, C Popp, B Thienpont, W Dean, W Reik. 2012. "The Dynamics of Genome-Wide DNA Methylation Reprogramming in Mouse Primordial Germ Cells." *Molecular Cell* 48(6):849–862. https://doi.org/10.1016/j.molcel.2012.11.001.

Smajdor A. 2015. *Artificial Gametes: Background Paper for the Nuffield Council on Bioethics*. The Nuffield Council on Bioethics.

Surani A. 2015. "How Close Are We to Successfully Editing Genes in Human Embryos?" *The Conversation*. https://theconversation.com/how-close-are-we-to-successfully-editing-genes-in-human-embryos-52326.

Testa Giuseppe, John Harris. 2005. "Ethics and Synthetic Gametes." *Bioethics* 19(2):146–166. https://doi.org/10.1111/j.1467-8519.2005.00431.x.

Thompson Charis. 2013. *Good Science: The Ethical Choreography of Stem Cells Research*. Cambridge, MA: MIT Press.

van de Wiel Lucy. 2020. "The Speculative Turn in IVF: Egg Freezing and the Financialization of Fertility." *New Genetics & Society* 1–21. https://doi.org/10.1080/14636778.2019.1709430.

von Meyenn F, W Reik. 2015. "Forget the Parents: Epigenetic Reprogramming in Human Germ Cells." *Cell* 161(6):1248–1251. https://doi.org/10.1016/j.cell.2015.05.039.

5

REPRODUCTION, SACRIFICIAL LIFE, AND THE LOGICS OF ATTRITION IN THE AFTERLIFE OF APARTHEID

Tessa Moll

Introduction: Scenes of Cyborg Littermates

This chapter is about the overlapping *logics of attrition* in reproductive futures in contemporary South Africa. I juxtapose two seemingly disparate contexts—toxic exposure along the rural Northern lowlands and urban fertility clinics—not as an exercise in alterity but to highlight intersecting logics and ways of thinking. My aim is to reflect on how these seemingly disparate spaces are tethered to each other through the racialized conjuring of surplus and sacrifice in the preservation of enumerated life. The two scenes/spaces I investigate here reflect how the economic, racialized values placed on reproductive life and death manifest via different technological interventions.

What is attritional in these contexts? For instance, how do we situate death in a context where embryos have come to stand for a "sacred image of life" (Franklin 1999:64) and the futurity of potential biographical life (Thompson 2005)? Sarah Franklin's examination of the controversies over "excess embryos" in the UK reveals a "sacralisation of life itself" (Duden 1993 in Franklin 1999:64)—the infusion of embryos with Christian-inflected images of sacredness and futurity. Yet, "little deaths" are also replete in fertility clinics, according to Aditya Bharadwaj and Marcia Inhorn, who explore the "life-death dialectic" (2015:79) in reproductive technology in India and the Middle East. There, "little deaths" take the form of embryos destroyed in stem cell technologies, fetal reduction in multiple gestations, and miscarriages following assisted conception.

The two scenes I describe here are part of our present and futures as techno-sapiens, cyborgs co-evolving with technology. In the first scene, I cover debates over DDT, an insecticide used to protect present life (from malaria), yet at the same time debilitating certain potential futures (via infertility). In the second scene, I describe reproductive technologies, including the production of surplus tissues and cells, the monitoring of embryos, and grading systems. In both contexts, the threat of toxic absorption manifests because of technological measures to protect against certain forms of harm. Both reveal a tension between protective measures that participate in the *logics of attrition*—what I describe as the braiding of present atrophies in the project of making potential future life—a feature of the biotech mode of reproduction (Thompson 2005).

Methods and Context

This chapter emerges from two interrelated ethnographic projects. In the first, I have explored reproductive potentiality in assisted conception in South Africa since 2014 via participant observation with embryologists, physicians, and patients in IVF clinics. In the second project, I am presently exploring the circulation of epigenetic knowledges—a broad field that focuses on understanding genetic and environmental interactions and their implications for health—in the Global South. Of particular interest in my early fieldwork has been the concerns over fetal exposure to endocrine disruptors, which includes the insecticide dichlorodiphenyltrichloroethane (DDT) due to malaria vector control in northern Limpopo province.

These two contexts are linked through the legacy of 350 years of colonialism and later apartheid: the creation of elite, urban, and formerly white spaces and of so-called "reserves" where DDT spraying takes place. Apartheid was the most recent of such systems (only formally deposed in 1994) that formalized a policy of racism that "demarcated humanity in terms of the categories fully human, not quite human yet and not human" (Erasmus 2017:53). In the era before apartheid and after the formal end of slavery, the Native Land Act of 1913 restricted ownership for Black people to just 8% of the land—places that would later be referred to as the "reserves" or "Bantustans." These reserves undergirded the system of cheap and exploited migrant labor, particularly in the mines, through social and biological reproduction (Wolpe 1972). They provided the "social services," subsistence food supply, and new populations that fed the capitalist accumulation of wealth in White South Africa. Thus, Black life had a seemingly contradictory value as both debased and as "productive sacrifice" (Mbembe 2004:380) for the creation of white wealth.

During the decades of the apartheid regime, a growing fear emerged that the "surplus populations" (particularly Black peoples) would eventually demographically envelop the minority and elite white population, thus fueling the state's impetus for direct intervention and management. By the early 1970s, the regime's increasing anxiety resulted in concerted and well-funded population policies involving public health education and birth control programs that targeted the Black population, resulting in a rapidly decreasing fertility rate (Moultrie 2001:131–146). This era of "family planning," forged in racist logics of lives best averted, laid down the infrastructure for today's anti-natalist state, which particularly maligns the reproduction of young, poor, Black women (Mkhwanazi 2014).

At the height of the apartheid regime, the white population was encouraged to flourish. For instance, the state offered tax relief to white people for having children. White immigration was encouraged, bringing more than a million white people to South Africa from 1945 to 1977 (Brown 1987). Shortly thereafter, the first IVF programs emerged, beginning in the university hospitals and subsequently in the private sector. The growth of private fertility clinics followed the trajectory of the larger healthcare system. Since the 1980s, the privatized healthcare sector has proliferated, increasingly urbanizing health infrastructure and absorbing the country's human healthcare resources (Coovadia et al. 2009).

The continued disparity in these contexts reflects the enduring legacies of colonialism and apartheid that differentiated and stratified spaces, bodies, and potential futures. In the US context, Saidiya Hartman describes the legacy of slavery as an "afterlife," as "black lives are still imperiled and devalued by a racial calculus and a political arithmetic that were entrenched centuries ago" (2007:4). The term "afterlife" connotes that racism endures long after the end of racist political and legal systems and expresses itself through the daily ongoing disparities between Black and white lives. Hartman's reference to "calculus" is significant, as these are enduring expressions of differential values of life. Many of the areas where DDT is sprayed today, such as the Vhembe district in northern Limpopo, were formerly Bantustans, and thus are marked by the enduring structural violences of apartheid's intentional deprivations—entrenched poverty, lack of basic infrastructure such as piped water and wastewater processing, and meager healthcare services (Abrams 2018). Since 1994, the restructuring of primary health care, the legalization of abortion, the guarantee of education, and domestic violence legislation all contributed to a dramatically different policy landscape for reproductive rights (Mkhwanazi 2014). However, anthropologist Nolwazi Mkhwanazi (2014) argues that despite the policy frameworks in place, young, poor, Black women experience only a negligible change in their material realities, enduring high rates of domestic and sexual violence, high rates of HIV transmission, and long-lasting social stigmatization of their sexuality and reproductivity.

These enduring disparities can also be viewed in today's private healthcare sector, which serves only an estimated 16% of the population that has private medical insurance (Coovadia et al. 2009), which largely does not cover fertility services. Today, the private fertility sector, which includes 12 of the 15 fertility clinics open during my research, remains distinctly urban, white, and elite. The cost of participating in reproductive technology is prohibitive for the majority of South Africans, but particularly for Black South Africans. Their historically entrenched geographic marginalization restricts access not only to formal employment or better paying jobs in urban areas, but also to the largely urban-based health and hospital systems (Coovadia et al. 2009) and fertility clinics, both public and private.

DDT Flows in Limpopo

Scholars have often traced the ways in which certain populations come to be deemed "surplus" and their biopolitical implications, such as those "surplus populations" subject to family planning programs in Bangladesh (Murphy 2017a). Such populations are made and made up through racial stratifications, political economic histories and geographies, and state borders. In *The Economization of Life*, Michelle Murphy (2017a) describes "surplus life" as that which is deemed sacrificial and non-valuable to the future economy. The reframing of life and value in relation to the economy, she argues, "has been composed by the necropolitical trilogy of death, not dying, and not being born" (ibid.:103). The same systems that would place some within frames of "surplus populations"— colonialism, racism, and global capitalism, for examples—are embodied at differential intensities when examining exposures to toxicity (Agard-Jones 2013). Endocrine disruptors, for instance, are hormonally active agents that interfere with endocrine systems. They are "in all of us" (see Murphy 2017b)—yet at varying degrees, different mixtures, and compounded by differing stressors, histories, and contexts. These varying intensities reflect embodiments of the differential value of life, thereby reproducing "racism [as] a transactional practice with radical implications for the distribution of death" (Mbembe 2004:381).

At a recent conference on endocrine disruptors in Africa, researchers presented a wide array of findings on various chemicals—DDT, pyrethroids, bisphenol A—that negatively affect human and non-human well-being via the endocrine system. Many presenters focused on Limpopo, one of three provinces in South Africa that use DDT to spray the interiors of homes as part of a state-run vector control program to eliminate malaria. Malaria is not widespread in South Africa; it is limited to lowland areas in the north and east. Despite the overwhelming focus on Limpopo, many also emphasized the universalizing dispersal of endocrine-disrupting chemicals. "Why should the Western world do this [take regulatory steps]?" one researcher asked rhetorically, then answered, "Because it's all our problems. It's in my blood; it's in all of us." Some also emphasized that DDT was likely impacting fertility at the individual level, as one of the most consistent findings of DDT effects in humans, both globally and in Limpopo, is the deterioration of men's sperm quality (Aneck-Hahn et al. 2006; de Jager et al. 2009). Researchers have also linked synthetic pyrethroid exposure—the alternative to DDT—to a reduction in women's ovarian reserves, which can also affect potential fertility (Whitworth et al. 2014). Thus whichever chemical is used, fertility could be negatively affected. Researchers speculated that the effects hadn't been registered at the level of population. Limpopo has one of the highest fertility rates in South Africa, at an estimated 2.8 children per woman (STATSSA 2019), yet this rate is much lower than in other countries in sub-Saharan Africa (at an average 4.7 children per woman).

Ostensibly, DDT is for indoor usage where the walls and roofs are sprayed, but anyone with a broom or who is barefoot can tell you that quite a lot of inside gets out and vice-versa. Researchers found high levels of DDT in gardens and play areas around these houses (Bouwman et al. 2011). Praised for its long-lasting insecticidal properties, DDT itself has a long afterlife: it further metabolizes into DDE, a known endocrine-disrupting chemical (Eskenazi et al. 2009), and has epigenetic and intergenerational consequences (Kabasenche and Skinner 2014). Far beyond homes, an extensive survey published in 2010 on Limpopo water-ways found that DDT had made its way into the rivers and streams of the prov-ince and back into humans through food systems (Bornman et al. 2010). It has been found in breastmilk, blood samples, chickens, fish, and soils; it also leaches into skin and is inhaled long after it has been sprayed (Eskenazi et al. 2009; Barnhoorn et al. 2009; Gyalpo et al. 2012).

The question of DDT's usage in malaria vector control is a controversial one. Very soon after its formulation in 1938, DDT was being used in South Africa as part of malaria prevention. Quickly, DDT was enrolled in the war machine of World War II. The dispersal of British and US military allowed for the global deployment of DDT for both agricultural and public health purposes, and spe-cifically for protecting troops abroad (McWilliams 2008). DDT's subsequent commercial success was similarly bound up in the post-WWII consolidation of US chemical corporations, which became major industrial players and for which insecticides accounted for a significant segment of profits. However, ques-tions quickly arose—concerns around toxicity, DDT's presence in breastmilk, and insects' increasing resistance to DDT—finally leading to the "transformative effect" (McWilliams 2008:194) of Rachel Carson's 1962 *Silent Spring*. Carson's work alerted readers to the fact that human life was swimming in synthetic chemicals.

Since then, DDT's usage has been severely curtailed, and this insecticide has become almost synonymous with environmental and human toxicity. By 1974, South Africa limited usage to malaria control, which was later discontinued by the late 1990s. The Stockholm Convention on Persistent Organic Pollutants, which came into force in 2004, banned DDT usage except for public health. South Africa led the appeal for a public health exception after a virulent malaria outbreak in the summer of 1999–2000, when 60,000 cases were reported (Raman et al. 2016). In 2007, after the return of DDT spraying, the state recorded only 6,000 malaria cases, proving its effectiveness in achieving the goal of saving lives.

At the same time, reports of health risks were dismissed by the then-Minister of Health, who said that the majority of research says that DDT is safe when utilized correctly (Parliamentary Monitoring Group 2010). Yet many research-ers have acknowledged the potential health risks from DDT—including breast cancer, impaired neurodevelopment in children, congenital birth anomalies, decreased semen quality, and diabetes (Eskenazi et al. 2009). Some also argued that the risk and impact of morbidity and mortality from malaria were greater than those from DDT (Bouwman et al. 2011). Malaria remains a significant pub-lic health threat, particularly in the Global South; it is one of the leading causes of death among children under 5 in sub-Saharan Africa. With eliminating malaria on the global agenda as part of the Millennium Development Goals and later the Sustainable Development Goals, DDT usage has increased in the last 15 years. Beginning in 2005, the US President's Malaria Initiative ramped up DDT usage through billions in funding in 15 sub-Saharan countries (not including South Africa) (Oxborough 2016).

The Sustainable Development Goals are what Murphy (2017a:30) would call "a dashboard for development." By this she means the indices produced through the global infrastructures of data collection that enroll countries into orienting and organizing their economies toward the limited purview of liberalism and capitalist accumulation. Such global infrastructures shape what gets counted and what remains uncounted. Undoubtedly, DDT spraying prevents deaths—and largely the deaths of Black people—from malaria; for a state, it is cheap and effective. Does that absolve it from critique for the harms it may cause? The barometer of malaria deaths averted due to the inexpensive containment strategy of DDT spray is enumerated and counted. We can know that lives are saved from DDT spraying to eliminate mosquitos—the vectors of malaria transmission. We do not know which lives are debilitated, harmed, averted, or injured from DDT spraying, largely because the infrastructure is not in place to count them. The deterioration of men's sperm from DDT spraying potentially exposes generations to the "externality" of "not being born," thereby offloading the cost of malaria prevention onto the same populations (see Murphy 2017a). Uncounted are the "not born" due to exposure to DDT. In the context of post-apartheid South Africa and the enduring infrastructural violence of its past (Abrams 2018), similarly uncounted would be the cases of breast cancer, cognitive development issues in children, and feminized fish. Many of the homes in Limpopo, often constructed of mud walls and thatched roofs, which receive yearly DDT sprays, index not only enduring poverty, but also the durational legacies of apartheid and colonial policies that restricted the mobility of the Black population away from areas that map onto malarial regions. While DDT leaching from such walls represents one kind of toxic threat, the borders of race that are etched into bodies and spaces represent yet another kind of toxicity and one equally, if not more, durational.

Attending to Embryos in Cape Town

At the same time that the apartheid regime formalized the Venda Bantustan in what is now Limpopo, researchers at Tygerberg Hospital in Cape Town, South Africa, were confounded by the persistent failure of their experimental mice embryos. In the late 1970s and early 1980s, researchers hoped to develop the first successful IVF program on the African continent. Yet in numerous attempts with novel techniques of in vitro fertilization (IVF), the experimental mice embryos died. A researcher later told me that he reviewed the Steptoe and Edwards protocol—the steps the famous British researchers used in the experiment that resulted in the birth of Louise Brown in 1978—and realized that the British team had not used gloves in the lab. "We removed the gloves, and the embryos grew," he said. A few years later in 1984, Falcon de Vos was born in Cape Town. He was named after the brand of petri dish used in the lab, which encased the embryo that would eventually develop into Falcon himself. What had hindered the development of mice embryos in vitro was the use of common lab gloves. Many brands of gloves used powder to make them easier to use and remove, powder that proved toxic to developing embryos. What is meant as protective cladding can in fact prove toxic.

This origin story contains many elements that social science researchers have highlighted over four decades of what Charis Thompson refers to as the "biomedical mode of reproduction" (2005). Thinking with the "sacred" and "profane" embryo, Thompson's conceptualization explores how this mode of reproduction aligns with contemporary capitalism. Among her many parallels, extra-corporeal reproductive materials, particularly eggs and embryos, are at risk of being alienated from the bodies from which they come. Thompson here alludes to the risks of being excluded from reproductivity due to the inaccessibility of IVF and the potential exploitation of those who contribute reproductive labor, such as egg donors and surrogates. Additionally, extra-corporeal reproductive material is more generally at-risk when outside of bodies. Embryos absorb their environments, including toxicity such as the powder from surgical gloves. As Elizabeth Roberts (2014) has noted, the acknowledgment of embryo porosity has led to investigations of the "nano-environments"—petri dishes and culture mediums—of techno-embryos. While "in vitro" literally means "in glass," most petri dishes are made of plastic, a material both less robust in keeping the external world out and even potentially harmful itself.

In Falcon's case, his naming echoes another of Thompson's reflections on embryos—that they are viewed in relation to their biographical potentiality. Embryos that could become persons, or in this case, the embryo that became Falcon, are related through that potential of biographical life. The "sacredness" of the potentialized embryo is held in tension with the "profane" embryo removed from biographical trajectories through techno-scientific means of embryo grading, becoming an everyday work object for embryologists (Thompson 2005; Arman and Styhre 2016).

Lab technicians working with embryos must navigate these two characteristics—the sacred and the profane. While embryo environments must be protected, embryologists must balance the need to ensconce embryos with the need to observe them. Embryos require very different environments than the people who attend to them. *Attending to* embryos means protecting them from environmental toxicity, but *attention to* embryos—observing, assessing, and recording their development and at times manipulating and intervening—also puts them at risk, threatening their trajectory toward biographical life. Monitoring and manipulating embryos means taking them out of their climate-controlled incubators for brief (and fastidiously timed) periods. Monitoring embryos, though risky, is done to assess a given embryo's potential to remain on the biographical trajectory—for it to become a live birth, a baby, a person. Morphological assessment—examining an embryo's form or structure—is the most common method for evaluating an embryo's potential viability. When assessing in the labs I observed, embryologists quickly removed each petri dish from the incubator, then examined and graded the embryos, recording the number of cells and the quality of several features, such as the inner cell mass, the size of the blastocyst, and the trophectoderm (the outer skin or shell of the embryo). Embryos were often then described as "pretty" ("good," developing well, likely to succeed as a pregnancy) or "ugly" (malformed and likely to fail). The best embryo would get transferred into a uterus, and the remaining would be frozen for subsequent attempts. Those embryos that score low, or whose development had ceased completely, become "waste."

The need to monitor embryo development and select the best among a given cohort has become increasingly important in light of a new scientific consensus that the fertility industry needs to address the problem of multiple gestations—twins or triplets. In earlier clinical practice, physicians would transfer multiple embryos in a single cycle, thinking that the greater number of embryos meant the greater the chance one would "stick." There is growing recognition that transferring multiple embryos does not increase the chances of success, but rather increases one's chances for multiple gestations, which are risky for fetuses and for the pregnant person. As a result, research in embryology has increasingly focused on ascertaining techniques for finding *the best* embryo among a given cohort. I would often hear among embryologists that, "You just need one." An assemblage of techniques, knowledge, clinical practice, and, what I argue here, logics, were congealed in the service of finding *the one*.

To get *the one*, nearly every doctor and IVF patient I worked with said that they try to start out with many. One patient I interviewed, who had six rounds of IVF before her "success," remarked on the loss of "potential children": "The amount of potential children, 40 already, have just died. But you can't think of them as kids. Cause for that little thing to turn into a baby… There's such a lot of stats it [the embryo] needs to overcome to be one." Starting with many eggs (ideally 12 to 15) was necessary because as the process proceeds, the numbers just go "down, down, down," as one patient I met put it. As Catherine Waldby (2015: 227) describes the scarcity economy of human eggs, "While treatment is centred on the hormonal production of multiple oocytes, the creation of abundance, the outcome is often an insufficient number to produce a pregnancy." During my fieldwork, for a patient going through IVF, the numbers did indeed just "go down": down from the number of oocytes to the number of fertilized eggs; then down to the number of Day 2 embryos; then finally down to the number of Day 5 embryos that were ready to transfer to the uterus. Many embryologists only froze those embryos that made it to Day 5, arguing that there was no use saving something if it ultimately could not offer the chance of a viable pregnancy.

Any fertilized embryos could be transferred into a uterus, but many embryologists I encountered argued instead that embryos should develop in vitro so that the "best" embryo could emerge—that it was better to allow the viability of the embryo to make itself known—better to have "nature" reveal its own selection. Thereafter, embryologists could intervene and attempt to select the best embryo through techniques such as morphology. Allowing embryos to develop in vitro to Day 5 facilitated a "natural" dispersal of viability to emerge. For embryologists to find the best embryo in a given cohort, not only would numerous embryos fail to develop, but many *should* in order for a seemingly "natural" dispersion of potentiality to emerge, thus braiding the logics of sacrifice into the production and potential of some reproductive futures. The multi-day in vitro development of embryos, rather than a creation of "profane" embryos removed from possible biographical trajectories, allowed for their reframing as "sacrificial." Acknowledgment of embryos' vulnerability—and the likeliness of "failure to develop"—is built into the system surplus of IVF technoscience. This is what I have come to think of as the "logic of attrition" in the biomedical, technoscientific mode of reproduction.

An Emerging Infertility Politics

How do these two scenes connect? Multiple threads, from racism and apartheid legacies to capitalist accumulation, toxic landscapes, and proximity to death, move through both sites. Both analogously reflect a spectrum of reproduction potential in relation to time, space, and death. But first, and more concretely, in Limpopo, exposure to DDT can render one infertile, a condition that would bring some to our latter scene of fertility clinics to attempt to remedy that state— should they be able to afford it. However, rather than simply being biomedical solutions to infertility, conceptive technologies are socially and politically situated in ways that *some* (read: the elite and mobile, via race, class, and sexuality) may experience remedy. Yet the minimal expansion of access does nothing to upend the stratifications and structures that render some more likely than others to be infertile in the first place.

Infertility is a greater problem in sub-Saharan Africa than any other region; some call it the "infertility belt" (Nachtigall 2006). Researchers attribute the high incidence rate compared to other regions to the high presence of co-occurring disorders—scarring and damage to fallopian tubes from untreated sexually transmitted diseases, and morbidities from previous pregnancies (Ericksen and Brunette 1996). Both factors result from inaccessible, uneven, and under-resourced medical infrastructures. Infertility and the reasons for its high rates in Africa cannot be divorced from the racialized political-economic histories and post-colonial legacies that have resulted in poverty, poor medical care, vulnerability to STIs, environmental toxicity such as DDT spraying, and the inability to move to non-malarial regions. And yet, for many well-meaning advocates who wish to counter racist depictions of African "overpopulation," the "fix" to the problem of infertility in Africa is perceived as more biomedical care in the form of "low-cost" IVF, despite the fact that it is clustered in inaccessible urban areas, remains expensive, and often carries extremely high failure rates. Advocacy for the relatively few able to access (largely unsuccessful) IVF treatment does little to challenge the reasons for which many are infertile in the first place nor to help the majority find solutions to their infertility.

Furthermore, these access arguments allow for the streamlining of pharmaceutical profiteering on the African continent, a largely untapped market for the multi-billion-dollar fertility industry. In recent years, the pharmaceutical giant Merck has, via its charitable foundation, launched the "More than a Mother" (Merk 2020) campaign to "de-stigmatize infertility on all levels...giving every woman the respect and the help she deserves to live a fulfilling life, with or without a child." Despite the campaign's ambivalence to reproductivity in this mission statement, the More Than a Mother campaign has trained nearly 150 fertility specialists and embryologists from countries in the Global South, predominantly in sub-Saharan Africa. While side-stepping the structural violences that render infertility one of the most unmet problems of sub-Saharan Africa, such campaigns use philanthropic imaginaries to offer biomedical "solutions"—which, again, remain largely inaccessible and unsuccessful. Ironically, philanthropic campaigns—the President's Malaria Initiative and More than a Mother—feature in both ends of this story. Investments of "soft" diplomacy, in the form of US funding for malaria vector control, and what we might call "soft" capital can, in the wording of Jaspir Puar (2017), debilitate many through infertility and capacitate few to have babies.

Conclusion: Logics of Attrition

According to Achille Mbembe (2004:381), "Superfluity consisted in the vulnerability, debasement, and waste that the black body was subjected to and in the racist assumption that wasting black life was a necessary sacrifice—a sacrifice that could be redeemed because it served as the foundation of civilization." The spatial arrangement of apartheid remains enduringly etched into sociality in contemporary South Africa, such that DDT spraying easily maps over areas once demarcated as "reserves" for the Black population. These regions have historically been viewed as "surplus" and thus, in Mbembe's formulation, also "sacrificial." In his depiction, apartheid encompassed a seemingly contradictory relation between the devaluation of Black life and its necessary reorganization to service capital accumulation in a "logic of productive sacrifice" (Mbembe 2004:380). The language of sacrifice invokes the horizon of the future, for the price paid now expects future recompense. Thus, and critically to my argument, he links the exploitation of Black life to the lavish aesthetics of the "unrepentant commercialism" of contemporary Johannesburg, a city notably built on Black labor in the mines. Superfluity is not only a characteristic of surplus populations, but also of the spaces of white wealth, the context for which the "sacrifice" is made.

How does this relate to IVF and embryos? Herein I have described how notions of sacrifice, the sacred and the profane, debility and attrition, surplus and waste, provide the scaffolding for overarching logics in seemingly disparate corners of contemporary South Africa. The urban, private, for-profit IVF industry similarly relies upon a system of surplus and sacrifice. Hormones are used to over-stimulate ovaries, seeking to produce a surplus of eggs and yielding an ever-decreasing stock of embryos. These ever-decreasing numbers—what I call IVF's *logic of attrition*—reflect the braiding of sacrifice in the making of ART's techno-babies. Embryos that fail to develop, that atrophy, are not framed as "deaths," but as "sacrifices" for achieving the "best" embryo that will potentially result in pregnancy and a child. The pathways from "excess" to "atrophy" are facilitated through techno-scientific techniques and knowledges of embryo monitoring, grading, and selection. The "best" embryo is thus a technological achievement, but one made at the cost of producing "surplus" and "excess" "profane" embryos. These atrophies in the present, the "sacrifices" for hope, produce expectations of sacred life in the future.

The logics of attrition, I argue, are part of a larger infrastructure linking race, political economies, "surplus" populations, notions of sacrifice, and the conjuring of superfluity that constitute "the dialectics of indispensability and expendability of both labor and life, people and things" (Mbembe 2004:374). What his notion of superfluity holds, then, are not only the dialectics of life and death, but also of "excess and exclusion" (2004:404)—the shifting of resources and vitality from one space to another. While these two scenarios hold together in logics of attrition, they represent different scales of population and differing geographies and temporalities of sacrifice and futures. In IVF clinics, present sacrifices of embryos intend to preserve a singular future life. DDT spraying frames present lives as saved, obscuring debility and the absence of those not-born. The logic of attrition connects these seemingly disparate scenes under the racialized landscape of reproductive potentialities in South Africa by demonstrating how attrition is braided into reproductive futures. This chapter points to underlying logics that connect superfluous lives as sacrificial lives, spaces of sacrifice as entangled with toxic barriers, and present sacrifices for differing techno-futures.

Acknowledgments

Thanks to Robbie Davis-Floyd for her careful edits and comments on this chapter and the curation of this book. Also many thanks to Fiona Ross, Jaya Keaney, Michelle Pentecost, Maurizio Meloni, Rasmus Bitsch, and Kelsey Draper for their care and intellectual labor in providing feedback for earlier versions of this chapter.

References

Abrams A 2018. *Wellbeing on the Edge: The Dynamics of Musundian Edge-Dwelling on the Boundaries of Protected Natural Areas in Limpopo, South Africa.* (PhD) thesis. University of Kent.
Agard-Jones V 2013. Bodies in the system. *Small Axe: A Caribbean Journal of Criticism* 17(3):182–192.

Aneck-Hahn NH et al. 2006. Impaired semen quality associated with environmental DDT exposure in young men living in a malaria area in the Limpopo Province, South Africa. *Journal of Andrology* 28(3):423–434.

Arman R, Styhre A 2016. The sacred and the profane in life science work: The case of assisted reproduction laboratories. *Culture and Organization* 24(5):348–364.

Barnhoorn IEJ et al. 2009. DDT residues in water, sediment, domestic and indigenous biota from a currently DDT-sprayed area. *Chemosphere* 77(9):1236–1241.

Bharadwaj A, Inhorn M 2015. Conceiving life and death: Stem cell technologies and assisted conception in India and the Middle East. In: *The Anthropology of Living and Dying*, eds. C Han, V Das. New York: Wiley-Blackwell, 67–82.

Bornman R, Barnhoorn I, Aneck-Hahn N 2010. A pilot study on the occurrence of endocrine disruptive chemicals in a DDT-sprayed area. *Water Research Commission Report* No. KV 220/09.

Bouwman H, van den Berg H, Kylin H 2011. DDT and malaria prevention: Addressing the paradox. *Environmental Health Perspectives* 119(6):744–747.

Brown BB 1987. Facing the "black peril": The politics of population control in South Africa. *Journal of Southern African Studies* 13(2):256–273.

Coovadia H et al. 2009. The health and health system of South Africa: Historical roots of current public health challenges. *South African Medical Journal* 374(9692):817–834.

de Jager C et al. 2009. Sperm chromatin integrity in DDT-exposed young men living in a malaria area in the Limpopo Province, South Africa. *Human Reproduction* 24(10):2429–2438.

Erasmus Z 2017. *Race Otherwise: Forging a New Humanism for South Africa*. Johannesburg: Wits University Press.

Ericksen K, Brunette T 1996. Patterns and predictors of infertility among African women: A cross-national survey of twenty-seven nations. *Social Science and Medicine* 42(2):209–220.

Eskenazi B et al. 2009. The Pine River statement: Human health consequences of DDT use. *Environmental Health Perspectives* 117(9):1359–1367.

Franklin S 1999. Dead embryos: Feminism in suspension. In: *Fetal Subjects, Feminist Positions*, eds. L Morgan, M Michaels. Philadelphia: University of Pennsylvania Press, 61–82.

Gyalpo T et al. 2012. Estimation of human body concentrations of DDT from indoor residual spraying for malaria control. *Environmental Pollution* 169(C):235–241.

Hartman S 2007. *Lose Your Mother: A Journey Across the Atlantic Slave Route*. New York: Farrar, Straus and Giroux.

Kabasenche WP, Skinner MK 2014. DDT, epigenetic harm, and transgenerational environmental justice. *Environmental Health: A Global Access Science Source* 13:62–67.

Mbembe A 2004. Aesthetics of superfluity. *Public Culture* 16(3):373–405.

McWilliams JE 2008. *American Pests: The Losing War on Insects from Colonial Times to DDT*. New York: Columbia University Press.

"Merck More Than a Mother." 2020. www.merckmorethanamother.com/ Accessed: February 2020.

Mkhwanazi N 2014. Twenty years of democracy and the politics of reproduction in South Africa. *African Identities* 12(3–4):326–341.

Moultrie TA 2001. *Apartheid's Children: Social Institutions and Birth Intervals during the South African Fertility Decline, 1960–1998*. PhD Thesis. London School of Hygiene & Tropical Medicine.

Murphy M 2017a. *The Economization of Life*. Durham, NC: Duke University Press.

Murphy M 2017b. Alterlife and decolonial chemical relations. *Cultural Anthropology* 32(4):494–503.

Nachtigall RD 2006. International disparities in access to infertility services. *Fertility and Sterility* 85(4):871–875.

Oxborough RM 2016. Trends in US President's Malaria Initiative-funded indoor residual spray coverage and insecticide choice in sub-Saharan Africa (2008–2015): Urgent need for affordable, long-lasting insecticides. *Malaria Journal* 15:146–154.

Parliamentary Monitoring Group 2010. Questions & Replies No 1451 to 1475. June 7. Available at: https://pmg.org.za/question_reply/202/.

Puar J 2017. *The Right to Maim: Debility, Capacity, Disability.* Durham, NC: Duke University Press.

Raman J et al. 2016. Reviewing South Africa's malaria elimination strategy (2012–2018): Progress, challenges and priorities. *Malaria Journal* 15(1):438–448.

Roberts EFS 2014. "Petri dish." *Somatosphere.* somatosphere.net/2014/petri-dish.html. 31 March.

Stats SA 2019. *Statistical Release: Mid-Year Population Estimates. Statistics South Africa.* Republic of South Africa.

Thompson C 2005. *Making Parents: The Ontological Choreography of Reproductive Technology.* Cambridge, MA: MIT Press.

Walby C 2015. The oocyte market and social egg freezing: From scarcity to singularity. *Journal of Cultural Economy* 8(3):275–291.

Whitworth KW et al. 2014. Predictors of plasma DDT and DDE concentrations among women exposed to indoor residual spraying for malaria control in the South African study of women and babies (SOWB). *Environmental Health Perspectives* 122(6):545–552.

Wolpe H 1972. Capitalism and cheap labour-power in South Africa: From segregation to apartheid 1. *Economy and Society* 1(4):425–456.

6

MAKING BETTER BABIES?

Past and Future State Fair Contests Evaluating Geneticized Worth

Meghna Mukherjee and Margaret Eby

Setting the Stage

From an imagined 1932 Iowa State Fair to a dystopian 2032 World's Fair, this story follows fictional antihero George Jamerson, eugenicist and physician, as he sees for himself the consequences of his legacy on the reproductive imaginaries of the 20th and 21st centuries. This work is informed by our joint research on direct-to-consumer genetic testing, as well as by our individual comparative research on the history of reproductive control and eugenics advocacy movements in Germany and the United States, and on egg donation in India and the US (Mukherjee 2019; Eby 2019). Our methodologies include in-depth interviews and ethnographies of fertility clinics in India and the US, and archival research on early eugenics movements and their contemporary ethical debates. With our exploration of these modern practices of speculative neo-eugenics, which advocates the use of repro-genetic technologies to improve human reproduction outcomes, we interrogate the perceived cultural values ascribed to technologically reconfigured identities and share a cautionary tale about the dangers of advancing reproductive technologies without reckoning with their problematic history. Our imaginary of the 1932 Iowa State Fair below is based on archival research about other, similar State Fairs of that era.

Iowa State Fair, 1932

The opening day of the 1932 Iowa State Fair dawned bright and crisp. Women pushing prams in their Sunday best jostled men in porkpie hats, countryside farmers mingling with Indianapolis society. Where better to plant the seeds of reproductive responsibility? The Iowa State Fair was the perfect place to gently push the public to concern itself with issues of heredity. The exhibition halls were packed with displays on soil treatments and award-winning watermelons, but the real draw lay beyond—the Better Babies Building. Inside, examiners weighed, measured, ranked, and graded babies; from birth marks to reflexes, each child was translated into data and scored (Figure 6.1).

Senior Director Dr. George Jamerson beamed. His fair was progressive, future-oriented. For over 10 years now, he had been running the annual Iowa Better Baby Contest—the highlight of the Iowa State Fair. He had worked tirelessly to ensure that the best physicians, scientists, and publishers would dedicate their Labor Day week to the betterment of future generations. As a man of science and a doting grandfather, George cared most about social progress that

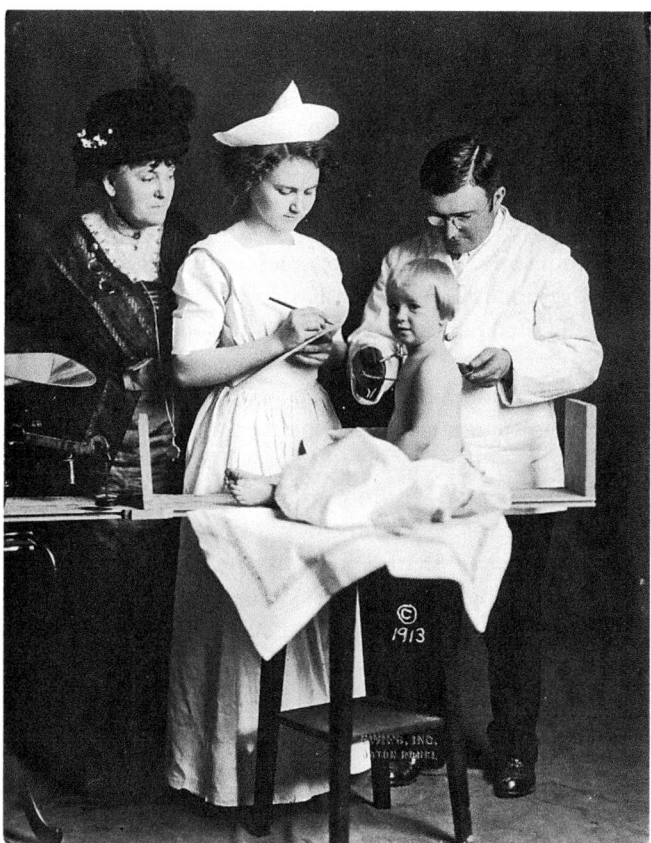

FIGURE 6.1 Anthropometric Data Collection, Better Babies Contest, Louisiana State Fair, 1913. Used with permission of Special Collections, University of Tennessee, Knoxville.

would ensure his grandchildren inherited the best and healthiest society possible. He personally congratulated each winning family and made sure to encourage less fortunate parents to intervene with nurture where nature had failed them. It was a moral responsibility, he felt, for society to do all that it could to ensure healthier futures through "responsible," calculated, reproductive choices (Savulescu 2001). George hoped the annual Iowa Better Babies Contest would lay the foundation for population health in America (Figure 6.2).

Well into his 50s, George knew clearly that this was his calling. He had spent his career pushing for public health "improvements" via eugenic interventions. In his youth, he had the opportunity to see Sir Francis Galton deliver his acclaimed Huxley Lecture at the Royal Anthropological Institute in 1901. Galton spoke of heredity and eugenics. He urged the scientific and medical communities to better understand human control over nature, reproducing success via conscientious combining of only "the best" bloodlines. George was immediately taken by what he perceived as Galton's message for public good. After all, if we sought a healthier population, shouldn't we begin at the very start by birthing better babies? The Better Babies Contest presented just that opportunity. It encouraged families to judiciously pair only the "fittest" parents and reproduce only the most capable babies. When President Roosevelt spoke in 1905 on the importance of white, educated women's fertility to prevent "race suicide," George knew that it was his patriotic duty to demonstrate the importance of heredity (Galton 1904).

Since the first competitions in the 1910s, the Better Baby Contests had spread the gospel of infant development and made a spectacle of eugenic standards. These contests represented only a small part of the eugenic fervor that permeated

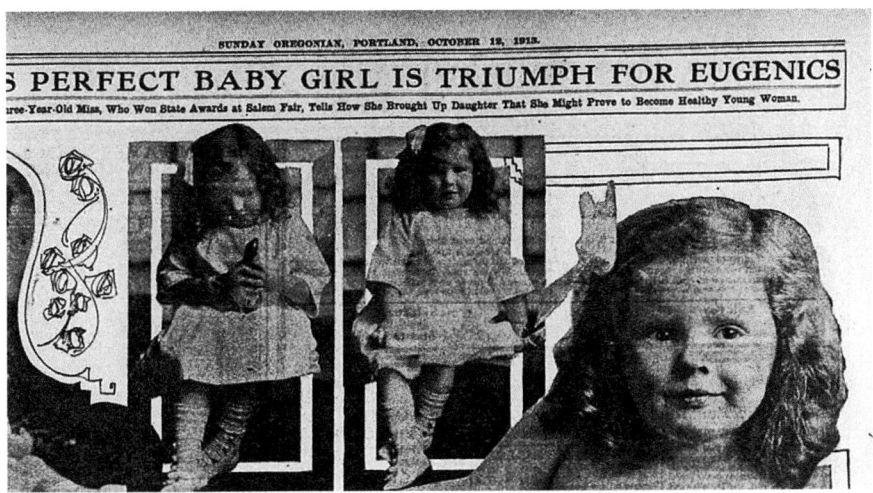

FIGURE 6.2 Sunday Oregonian newspaper headline, 1913. Public domain.

scientific, political, and feminist arenas at that time. While Theodore Roosevelt warned against white race suicide, reproductive rights activist Margaret Sanger sought contraceptive access for immigrants, and physicians urged state-sanctioned sterilization of targeted, non-white populations (Chesler 2007; Reilly 1987; Eby n.d.). Further, population control advocates were grappling with the tensions of the interwar period, which manifested in an increasing orientation towards the designation of a certain (whiter, ableist) national makeup with tightening immigration policies (Ngai 1999) and the policing of white reproduction (Bridges 2019). White babies symbolized the purity and potential of the ideal Anglo-Saxon American population.

Onlookers crowded to watch babies ranked and compared. Babies were measured for physical and intellectual growth and development through five sections: Mental and Developmental; Measurements; Physical Examination; Oral and Dental Examination; and Eye, Ear, Nose, and Throat. Entrants were then awarded a score out of a possible 1,000. For each section, a nurse or physician recorded slight defects (bad-tempered during examination, delayed teething) or more significant concerns (unable to stand or sit alone, bowlegged) and signed off, passing the baby onto the next station (Figures 6.3 and 6.4). George wanted to make sure his contest held participants to the highest of standards for the brightest of futures. What George, the physician eugenicist of 1932, could not foresee was the advent of *genetic* intervention, or the Nazi genocide that would occur in pursuit of a racially pure population (Chalmers 2015). The next decades would see these programs carried to their extreme eugenic conclusions.

Each year's Better Babies Contest ended with a much-anticipated award ceremony—George's favorite part. "With a near perfect score of 980, little Peter Nelson!" (Figures 6.5 and 6.6). The family made their way up to the stage, holding little Peter—their perfect creation—close. Peter was everything a parent could ask for. At a mere 12 months, his physical stature was strong. He could walk almost unsupported. He knew more than just a few syllables. And he clung to his mother, showing how cleverly he recognized his own. Having demonstrated utmost health, intelligence, fitness, and whiteness, Peter was the embodiment of the eugenic dream. Of course, Peter would need a suitable upbringing to make him an upstanding citizen—one who valued family, hard work, and his country—but he had every genetic advantage.

As George handed Peter's diploma to the proud Nelsons, he felt an unexpected jolt in the back of his head. A sharp pain ran down his neck. His vision blurred, he struggled to draw breath. The last thing he saw as he fell was Peter in his mother's arms.

The crowd stood silent as Iowa State Fair authorities and physicians rushed to George's side, but he was already dead. Many years earlier, George had seen his mother pass in a similar unfortunate moment. Though he championed Galton's legacy of "judicious" reproduction via genealogical heritage patterns, George had succumbed to this very logic.

Test I—Mental and Developmental

These tests are based on the F. Kuhlmann revision of the Binet Simon System.

The examiner should mark "x" after each test in which the child fails to qualify. Examiners do not compute any of these tests. This work is done by the Scoring Committee.

SIX MONTHS. Sits alone (40)_____ can balance head (40)_____ bears (looks in direction of unexpected noises) (40)_____ eyes (follow bright object (40)_____ reaches for bright object (20)_____ will grasp and hold it (20)_____

TWELVE MONTHS. Stands (momentarily unsupported) (40)_____ walks with support (40)_____ can repeat few syllables—da, ma, bye (40)_____ plays with toys (40)_____ knows mother (will cling to her) (40)_____

EIGHTEEN MONTHS. Stands and walks without support (40)_____ says few words: mama, baby, go (40)_____ obeys simple commands (40)_____ imitates simple movements (clapping of hands, etc.) (40)_____ points to common animals in picture-book (40)_____

TWO YEARS. Runs (40)_____ imitates movements (puts hands on head, above head, makes circle with hands) (40)_____ obeys simple commands (hand me the pencil; throw me the ball; sit down here) (40)_____ can recognize simple objects in surroundings (hand, dog, ball) (40)_____ will use paper and pencil (40)_____

TWO AND ONE-HALF YEARS. Talks in short sentences (40)_____ can point to eyes, ears, nose (40)_____ knows names of members of family (40)_____ will use paper and pencil and will try to copy a circle (40)_____ can recognize self in mirror (40)_____

THREE YEARS. Talks distinctly (40)_____ can repeat sentences of six simple words (40)_____ can repeat up to three numerals (40)_____ recognizes his full name (40)_____ tries to describe a picture showing common objects (40)_____

FOUR YEARS. Knows sex (40)_____ names simple objects (match, key, penny, ring, closed knife) (40)_____ compares two sticks (can select the longer) (40)_____ compares two horizontal lines (can select the longer) (40)_____ can discriminate forms, round, square, etc.) (40)_____

FIVE YEARS. Can count four pennies (40)_____ can copy a square or circle (roughly) (40)_____ compares two weights (identical in appearance, one several times heavier than the other) (40)_____ can put together visiting card cut diagonally (40)_____ can repeat or tell a short story (40)_____

Maximum total _____

Actual total score in Test I _____

Examiner _____

Test II—Measurements

The examiner should insert actual measurements only. The Scoring Committee will compute the score as per leaflet, "Special Instructions for Scoring."

		Maximum Score	No. Points Deducted for Defects
Height	_____ in.	20	
Weight	_____ lbs.	20	
Circumference of head	_____ in.	15	
Circumference of chest at nipple line	_____ in.	15	
Circumference of abdomen at umbilical line, taken with child standing	_____ in.	10	
Diameter of chest ant-posterior, taken with calipers at level of nipple line in mid-sternal line	_____ in.	5	
Lateral diameter of chest taken with calipers at level of nipple line in mid-axillary line	_____ in.	5	
Length of arm from tip of acromion process to tip of middle finger	_____ in.	5	
Length of leg from greater trochanter to the sole of the foot	_____ in.	5	

Maximum Total 100

Actual total score in Test II _____

NOTE: *Physicians have asked that the following measurements be made for statistical purposes, but they do not score for or against the baby.*

Sitting height, to be taken with the baby seated on the table; measurements to be made from top of table to top of baby's head _____ in.

Antero-posterior diameter of head (glabella to occipital protuberance) _____ in.

Lateral diameter of head (calipers above the ears) _____ in.

Examiner _____

Table of Standards

IMPORTANT: *To score babies whose sizes fall between standards given below, see "Instructions for Scoring."*

Test III—Physical Examination

The examiner marks "x" for each defect as listed in this test. Where no defect is found, leave the space blank. The Scoring Committee will figure the score from the penalties noted at "x."

	Minimum Points for Defects
1. HEAD. Abnormally small (5) _____ abnormally large (5) _____ asymmetrical (5) _____ Box-shaped (5) _____	20
2. HAIR. Scanty (5) _____ brittle (5) _____ bald spots (5) _____	15
3. SCALP. Poor condition (5)	5
4. FONTANEL. Delayed closure (should be closed at 18th month) (10) _____ abnormally large (5)	15
5. FACE. Features irregular (10) _____ chin receding or projecting (10)	20
6. NECK. Enlarged glands (consider small, palpable glands not abnormal) (10) _____ scars of glands (10)	20
7. CHEST. Inspection: Poor development (10) _____ asymmetrical (10) _____ abnormal shape (pigeon breast, barrel or funnel-shaped) (10) _____ rickets, beading (10) _____ With stethoscope: Heart irregular (10) _____ murmurs (10) _____ lungs diminished or bronchial breathing, rales (10)	70
8. BACK. Spine: Curvature lateral (10) _____ curvature antero-posterior (10) _____ Scapulae Winged (5) (10)	30
9. ABDOMEN. Abnormal distention (normal abdomen is protuberant in infancy (10) _____ enlarged liver (10) _____ enlarged spleen (10) _____ hernia at navel (10) _____ hernia at groin (10)	50
10. ARMS. HANDS and FINGERS. Enlarged epiphyses (10) _____ asymmetrical (5) _____ clubbing of fingers (10)	25
11. NAILS. Defects (5) _____ discolored (5)	10
12. GENITALIA. Male: Adherent prepuce (5) _____ inflammation (5) _____ testicles, non-descended (above scrotum) (5) _____ serous abnormalities (5) _____ Female: Congenital defects (10) _____ discharge (5) _____ inflammation (5)	30
13. POSTURE and GAIT. Incorrect posture (round shoulders, head held forward) (10) _____ gait (waddling or spastic) (10) _____ pigeon toes (10)	20
14. FEET. Flat-footed (10) _____ deformed (10) _____ knock-kneed (10) _____ bow-legged (10) _____ curvature of thigh bone (10) _____ enlarged epiphyses (10) _____ flat or weak feet (10) _____ toe nail defects (5)	25
15. SKIN. Pallor (5) _____ skin rough (5) _____ Membranes (5) _____ baby fat (10)	65
16. NUTRITION. Abnormally thin (10) _____ abnormally fat (10)	30
17. MUSCLES and NERVES. Flabbiness of muscles (10) _____ muscular in-co-ordination (10) _____ nervous instability (twitching, extreme nervousness) (10)	20
18. DEPORTMENT DURING EXAMINATION (Bad temper); uncontrollable or lacking in self-control)	30
19. DEFECTS or EVIDENCES OF DISEASE NOT LISTED	20

Maximum total _____

Actual total score in Test III _____

Examiner _____

FIGURE 6.3 Better Babies Scorecards, 1920. Used with permission of Collection of Wendy McClure.

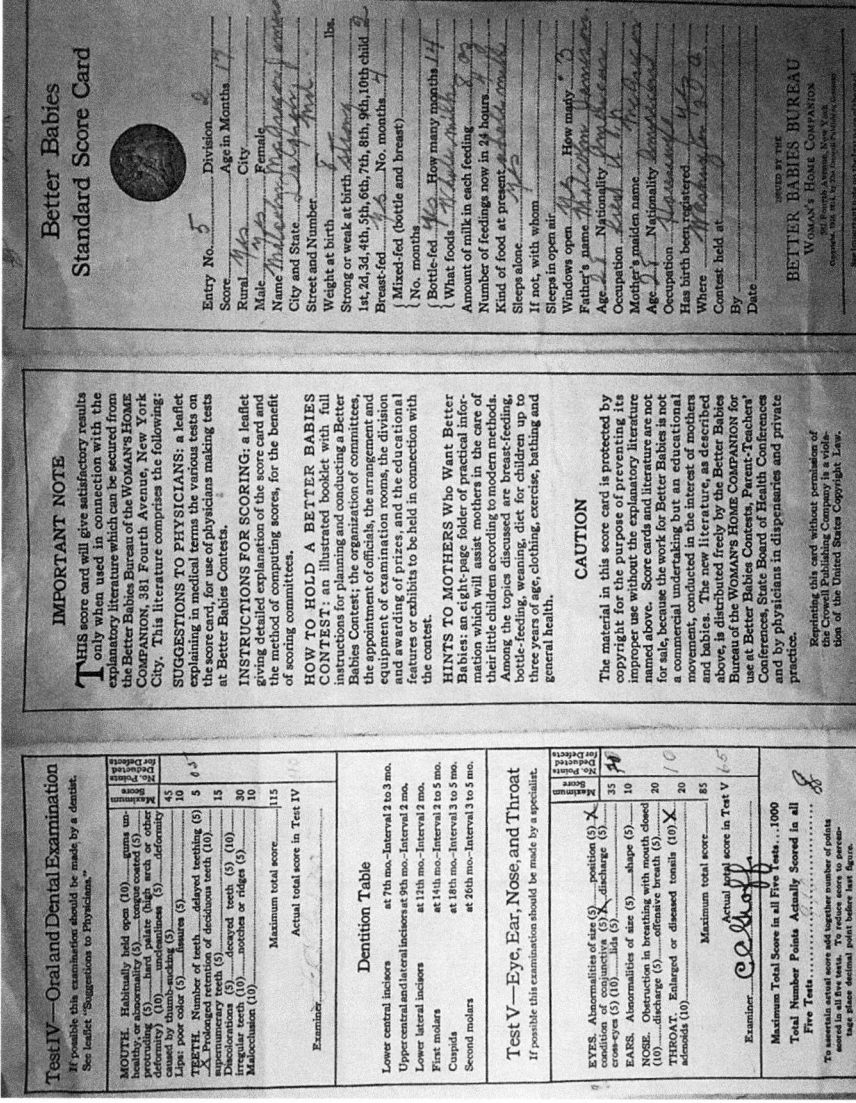

FIGURE 6.4 Better Babies Scorecards, 1920. Used with permission of Collection of Wendy McClure.

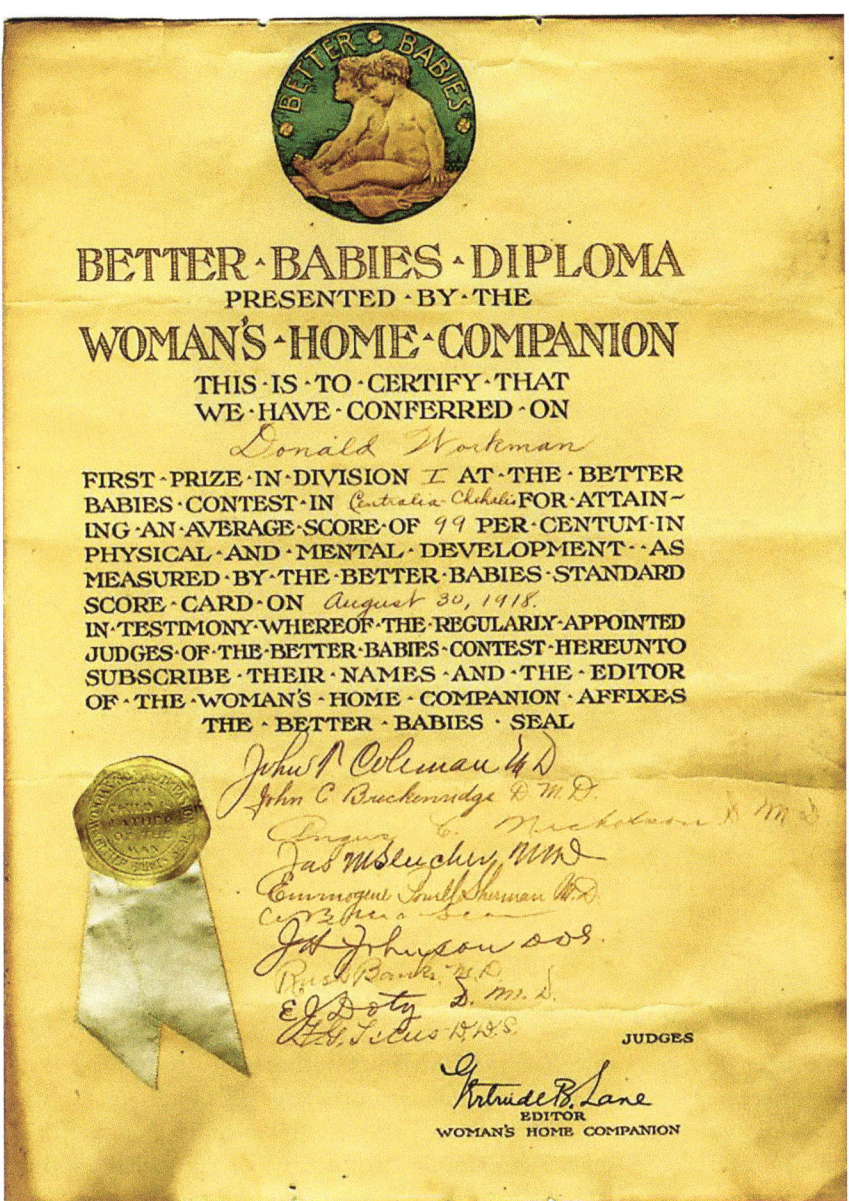

FIGURE 6.5 Better Babies Diploma, 1918. Washington GenWeb Project. Used with permission of Tracy Workman.

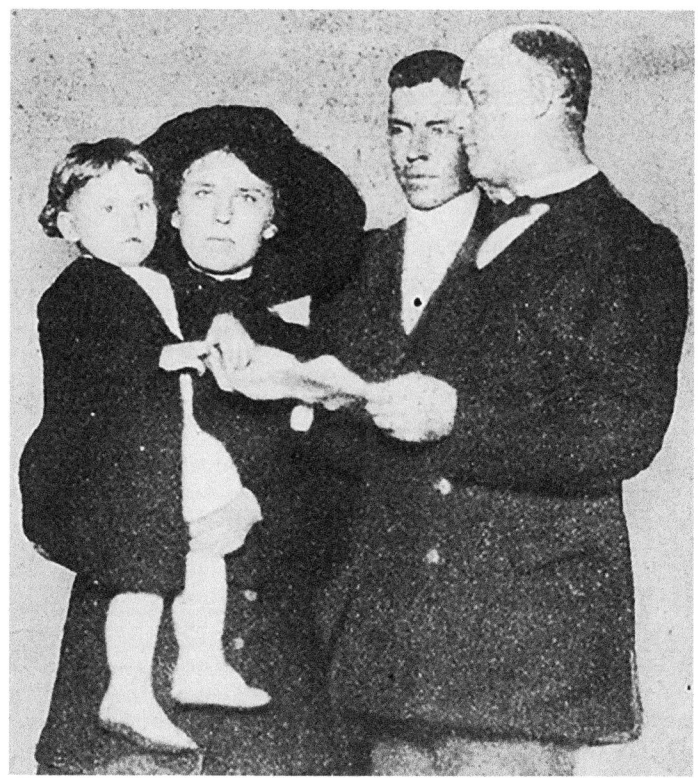

FIGURE 6.6 Champion baby Robert Royal Smithwick receiving gold medal from Secretary of State J. Bryan Grimes, 1913. Used with permission of Louis Round Wilson Special Collections Library, University of North Carolina, Chapel Hill.

World's Fair, 2032

It had been 100 years since George Jamerson's untimely death. In place of the stage where he had lived his final moments stood a large glass encasement. Inside was a tank, with a host of multi-colored wires and tubes spilling outward. The Annual World's Fair Director announced, "Today, we celebrate the life and legacy of our dear George Jamerson, former Director of our 'Genetics and a Secure Future' convening." The crowd cheered (or played their "clap" effect, if they were attending via bot). "Now, scientists will debut our first ever cryopreservation success, reconceptualizing longevity and a new generation of techno-sapiens." On cue, he flipped a switch. The tank opened up, and George Jamerson, not a day over 57 years, gasped his first breath of the new millennium.

Doctor Sheila Chakravarti, the cryo-team's lead scientist, exclaimed, "Welcome to your legacy, George!" The crowd was dumbfounded. Some used their digital "Hurrah" effect. Others stood paralyzed by this feat of rebirth. Dr. Chakravarti quickly led a stunned George off the stage to complete his orientation before he entered irreversible shock.

For the next hour, after the hungry George was provided with a meal, Dr. Chakravarti and George went through virtual history simulators, confused questions, and consent forms. George was coming around to the idea that he had been "genetically mended" and "reawakened" 100 years after his passing, as a tribute to him and his Better Babies vision. As he looked around and took his first paces into the World's Fair, Dr. Sheila addressed all his questions and proudly conveyed what the Better Babies Contest had evolved into: Genetics for a Secure Future. It took a moment for George to see, through the bright lights and electronic cacophony, that this was hardly the fair of yesteryear. An event that once called for one's Sunday best now had only a few humans in attendance. Instead, rectangular screens mounted on steel frames zoomed around. Where presenters might have stood, shimmering mirages of scientists in lab coats took their place. "Holograms," Sheila explained, "it all started in 2012 at this music festival, Coachella—Tupac—never mind." She gestured to physical patrons passing through a security checkpoint. "Not everyone is on board with the new technology. We still allow in-person attendance, but it must be limited. They get fitted with sensors. Any biological intrusion within six feet sets off an alert to move." George felt he should nod here, so he did.

The 2032 fair had gone far beyond Iowa. Representatives from countries from around the world gathered to showcase their latest biotechnologies, promising ever-better health security. Winners would receive funding to manufacture and distribute their products worldwide. One of the largest prizes—upwards of US$6 billion—was allocated to the "Genetics and a Secure Future" convention. Countries where scientists had been especially well-funded and state-backed displayed as many as 20 repro-genetic technologies. Some could take a few drops of blood or a fingernail clipping and predict one's health trajectory and likely cause of mortality. George dared to consider what this would have meant for him a century ago. There were "selection programs" where one could purchase desired gametes, with so-called "full insight" into offspring's outcomes. (The possibility of making artificial gametes via *in vitro* gametogenesis (IVG) is discussed in Chapter 4.) Some were pitched as "dating aids," illuminating one's partnership compatibility with regard to judicious reproduction. Replacing rudimentary developmental tests, there were electrodes measuring brain activity, and sequencing displays rapidly testing for disease carriers and genetic mutations. Genetic science had therapies for more illnesses than George had known to exist. All these technologies aimed to build a techno-sapiens (by then, a widely used and familiar term) future, where humans could transcend their only remaining limitations: health, heritance, and mortality (Bostrom 2003; Koch 2010). Clearly, improvements had been made while George slept. These were a more scientific, enlightened people. With pride and embarrassment, George realized that even lay understandings of science had surpassed him.

Much of George's mission at the Better Babies Contest had been to convey some simple understanding of heredity and encourage people to reproduce responsibly. Now, he could see that his mission had outgrown these limits. He noted this with growing trepidation; without knowledge of more complex heredity, might he have unknowingly passed "bad genes" on to his children? Were the basic measures used to rank babies accurately interpreting their potential? He recalled Galton's 1904 closing statement: "The first and main point is to secure the general intellectual acceptance of eugenics as a hopeful and most important study. Then let its principles work into the heart of the nation, which will gradually give practical effect to them in ways that we may not wholly foresee."

Sheila told George of a past and present he could barely fathom: "After the pandemics, scientists worldwide committed to strengthening our uses of genetics. If you put all these booths together, you'd have a cure for every parasite, infectious virus, and innate biological flaw there is." As he gazed in awe at the promise of what reproduction had become, a part of George wondered why these technologies remained necessary. If Galton was right about heredity and judicious reproductive choices, wouldn't we have "naturally" evolved into our most perfect version without necessitating technological assistance? (Jasanoff et al. 2015).

As they reached the end of the hall, Sheila stopped and gestured to the arena ahead. "Here it is, Dr. Jamerson—after 100 years, we're bringing back your legacy." Emblazoned above the entrance to the arena were now-digitized banners he recognized from his own fairs. "The judging has been going on all morning." Sheila tilted her handheld screen towards George. "Here's the scorecard we use now. All of the physical categories are weighted according to ethno-racial standards. We've gotten a lot of complaints that it's impossible to create guidelines that aren't informed by scientific racism and white American benchmarks, but we had to start somewhere." Then come the genetics categories, which account for more points. As Sheila described, "Standard gene sequencing determines health histories and projections, while electrodes substantiate intellectual development measurements."

"Does everyone reproduce this way?" George asked. "One day, hopefully," Sheila replied. "But this is all tremendously expensive. We'd like to see more nations here, but only a few could afford to submit embryos—the United States, although that's mostly through private investment and biotech companies, Canada, most of Western Europe, Russia, China, India—anywhere wealthy, or who sees this as the next Olympics. Our goal is to expand the entrant pool and extend the competition, tracking these 'perfect babies' through adolescence. That could identify key advantageous genes we can engineer for, or indicate screening sites as unnoticed mutations manifest."

George wondered anxiously if being screened throughout adolescence might have caught his genetic predisposition to aneurysms. "And if some mutation were to manifest?" he asked. "By that stage, most people would choose not to reproduce. After all, who would subject their child to a life of medical uncertainty like that? New treatments do develop, but that's a big risk to take" (Timmermans and Buchbinder 2012).

Inside the Genetic Futures Competition

They continued into the Genetic Futures Competition Arena, and George thought of how far Better Babies had come. Reproductive risk and reward were not judged based on babies, per se, but rather on the molecular level of intricate DNA information preceding these babies (Rose 2001). There were three distinct stations. Lab coats and cyborg-bots observed vigilantly as the Virtual Reproductive Technology (VRT) systems—the latest version of Assisted Reproductive Technologies—appraised each contestant.

The first station was the Embryonic Simulator. There was a small hatch and compartment, just big enough for a petri dish or two full of embryos. Sheila had explained in-vitro fertilization (IVF) during their tour. "They'll take eggs, fertilize them with sperm, allow them to develop for a few days, and then freeze in time the ones that look good—kind of like what we did to you! The good embryos are later thawed and implanted into a human or womb-tech, or in some cases we get to use them for research." George listened to the story of Louise Brown—the first IVF baby born in 1978, almost 50 years after his death. As Sheila explained, Louise paved the way for what is today's norm. "Creating" in the petri dish was safer, more efficient, and enabled much more selectivity (Greely 2016; Dow 2019).

Some contestants came to the Embryonic Simulator with their own biological materials; those who could afford to brought "top-notch" gametes that they had purchased. The simulator was the most advanced iteration on prenatal genetic testing (PGT). When PGT was first developed for humans in 1988, embryos could only be screened for irregular chromosomal development or sex. Embryos could be diagnosed with hereditary issues and genetic mutations, most often if traits in question were well-known from both parents (Greely 2016). Today, these embryos could be screened and diagnosed for just about anything. At the basic level, the simulator provided results for general health outcomes, developmental potential, and common reasons for mortality. For an extra fee, contestants could access the Virtual Futures add-on, which projected the physical appearance of each embryo as well as future strengths, weaknesses, and higher-level health outcomes. For an additional price, one could see up to three generations ahead. Such insight enabled participants with sufficient capital to select their most promising embryos and fix remaining flaws in the genome engineering lab. Contestants used the simulator to make judicious reproductive choices, selecting only the "best" embryos to enter into the Genetic Futures Competition—and eventually, to be implanted in a uterus.

Second, the Demographics Database. Here, people could input the social outcomes they desired from offspring: intended college, profession, athletic ability, personality traits, even their sense of humor. The Database provided a best estimate of the necessary biological configurations that would enable the desired social outcome. Contestants could then make decisions about their partners and embryos, and could purchase the right gametes to bring their reproductive visions to life. George was intrigued; however, he did question to what extent biological traits could precisely predict certain social outcomes (Mukherjee 2019). He remembered that, even back in 1904, social scientists had been hesitant to take Galton's claims at face value. Of course, additional levels of insight from the Database came with incremental price points. Back in George's day, especially if the woman birthed at home, one could reproduce almost for free. Today, reproducing judiciously could cost a fortune. One could opt out—though, as Sheila put it, "a lower upfront reproductive investment would risk one's future hereditary rewards."

Finally, The BioBank, the largest of its kind. "This one is special," Sheila noted. "This station captures your idea: health as a moral obligation" (Savulescu 2001; Rose 2001; Clarke et al. 2003). In this station, contestants did not compete; they contributed. If there were remarkable gametes or embryos that contestants did not intend on using, they could donate them to the BioBank. "Better" biological materials entailed higher remuneration. This global BioBank comprised unparalleled genetic diversity. From it, scientists (in countries where this was permitted) could source biological materials for novel experiments. Intended parents could find just the right composition for their future children. Sheila boasted that just the massive amount of data amassed could push forward genetic predictability about health and heritance from estimations to guarantees. With every contribution recorded in their E-Scorecard, contestants showcased their genetic and health potential toward the competition.

"I want to express how grateful we are to you. Without your work, we would never have had this critical 'Genetics and a Secure Future' portion of The World's Fair." George knew he might have had a vision, but he wasn't sure he could be credited for envisioning all *this*. Sheila motioned George toward the Competition Arena, "If you have questions, do ask, but please wait for the VRT to finish examining, so moderators are not distracted. It's rare, but we have had hacker contestants falsify bio-data input."

The Competition Arena

Life in 2032 could be assessed, projected, and, if needed, precluded without babies ever entering the Competition Arena. In fact, if things went according to plan, no undeserving baby would enter the Arena grounds. Judicious reproduction meant control and selectivity at the earliest intervention possible. Those were the principles driving the Embryonic Simulator. Contestants who were confident they had found an ideal match of high-quality gametes brought fertilized embryos. Others brought unfertilized gametes, either their own or prized BioBank purchases. Contestants vied for the highest possible results: favorable outputs from the Simulator and top-notch marks from the examiners.

As the guest of honor, George was invited to observe from the examiners corner. A young woman approached the Simulator. "Fertilized or unfertilized?" "Unfertilized. These are mine. I've been told that they'd do well here." One of the lab coats began rebooting the Simulator for this new entry. The young woman remained stoic. She couldn't show signs of anxiety, as examiners would down-mark her eggs' mental health potential. "I've donated blood three times this year, so these children will be 'altruistically minded.' I also learned the violin. I remember last year they told me that liking music wasn't enough. These kids, they'll be driven" (Mukherjee 2019). The examiner opened the hatch, the woman placed the petri dish containing her gametes inside, and added, "Oh, and I paid for Level 2."

The Simulator screen lit up and examiners began their copious notes and discussion. George stood by, doing his best to follow the assessment. "Health is okay, with a moderate risk of cardiovascular conditions and potentially a breast cancer episode. But it's all quite low and does not detract much from the longevity score." "Yes, but 5'1. Short." "Very short. The lineage too." "Right, very short hereditary pattern. Even if these were paired with the 6-foot and above options, the resulting offspring wouldn't be what we are looking for, aesthetically" (Mukherjee 2019). George leaned over to Doctor Sheila and whispered, "Does that really matter?" Sheila reassured him, "Height is much more impactful than we've realized. Taller people do better in life. Studies even show that taller people are more likely to be selected for jobs. We want these next generations to have the best chance at life" (Stulp et al. 2015). Unsatisfied, George wondered, was children "needing" to be taller to get jobs a question of reproduction? He questioned why his Better Babies Contests so diligently measured height in the same way.

They turned to the Level 2 insights. "Education potential is good. Slightly above average with a good reading score. Decent athletic potential. Aesthetics overall strong with blue eyes, off-brown hair, North European appeal. Not a bad addition to society" (Mukherjee 2019). The examiners continued scrolling through the Simulator's output as they decided the supposedly inevitable fate of this potential offspring. Throughout, the young woman remained composed, averting being docked for low affect control response. "Some of these traits are challenging. The offspring could be highly extroverted, which bodes poorly for social decorum." "There is risk here." "I think we have a decision." The young woman looked down at her updated E-Scorecard. With a heavy exhale, she exited the tent. George recalled advising parents to intervene with nurture when possible. But here, it seemed like even extroversion was treated as genetic. Surely upbringing must have something to do with personality—and shouldn't there be some extroverts in the world?

George had been doing his best to follow, nodding during pauses while his mind scrambled to make sense of 2032's reproductive logics. He couldn't help but wonder what the world outside this tent looked like—was it inhabited only by tall, white, musical superhumans? If everyone was like that, what advantage did any one of them have? Then he remembered what Sheila had said about the cost and realized that this homogeneity was likely only to exist among the urban wealthy. The farm fields of Iowa seemed very far away.

This next station was yet another large screen—the Demographics Database. It had cutting-edge computing and predictive power, which was a significant boon in facilitating judicious reproductive choices. George noted the long line of contestants. Of those there in-person, he was struck by how different each contestant seemed. Back in his day, it was unheard of for those of color to stand this close to the white folks, let alone utilize the same services and events. Indeed, much had changed since the 1930s.

The examiner was dressed in a smart suit and sat before a commodious sofa set. "Okay, who's next?" A set of hopeful parents walked up and took a seat. "So, tell me, who are you and why are you at the Database?" "I'm Gina. He's Carlos. From El Salvador. We want to have a girl. We need to purchase better eggs based on the Database's results. Mine were a poor match with his." They went on to detail their desires for a daughter-to-come, as the examiner fed the Database. "How important is ethnicity to you? How important is it that the donor be Hispanic?" Gina replied, "Not that important honestly. We just want her to be tall and have his complexion. He wants her to be fair." She continued, "Maybe she could have blue eyes, or light eyes at least, and dark hair." Carlos chimed in, "She should like soccer, because I love it. And we want our daughter to be a teacher. So, she has to be intelligent" (Mukherjee n.d.).

The examiner diligently captured each of their requests. She reminded them that they had only paid for the Level 1 insights, so their outputs would not include the most coveted purchasable gametes. Alas, Gina and Carlos knew that was all they could afford. The examiner provided several options. "I've got one donor here. She sent in a picture—see? The Database shows that if her eggs were paired with Carlos' sperm, we could see a child that grows to be 5 feet 10 inches at her best. She's blonde, but Carlos' darker hair gene would likely be dominant. The donor also has blue eyes and for a little extra you could ensure your daughter will inherit those." "What does she do?" asked Carlos. "Teacher. Intelligence score is great." Gina and Carlos seemed extremely satisfied (Mukherjee 2019). George, on the other hand, was deeply unsettled. Per the donor's photo, she was white. Better Babies had always prioritized whiteness. But this seemed unfitting; a darker-skinned couple from El Salvador could have a white daughter? A part of him rejoiced at the whitening of the next generation, while the other struggled with not having foreseen the racial complexities of an assisted reproductive agenda that transgressed global borders.

"There's two others. This one is from Mexico, so you'd get a closer genetic ancestry. But the projected child would only be 5 feet and 4 inches, and these predictions show her to be on the heavier side. A bit plump. She's—" Gina interrupted, "No." Moving on, the examiner presented a final option: "This one would give you a very high aesthetic score. She's 5 feet 6 inches, but the eggs have a Middle Eastern heritage. So, your daughter's skin may not be as fair as you'd like, but she would look more like you. She also loves soccer." Carlos turned to Gina, "Why don't we get a dish of the first and the third? We can fertilize both. If we refinance the house, we can do genetic testing and pick the best. It'll pay off" (Mukherjee 2019). The couple agreed and the examiner uploaded their E-Order card. It was as Sheila had said: invest upfront in judicious reproduction to secure one's future.

As Gina and Carlos left the station, the examiner said to George, "They were so open-minded." "What do you mean?" asked George. "They only had a few requirements and barely cared about her race or ethnicity. They took the Middle Eastern ones." "But didn't they say they wanted a fair child?" "Ah, yes. Who doesn't?" the examiner laughed. She continued, "I'm not surprised. I find that people are more open to having light-toned or white donors, even if that doesn't match their ethnicity. I've seen people crossing ethnic and race lines to take Hispanic donors, even half-Asian donors. But never African American. There's a certain resistance to African gene heritage. People all over the world have this preference for fairer skin (Mukherjee 2019; see Conclusions). Those are the eggs we charge the most for in any case; when we do have Black parents who want Black children, we have to explain that there's simply less material to choose from." It was starting to click for George. Whiteness was no longer only for the white, but could be purchased. It was part of judicious reproduction, ensuring that your child presents favorably. While the Better Babies' judges prioritized white babies, the contestants and examiners of today were able to start earlier, placing higher reproductive value on whiter gametes (Almeling 2011; Mukherjee 2020).

The next couple came over. "We are from India. We need to purchase embryos, sex doesn't matter." The examiner asked them to list their requests. Shalini spoke first, "I want the child to be like me. They should grow up to have my kind of mentality, good education, culture, and a good family background. We have to make sure the embryo doesn't present any health complications. That means making sure the providers are well-socialized, from good genetic heritages." Raj added, "The child also has to believe in Hinduism. We believe that will also come from a donors' good genetic bloodline." The examiner paused, "What about skin color?" Shalini responded, "She should be fair. She should look good. But not too good. No one should be able to question whether this is our child or not" (Mukherjee 2019). Finally, Raj noted, "We'll pay for Level 2 insights." The examiner seemed relieved. "With all these characteristics, you're going to need Level 2. In any case, more insight is more responsible."

While the emphasis on health outcomes did resonate with George's intended vision, the thought of projecting desired social, physical, and behavioral outcomes from the most basic, cellular levels of fertilization was almost unbelievable to him. Though he did not understand how, he marveled at social traits being predicted and selected for in embryos, let alone gametes. It also sounded like the hopeful parents had their own conceptions about nurture versus inheritance; Raj and Shalini thought bloodlines contributed to a well-cultured child. Had the eugenics movement solidified the linkage between the social and biological? Had they heeded the genetic advantages of whiteness? He was perplexed that people of all shades were utilizing these technologies. Yes, they were reproducing better, fairer babies, but his vision was never for *them*. The incorporation of non-white parents, donor material, and genetic engineering expanded the judicious reproduction vision beyond George's scope. Perhaps this was contemporary science's approach to creating hope for everyone in this eugenic utopia.

As they left the Demographics Database, Sheila quietly remarked, "This thing is great, but they hesitate to mention that we're still working on reliability. Genes are powerful tell-tales, but we don't always get those social predictions right. We're still figuring out the exact links and combinations" (Lippman 1992).

They were now at the third and final station. George's head was swimming with the scientific revelations of the past century. Something more was growing here, almost akin to a religious fervor, a belief in the transcendence of flawed human imagining. He was pulled from his musings by Doctor Sheila's introduction of the BioBank. Lab assistants were taking cheek swabs from a few in-person attendees. The display near the front advertised the "world's largest genetic database." The screen next to it cycled through names and logos he didn't recognize. "Pharmaceutical companies," explained Sheila. "It's been tremendously difficult for public health to compete with private collections. A few years ago, we launched a multinational partnership with some big pharmaceutical companies, just to have a fighting chance. We supply the training, employees, and the public face, and they provide the funding to make it a more attractive deal for donors. Compensating donors might not seem like much, but it's made a huge difference for our data collection. We estimate that 60% of the U.S. can be partially sequenced."

"Why do all this?" George interrupted.

"Why not?" laughed Sheila. "Imagine if you could have been targeted for drug trials before you knew you were at risk for an aneurysm—or your children, before they started developing epilepsy. With the cooperation of the drug companies, we can tailor medications for mood disorders, create drugs with minimal harmful gene interactions or side effects, and begin treatment before problems even start. We can also target genetic health dispositions per race, like high blood pressure in African Americans. Science has yet to prove that race is genetic; still, why not treat it as such, just in case?" (Roberts 2009, 2011a)

George watched as one attendee waited at the counter after giving a swab. When a light at the station began flashing, attendants emerged from the rear. The attendee watched as lab assistants directed him to sign a form before escorting him away. "What's happening?" asked George.

"He must have registered as having some irregularity. When we do a DNA intake, we scan for basic mutations. If anything looks suspicious, we offer a full sequencing to try and figure out what's going on. It's how we get our most valuable data."

"And if something *is* wrong? With the DNA, I mean."

"It's rare, but it does happen. Usually people are just glad we caught it sooner rather than later. We do offer various forms of birth control, if people are worried about passing it on, or editing services if they are thinking about starting a family. They get healthier children; we get better data."

From Iowa to Global Public Health? George wondered how they managed such a large-scale endeavor. "I never imagined so many people being involved in what started as a state fair event. What if something goes wrong?" Doctor Sheila paused. She didn't want George to focus on the impediments of repro-genetic advancements, but she wasn't one to be insincere. She found a nearby bench and motioned him to sit next to her.

"There have certainly been issues. A little over a decade ago, direct-to-consumer genetic testing companies took off. Anyone could send in a cheek swab and get comprehensive insight about their genealogy and health predispositions. They weren't very accurate, but people signed on. There were benefits, surely. We got the foundation for mass genetic data collection and polygenic risk scores, which enabled today's technologies. However, we also faced huge challenges with how genetic information was collected, stored, and managed. Data was sold to private companies that used it to deny people basic medical services, insurance, and employment. Governments bought data to increase state surveillance and target people they labeled 'societal threats,' which was almost always inaccurate. Of course, most were Brown and Black. People really stopped trusting us, the scientists, for a while. There was too much politicization and corporatization, which we unfortunately still see today" (Roberts 2009, 2011b).

Sheila took a moment, allowing George to absorb the historical overload. George stared blankly at the space between his feet on the ground. She went on, "I should also mention the case of the scientist in China, Dr. He. He started collecting genetic data without consent. He edited the genes of twin embryos, had the mother give birth, and then tracked the outcomes of each child. The parents had no idea what he was doing, and they didn't have the money nor the education to contest him. They just wanted those two baby girls. Now, from him, we have hugely controversial data on polygenic risk scores and complex genetic factors. We use a lot of that in our technologies, especially in that Demographics Database. It's terrible how he went about it, but over time we decided we couldn't let those advancements go to waste" (Molina 2019; Chapter 7).

"Advancements"—weren't those supposed to be positive? What Sheila relayed seemed antithetical to the value of progress. George asked, "What did you do about it?"

"We're working on it. The scientific community has been trying to do better for decades. We are committed to weeding out the 'bad apples' among us. There's not much to 'do' in terms of repercussions, except make sure we regulate ourselves more responsibly and make better rules for ourselves." Although it had been proven highly ineffective time and again, genetic scientists had managed to hold on to the power to regulate themselves, creating convenient loopholes and narratives to justify the transgressions of (what grew to be far more than) a few "bad apples" like Dr. He (Molina and Pherribo 2019; Pherribo and Molina 2020).

The Past Is the Present

George leaned back against the wall behind him, closing his eyes to the bright lights of the arena. A mechanical whirring announced the arrival of a bot-attendee, which clicked to a stop in front of him. "Doctor Jamerson? Doctor Sheila told me I might find you here." George opened his eyes and looked through the screen at the wizened face of a man lying in a hospital bed, a tube running across his face, white hair fanned out across the pillow.

"The name's Peter Nelson. I know you don't recognize me, but I was your 'Best Baby' in 1932."

"I do!" said George. "Of course I remember you. You were the last baby I held before—" he waved his hand at the arena, "all this."

"Incredible, isn't it?" said Peter from his faraway hospital bed. "Bet you couldn't have dreamed it up! A lot's changed. Some hasn't. People are still worried about their babies and other people are still trying to make a project out of it."

George understood. "It doesn't all seem to be good," he agreed. "When I was doing all this, I had some idea about wanting to make a better population. It seemed so important then, for the future of America."

"But what kind of future?" objected Peter, suddenly serious. "You might have had good intentions, but things got a lot worse. All that about individual repro-ductive responsibility—it only lasted so long before the government decided it was their problem. We fought a war with Germany to supposedly stop genocide and 'racial purity,' but Germany got those ideas from *us* (Kevles 1995). Making sure the 'right' people have babies also means making sure the 'wrong' people don't, all while conflating individual health with population health. It's been exactly a hundred years, and we still don't have it figured out. Do your science to cure disease, but know that 20 years ago they were sterilizing folks in prisons and 'unwanted' communities. It still happens today. This is the mess we've made."

George felt shame settle in his stomach. He didn't know enough about the past century, but he could tell instinctively that Peter's words were true. How could such a project not follow through to its logical conclusion? He opened his mouth to speak, but all he could find was, "Did it matter for you? Being the 'best' baby?"

"Not too much, I'm afraid—I lost my legs in Korea in 1951. That height advantage disappeared pretty quick!" Peter laughed, and then began coughing. "Now, cancer. Too many damn toxins in the air. Turns out the environment we live and breathe in plays a huge role alongside genetics" (Shostak 2003). The confusion George had been feeling all day was coming to a head—not only was his legacy diverging from what he had intended, but the project itself was flawed.

George found himself ruminating on Peter's words: "this mess we've made." From defining American nationalism as exclusively white, to punishing diver-gence and disability, George knew that the "we" was referring to ideological per-petrators like himself. Their work bound the possibility of genetic intervention inescapably with the atrocities of the past. Was there good, or the capacity for it, in this convention?

Intended parents responsibly choosing their reproductive material gave George hope. But it also highlighted that this choice revolved around ideals that harmed all those deemed "lesser than." Science doesn't care about problematizing the concept of "progress." Professional self-regulation could not be trusted, especially as it granted scientists immunity to pursue racist and ableist nationalist agendas. George imagined the world outside the tent, populated by technosapiens emerging from algorithms and speaking from screens. If eugenic "perfection" and judicious reproduction had seized the minds of the masses, what kind of meta-human was currently sowing the seeds of its ascent?

Peter interrupted, "I want to show you something." He virtually led George to the tent's emergency exit. As his eyes adjusted to the dusk outside the tent, George saw flashing cameras and a large group surrounding the pavilion. They hoisted signs proclaiming alternative, equitable visions. "There are Black People in the Future!" "Disability Rights are Human Rights." People in bodies and on screens raised their voices in clamorous unison. George looked out in awe and relief. Although science continued pursuing its flawed agenda, there *was* dissent here. There was action toward a radical, just future. These change-makers demanded an interrogation of reproduction, of its past shortcomings and future utopias.

George's chest filled with purpose and responsibility for the first time that day. He had to find Dr. Chakravarti, tell her they had it wrong. As George turned back to the tent, he felt that jolt in his head again. A sharp pain ran down his neck. His vision blurred, he struggled to draw breath. The last thing he saw before he passed out was Peter, not in the arms of his mother, but through the lens of infinite technological possibility.

References

Almeling R. 2011. *Sex Cells: The Medical Market for Eggs and Sperm*. Berkeley: University of California Press.

Bostrom N. 2003. "Human Genetic Enhancements: A Transhumanist Perspective." *The Journal of Value Inquiry* 37(4):493–506. https://doi.org/10.1023/b:inqu.0000019037.67783.d5.

Bridges KM. 2019. "White Privilege and White Disadvantage." *Virginia Law Review* 105:449.

Chalmers B. 2015. *Birth, Sex and Abuse: Women's Voices Under Nazi Rule*. United Kingdom: Grosvenor House Publishers.

Chesler E. 2007. *Woman of Valor: Margaret Sanger and the Birth Control Movement in America*. New York: Simon and Schuster.

Clarke AE, L Mamo, JR Fishman, JK Shim, JR Fosket. 2003. "Biomedicalization: Technoscientific Transformations of Health, Illness, and U.S. Biomedicine." *American Sociological Review*. https://doi.org/10.2307/1519765.

Dow K. 2019. "Looking into the Test Tube: The Birth of IVF on British Television." *Medical History* 63(2):189–208.

Eby M. 2019. *Development and Divergence of Feminist-Led Reproductive Control Movements in Germany and the United States, 1907–1942*. Paper presented at the Annual Meetings of the American Anthropological Association.

Galton F. 1904. "Eugenics: Its Definition, Scope, and Aims." *The American Journal of Sociology* 10(1):1–25.

Greely HT. 2016. *The End of Sex and the Future of Human Reproduction*. Princeton, NJ: Harvard University Press.

Jasanoff S, JB Hurlbut, K Saha. 2015. "CRISPR Democracy: Gene Editing and the Need for Inclusive Deliberation." *Issues in Science & Technology* 32(1):37.

Kevles DJ. 1995. *In the Name of Eugenics: Genetics and the Uses of Human Heredity*. Princeton, NJ: Harvard University Press.

Koch T. 2010. "Enhancing Who? Enhancing What? Ethics, Bioethics, and Transhumanism." *The Journal of Medicine & Philosophy* 35(6):685–699.

Lippman A. 1992. "Led (astray) by Genetic Maps: The Cartography of the Human Genome and Health Care." *Social Science & Medicine* 35(12):1469–1476.

Molina S. 2019. "The Banality of Scientific Progress: An Etiology of the #CRISPRbabies Controversy." *Paper Presented at the Meeting of the American Sociological Association*, New York.

Molina S, G Pherribo. 2019. "'Democratizing' Biotechnology: Institutional Constraints on Participatory Governance in Genetic Engineering." *Paper Presented at the Meeting of the Society for the Social Studies of Science*, New Orleans, LA.

Mukherjee M. 2019. *How Do You Want Your Eggs? Kin-Making in the Clinic and the Medical Management of Social Reproduction in the Bay Area and Kolkata*. Paper presented at the Annual Meeting of the American Sociological Association.

Mukherjee M. 2020. "The Management of Unequal Patient Status in Fertility Medicine: Donors' and Intended Parents' Experiences of Participatory and Imposed Enrollment." *Social Science & Medicine* 247:1–8.

Mukherjee M. n.d. "How Do You Want Your Eggs? Kin-Making in the Clinic and the Medical Management of Social Reproduction in the Bay Area and Kolkata." M.A. thesis, University of California Berkeley.

Ngai MM. 1999. "The Architecture of Race in American Immigration Law: A Reexamination of the Immigration Act of 1924." *The Journal of American History* 86(1):67–92.

Pherribo G, S Molina. 2020. "Backstage Decisions and Front-Stage Experts: The Politics of Genome Editing." *Presentation Delivered at the Plant Genome Engineering Symposium*, University of California Berkeley, May. https://pges.berkeley.edu/.

Reilly PR. 1987. "Involuntary Sterilization in the United States: A Surgical Solution." *The Quarterly Review of Biology* 62(2):153–170.

Roberts D. 2009. "Race, Gender, and Genetic Technologies: A New Reproductive Dystopia?" *Signs: Journal of Women in Culture & Society* 34(4):783–804.

Roberts D. 2011a. *Fatal Invention: How Science, Politics, and Big Business Re-Create Race in the Twenty-First Century*. New York: New Press/ORIM.

Roberts D. 2011b. "What's Wrong with Race-Based Medicine: Genes, Drugs, and Health Disparities." *Minnesota Journal of Law, Science & Technology* 12(1):1–21.

Rose N. 2001. "The Politics of Life Itself." *Theory, Culture & Society* 18(6):1–30.

Savulescu J. 2001. "Procreative Beneficence: Why We Should Select the Best Children." *Bioethics* 15(5–6):413–426.

Shostak S. 2003. "Locating Gene–Environment Interaction: At the Intersections of Genetics and Public Health." *Social Science & Medicine* 56(11):2327–2342. https://doi.org/10.1016/s0277-9536(02)00231-9.

Stulp G, AP Buunk, S Verhulst, TV Pollet. 2015. "Human Height Is Positively Related to Interpersonal Dominance in Dyadic Interactions." *PLOS ONE* 10(2):e0117860.

Timmermans S, M Buchbinder. 2012. *Saving Babies?* Chicago, IL: University of Chicago Press.

7

HUMAN GERMLINE GENOME EDITING AND ITS TECH-SUMPTIONS

Amarpreet Kaur

Introduction: CRISPR-Cas9

This chapter explores whether understanding the human genome will create possibilities for "redesigning" humans, and, if so, how plausible these possibilities are. The term "genome" refers to all of the DNA in a cell. Genome editing is a technique that can be used to make changes to a cell's DNA by deleting existing, adding new, or replacing DNA sequences (Ormond et al. 2017:168). DNA consists of three components, each one of which is called a "base." There are four types of bases, each of which is represented by a letter: adenine (A), thymine (T), guanine (G), and cytosine (C). The sequence of these bases forms instructions for the various cells in our bodies and determines how they function. This chapter will discuss changes that could be made to the human genome via egg, sperm, or embryo cells. These cells are heritable and are therefore referred to as *germline cells*. Cells that are not heritable are called *somatic cells*, and edits to such cells cannot be passed on to future generations.

The plausibility of human germline genome editing (hGGE) has received renewed and growing attention since 2012 due to the discovery of a new editing technique called CRISPR–Cas9 (Jinek et al. 2012). CRISPR is an acronym for "clustered regularly interspaced palindromic repeats," which is a reference to the unique organization of DNA sequences found in the genomes of microorganisms; this is simply a guiding system for Cas9. Cas9 is an enzyme that can be programmed to identify a specific DNA sequence so that it can create a break in the DNA to enable edits to be made at a targeted point (Ormond et al. 2017). This technique is far more efficient, accessible, and safer than preceding genome editing techniques (Cavaliere 2018; Morrison and de Saille 2019), making it easier to develop and use for a variety of applications. Considered applications include those for agriculture, bioeconomy, and military purposes, such as "to enhance or augment friendly forces, or target enemy forces" (Heslop and MacIntyre 2019:169), in addition to those upon which this chapter focuses: the prevention of disease and enhancing biological characteristics in humans. As this technology continues to develop, its potential applications continue to evoke considerable excitement and concerns from scientists, stakeholders, and the wider public across the globe.

In this context, this chapter aims to unravel the assumptions surrounding this technology—its *tech-sumptions*, and to examine the plausibility of them being realized in future reproductive practices. This chapter will draw upon findings from a 3-phase design of primary research, conducted between March 2018 and October 2019. The first phase consisted of a mixed-methods online survey of 521 UK citizens aged 16–82 years on "Understandings of Genetic Editing and its Potential Uses within Human Reproduction." The second phase was comprised of semi-structured interviews with 13 experts and professionals involved in the future of human germline genome editing, and the third and final phase of my research entailed structured interviews with 21 people affected by genetic conditions. The discussions surrounding my findings in relation to published literature address several tech-sumptions of hGGE technology to offer clarity to its potential.

Redesigning Humans

In 2002, Dr. Gregory Stock, an American biophysicist, authored a ground-breaking book titled *Redesigning Humans: Choosing Our Children's Genes*. In this book Stock detailed the future power we may have to manipulate human genetics to alter our biology in meaningful, predictable ways. Considering that the specific technology that could enable hGGE, CRISPR-Cas9, did not emerge until a decade later, Stock's book was quite prescient. Stock (2002:2) claimed that we were no longer questioning whether we will manipulate embryos, but rather when, where, and how. Although Stock did not know when reliable germline editing technology would be discovered, he argued that it would signal the beginning of human self-design (2002:3). He hypothesized that hGGE would come into being not as a replacement for existing technologies like embryo screening, but as an extension of them (2002:61). Stock made several valid arguments in his book before turning to suggest that germline editing could mean intentional human enhancement (2002:116).

Stock (2002:114–115) explained that some traits and diseases would not make compelling targets for hGGE due to the underlying processes that would enable it. I will discuss these processes in greater detail below. Here I note that he leaped from suggesting that the distinctions between unwanted traits and disease may fade, along with people's opinions on what diseases are severe enough to avoid, to the possibility of genetic enhancement. He clarified that "enhancement" did not necessarily mean pushing beyond possible human capacities, but that aspiring parents would seize the opportunity to insert traits into their possible child's genome that their child may not have otherwise had (Stock 2002:116), such as eye and hair color, and musical and/or sporting abilities. These "redesigning" traits differ from traits that are currently considered as enhancements, such as greater intelligence or greater tolerance to heat. Herein, I contend that Stock's notion of redesigning and enhancing humans is implausible for the foreseeable future.

Utilizing hGGE

Currently, in order for edits to be made to germline cells, they would have to be extracted from the prospective parents or donors and undergo in vitro fertilization (IVF). While procuring sperm cells may be relatively easy, acquiring human egg cells is not. For women, egg retrieval usually entails a period of self-administered intramuscular hormone injections, ultrasound monitoring, and then retrieval under sedation or general anesthetic (Franklin 1997)—an unpleasant process. Parts of this process, particularly the hormone injections, carry several notable side effects, some of which, although rare, can be fatal (Fauser and Devroey 2003). Later, if a suitable embryo is produced (the suitability of embryos is defined by their morphology, and if they are being screened, whether they are found to be affected by the condition being screened for (Franklin and Roberts 2006:32)), it can be transferred into a uterus to try to establish a pregnancy. The use of IVF technologies increases risks of ectopic pregnancy, miscarriages, and congenital defects (NHS 2017b), which contribute to IVF having a very modest success rate with an average of only 25%. This average steeply declines as maternal age advances (HFEA 2018). Such factors do not make this process inviting.

Furthermore, the cost of IVF varies around the globe, with a single attempt costing an average of £5,000 in the UK (NHS 2017a), around $20,000 in the US, and approximately Rs.155,000 (£1,635/$2,000 USD) in India (Sarojini et al. 2011). According to Stock (2002:142), the risks, costs, and low success rate of IVF could therefore be disincentives for many people who may consider accessing hGGE. They could also be effective deterrents for those who are not dependent on the technology to conceive a child, those who have alternatives, or those who may not be able to afford the expense (Inhorn 2015). In this respect, going through this process so a child can have green eyes or musical talent, as Stock argues, does not seem to hold much imperative.

However, should people be willing to go through IVF to utilize hGGE, whether to prevent disease or for enhancement purposes, they would also have to subject their embryo(s) to the technology being injected into it, hoping that it works, and then have preimplantation genetic testing (PGT), which Stock referred to as "embryo screening." PGT involves removing several cells from the developing embryo to test them for specific genetic traits. In many cases, embryos are frozen while the test results are pending. This means that embryos also have to be thawed if they are suitable for transfer. In theory, if hGGE works, then all morphologically sound embryos should be suitable, but would first have to withstand several complex interventions. I therefore argue that hGGE is only likely to be sought by people who have no other option to secure a healthy child, rather than as an expensive option for desirable traits.

The Genetic Origins of Traits

Nonetheless, for a disease or trait to be a candidate for hGGE, the genetic origin for it (if one exists), i.e. its gene, must be known and identifiable, so that tests can identify it. If the gene for any given disease or trait is not known, neither PGT nor hGGE would be possible, because the trait would not be targetable for any form of editing or screening. In this vein, there are several projects around the world sequencing human genomes. One such project is the 100,000 genomes project in the UK, which aimed to find associations between symptoms and disease traits and their genetic variants. In 2018, the project finished sequencing 100,000 genomes from people affected by rare diseases and/or cancers in the hope of identifying genetic traits among them (Ipsos MORI 2019). While many people who participated in the project have been told that a genetic link for their disease is yet to be found, the UK's NHS is hopeful that new discoveries will be made if they periodically re-sequence the genomes they have collated.

The project focused on finding genetic variants for diseases with an aim to advance treatments and interventions for these diseases. The same cannot be said for finding non-disease related traits, nor is an effort to do so likely to be launched in the foreseeable future. Interestingly, Stock (2002:60) acknowledged that "abuses" of germline interventions such as hGGE technologies, for purposes such as enhancements or "redesigning," are not nearly as likely as some critics imagine. He reached this conclusion because such interventions would have too few users to command the funds required to bring them into open use, and thus are not likely to be possible for a very long time, if at all. Yet he still felt the need to caution against such prospects. Findings from the 100,000 genomes project reinforce that a greater understanding of the human genome and its complexities is needed before advances with treatments and/or interventions can be made. The function of each gene and its relation to other genes must be known before any gene could be considered suitable for hGGE. There are currently few genes for which such information is reliably known and these are all primarily associated with diseases, not with enhancements or aesthetic traits (Keller 2015).

In May 2019, I was fortunate to interview Professor Robin Lovell-Badge, a prominent biologist at the Francis Crick Institute in London, on this matter. He shared the following:

> [For a gene to be considered for hGGE] we would need to know and understand enough about different variants of a gene to be able to predict with a high degree of certainty what the outcome of the editing will be. [...] We need to know that correcting a particular variant of a gene associated with a genetic disease would not have any deleterious effects. For example, we

know enough about the mutations that lead to Huntington's Disease to say that if we were to correct that back to a normal version, that should not give any bad effects and should be reasonably safe; similar for Sickle Cell disease and Thalassaemia. We know some variants can confer some risks to disease or some protection towards getting a disease, to change or correct that gene is much more of a gamble. For some small numbers [of disease causing genetic variants] we know a lot, for the rest we have to wait for things like the 100,000 genome project, which is many years away because there is a lot of work to do on that, for sufficient knowledge.

In this regard, if there is still insufficient knowledge and understanding of the many genes associated with genetic diseases, and this search is a priority for geneticists, then diverting attention to understanding non-disease traits seems highly unlikely. This said, *what is considered to be a disease is socially constructed*, and this construction differs across time and space (Kerr 2004). What may be considered a disease today may not be tomorrow, and vice versa. Thus, arguably, any trait could be framed as a disease if there were motivation to do so. The late epidemiologist Professor Abby Lippman (1991:17) wrote that genetics are increasingly identified as the way to reveal and explain disease and normality. She argued that there is an ongoing discourse in society on reducing individuals to their DNA sequences to define differences, such as diseases and physiological variations, as being, at least in part, genetic in origin (Lippman 1991:15). Lippman termed this discourse "geneticization."

As a result of geneticization, Stock's argument assumes that there are genetic origins for the traits for which he imagines humans could be redesigned. While I recognize that there are genetic origins for eye, hair, and skin color, there may not be for musical or sports-based talents (Duster 2003). Additionally, these are likely to be polygenic traits, making editing using current technologies nearly impossible. The search for, ascertaining knowledge of, and understanding such genes (should they ever be found) would take considerable resources that at present, no one seems to be compelled to invest in at a governmental level (Briggs 2017). But a private company with significant expendable resources may be willing to do so should such a desire manifest. However, a lack of reliable information on genes evidently does not deter some scientists from using them in human germline interventions, and if not prohibited, may not prevent them from experimenting with non-disease related traits.

The Assumed Consensus

In May 2019, Angela Douglas, the Deputy Chief Scientific Officer for England's National Health Service (NHS), shared the following with me:

> There is an international consensus at present that no changes should be made to human germ cells or embryos, and if in the process of research,

early human embryos or germline cells undergo gene editing, the modified cells should not be used to establish a pregnancy.

However, unbeknownst to her and the world at the time, Chinese scientist Jiankui He and his team had already used such cells to establish a pregnancy (Regalado 2019). Twin girls, Lulu and Nana, born in October 2018, were the result of this experimental research (Lovell-Badge 2019:2). A month later, He leaked the news of the twins' birth on the eve of the Second International Summit on Human Genome Editing in Hong Kong (ibid.). As a first-hand witness to his presentation at the summit and the interrogation that ensued, I can testify that no other scientist present supported He's research, which was swiftly and openly condemned at the summit and by scientists across the globe in its wake (Daley et al. 2019). Much to their dismay, the assumed consensus had been broken.

In addition to being unwelcome, He's research did not achieve its intended aim of generating resistance to a disease (HIV). His research was widely criticized for being premature, unjustified, and unethical, and was later outlawed by the Chinese government (Daley et al. 2019; Regalado 2019), but the consequences of his research are ongoing. He's three-year prison sentence, fine, and lifetime ban from conducting research constitute a warning to other scientists. The condemnation of He's research indicates that there is zero tolerance for misusing genome editing technology, even if it is in the pursuit of attempting to prevent disease, let alone human enhancement. In this regard, Stock's arguments on redesigning humans fall short. If the premature use of hGGE to try and prevent disease is still condemned, the use of such technologies to instill non-disease traits would be even more so. However, legislation and regulation vary among countries (Yotova 2017). Thus the globally non-unified approach to research involving hGGE could enable Stock's (2002) hypothesized enhancement and redesigning theories to come true, should there be an appetite for them.

International Regulation and Ethics

When I interviewed Dr. Rumiana Yotova, a lecturer in Public International Law at the University of Cambridge, in September 2019, she explained to me that no country explicitly allows hGGE for clinical applications—i.e., for pregnancies to be established from edited germline cells. However, she added that many countries have nothing that prohibits it either. This diversity in legislation and regulation of hGGE is concerning, considering that travel to access reproductive technologies, called "reproductive tourism," is a growing phenomenon (Inhorn 2015). Thus national borders are becoming less obstructive in the promotion of reproductive technologies; as soon as techniques are outlawed or applications are banned in one country, it is not uncommon to see an exodus of women to countries where they are still allowed (Inhorn 2015). Diversity in legislation and regulation could therefore lead to citizens from cautious countries, such as the UK and Europe, where research applications involving hGGE have been restricted, to travel to access the technology in countries where they have not, such as the US and Mexico (Kaur 2020).

In this regard, scientists in countries where legislation and regulation are unclear, as was the case in China, have called for a global moratorium on research involving hGGE (Lander et al. 2019). This could prevent further misuse/premature use of hGGE technologies. However, a moratorium could perhaps be too little too late (and is not supported by countries with relatively sound legislation and regulation, such as the UK). This is because such countries do not share the same concerns or ethical dilemmas, nor have need to. For example, in the US, "biohackers" (lay people who experiment with biological material) have used somatic genome editing in a variety of experiments in both humans and animals. This unregulated use has generated concerns around similar experiments being translated to germline genome editing. But biohacking is also relatively expensive and is not as accessible as the media portrays it to be (Briggs 2017). Nonetheless, as previously mentioned, the latter use has more profound consequences insofar as any effects could transcend into future generations. This could mean that any unintended, adverse side effects would not only affect the person who undergoes hGGE, but possibly their descendants as well. Such research is prohibited in the UK; hence it does not support a moratorium on germline genome editing research. But prohibitions in the UK and other countries do not extend to their citizens traveling abroad to seek and access interventions to circumvent them (Kaur 2020). Thus, such practices pose several ethical dilemmas.

First, if only affluent people can afford the travel and service fees etc. to access hGGE, this could further inequalities within societies (Briggs 2017; Coller 2019). This concern was cited by respondents to my survey as being influential in whether they would consider traveling abroad, should that be allowed. Respondent 307 stated:

> If their reasons are valid then maybe, but [traveling abroad] could be used to exacerbate social inequality/eugenics. (Male, 17, college student, not affected by a genetic condition)

Second, considering the commercialization of IVF and its associated services, if hGGE were to be added, promoted, and accessed before it is safe, this could have several, wide-ranging welfare implications on both the aspiring parents and children born as a result of utilizing hGGE (Morrison and de Saille 2019). For example, if complications were to arise, health professionals may have difficulties tracing and dealing with interventions undertaken in other countries, and this in turn may affect the treatment they are able to provide. Third, if Stock's notion of redesigning humans and/or enhancements were to be realized, these could drastically change humanity as we know it, and/or commercialize children (Rose 2006). This was listed as a possible consequence of not limiting the applications of hGGE by respondents to my survey.

Respondent 258: That people would edit out "less desirable" characteristics e.g. eye colour, hair colour or maybe skin colour (if this is possible) – I fear this could be misused certainly in other countries where ethics and relevant legislation might not be strong. I feel it's too close to eugenics. (Male, 26, counselor, not affected by a genetic condition)

Respondent 484: It could therefore be used on extremely minor things, and become more eugenics-based whereby all undesirable traits are eradicated. Not just traits which would affect a quality of life, but any traits whatsoever. (Male, 24, unemployed, not affected by a genetic condition)

Additionally, there are concerns that the use of hGGE could exacerbate stigma and discrimination towards people who are living with genetic conditions (Boardman 2019). Such concerns are evidenced in quotes from a participant in my structured interviews and from a respondent to my survey:

Haifa: There are still generations of people living with these conditions. And so, will it [hGGE] actually mean that we are more discriminated against because we are seen as these people who are out? We will be edited out at some point. (Female, 38, has Beta Thalassaemia)

Respondent 158: [re. consequences of not limiting hGGE] In any case, fostering discrimination against people choosing not to use genetic editing for any reason. If cosmetic editing is allowed—fostering discrimination against people with certain physical characteristics by encouraging fashions and trends to form around the "preferable" characteristics. A rebirth of eugenics through trying to make "better" people. Greater inequality between those who can and can't afford the treatments. (Male, 28, administrator, has Ichthyosis Vulgaris)

Such concerns indicate that indeed there is no longer an assumed consensus and that because of He's research, there are wariness and fear on the part of other scientists also prematurely attempting similar research (Cyranoski 2019). While a moratorium has not been honored, other, more pragmatic, global initiatives have been launched.

One such initiative was instigated by the World Health Organization (WHO) in December 2018. It established an 18-member Expert Advisory Committee on Developing Global Standards for Governance and Oversight of Human Genome Editing. The committee aimed to advise and make recommendations on appropriate governance mechanisms for hGGE, following its current examination of the scientific, ethical, social, and legal challenges associated with hGGE in 2020. But meeting this objective was delayed due to the coronavirus pandemic. In the interim, Dr. Tedros Adhanom Ghebreyesus, the WHO's Director-General, urged countries not to allow any further work on hGGE in human clinical applications until the technical and ethical implications have been properly considered

(WHO 2019). But countries and scientists are not obliged to heed his plea, nor may they be inclined to do so.

The WHO's committee recognized that research is likely to continue, and so, in August 2019, it launched a registry, hoping to track all research and clinical trials that involve hGGE. In parallel, in 2019, the UK's Royal Society—its national academy of sciences—and the US National Academies of Science and Medicine convened an International Commission on the Clinical Use of Human Germline Genome Editing (The Royal Society 2019). The commission aims to develop principles, criteria, and standards for the clinical use of genome editing of the human germline (Kaur and Border 2020:2–3), should such applications become approved. Such initiatives should eradicate assumptions that applications of hGGE may not be closely regulated and/or monitored, and extend recognition to the fact that there are widespread limitations on applications involving hGGE, even if these limitations could be tightened. This is because, despite ethical concerns regarding hGGE (and Stock's arguments), the science behind it continues to develop, and hGGE as a whole remains largely desired for the prevention of genetic disease at the very least.

Public Opinions on hGGE

Findings from a nationally representative quantitative survey commissioned by the Royal Society reveal that 76% of the UK's population feel that using hGGE to correct a genetic disorder would be positive to some extent (van Mil et al. 2017:63). Further to this, findings from the mixed-methods online survey I conducted with a similarly representative sample reveal that 69% would either use or consider using hGGE if the technology were available to prevent heritable disease (Kaur 2019:70–71). Additionally, a survey of 152 people affected by genetic conditions conducted by Genetic Alliance UK found that around 80% of their respondents approve of hGGE to correct a faulty gene (Wipperman and Campos 2016:20). Such high levels of support for using hGGE to prevent disease indicate that the development of the technology for such purposes is likely to be driven by those affected by genetic diseases. Participants in my interactive interviews, which, again, included people affected by various genetic conditions, shared why they feel that hGGE should be legalized as a preventative intervention for disease:

> Abdullah: Yes [hGGE should be legalized as a preventative intervention], because it is beneficial, especially because there are not many treatments for rare disease, like Primary Ciliary Dyskinesia itself. The treatment is often in the long-term not effective, so if there is a way to stop these kinds of diseases from spreading, and to stop them from occurring in the long-term future, it would be beneficial. (Male, 20, has Primary Ciliary Dyskinesia)

> Virginia: [hGGE] should be legalised. The key reason why I hold that opinion is because I am disabled myself, I have a genetic condition, and

> personally I would not want to have a child or bring another person into this world with the same genetic condition as myself. I think life with this disability is a struggle in this ableist world. Frankly, I would not choose to have this condition if I had the option, therefore I would not choose it for someone else either. (Female, 21, has Muscular Dystrophy)

In contrast, the utilization of hGGE for alternative purposes such as those conveyed by Stock for enhancements or redesigning humans, such as changing eye or hair colors, received far less support.

Additionally, other findings from the survey commissioned by the Royal Society indicate that only 24% of their respondents feel genome editing should be used for cosmetic reasons (van Mil et al. 2017:50). This suggests that the desire to "redesign" humans is largely non-existent, contrary to Stock's arguments. Rather, these findings imply that society would prefer to have restrictions placed on the applications of hGGE and that the prevention of disease would be the only widely acceptable use. Hence, such preferences may benefit from being overtly legislated and regulated to avoid assumptions and gray areas that maverick scientists may err into.

The tech-sumptions addressed above are not unfounded. Throughout history, people have sought to secure or avoid having offspring with certain characteristics for both social and personal reasons (Nuffield Council on Bioethics 2018:13). While these characteristics have not been limited to securing health and/or avoiding disease, they have also not involved altering genetic sequences. But, in this context, there are also concerns that prospective parents, as opposed to scientists, as Stock (2002:9–10) argues, may seek hGGE for reasons beyond preventing disease even if this desire generates ethical issues. Such concerns also include people feeling obliged to "create the best children" or children being commercialized (Rose 2006; Ormond et al. 2017). However, these concerns seemingly overlook the fact that hGGE would be contingent on IVF and its many risks, and that the genetic variants for traits must be known, which many are not (Doudna 2020). These concerns also overlook the fact that people have understandable reservations surrounding the use of such technologies and what they mean for future generations, as indicated in the following quote from a participant in one of my interactive interviews named Sally:

> I think I would like to see if one could naturally, I say "naturally," occur on its own without needing an intervention. I would have more faith in that embryo than in one that had had a gene spliced because of my sci-fi sort of fears about what might happen to that child in the future. Like they become telepathic to another, you know, and we've created the x-men. (Female, 55, has Stickler Syndrome)

I therefore maintain that while using human germline genome editing for "redesigning humans" and enhancement purposes may be possible, it is not plausible as a routine reproductive choice.

Conclusion: Tech-Sumptions

In this chapter, I have detailed several prominent assumptions made about the applications of hGGE technologies in order to clarify their validity, using evidence from my own research and from published literature. These tech-sumptions have included considerations of the science behind hGGE; the processes that will enable it; and the required genomic information. They have also covered legislative, regulatory, and ethical concerns, and public attitudes towards the potential applications of hGGE. As explored herein, there is weak impetus to redesign or enhance humans in the foreseeable future, due to the unpleasant nature and expense of IVF—the process that would enable hGGE, and to the minimal desire, if any, to use hGGE for applications that extend beyond preventing disease. Even if such desire did exist, the genomic data needed to secure such applications is not being prioritized by geneticists, most of whom are focused on finding genetic traits related to disease.

Furthermore, while legislation and regulation differ among countries, the ethical concerns and vast expense of developing the technology are largely universal and this potential development is widely condemned (Daley et al. 2019; Kaur and Border 2020). These factors are not likely to soften in the foreseeable future. To this end, I assert that although using hGGE to redesign or enhance humans could become possible, implementing it as a reproductive option is implausible. Therefore I conclude, in keeping with the theme of this book, that although we are co-evolving with our technologies, gradually becoming "techno-sapiens," and that ongoing co-evolution may well encompass efforts to eradicate genetic diseases, this will not involve genetic enhancement for decades to come, if ever.

Acknowledgments

My research is funded by a full Studentship from the Economic and Social Research Council's Doctoral Training Partnership in Cambridge, UK. Several parts of my research activities have also been supplemented by grants from Christ's College in Cambridge, UK. I thank both of these institutions for their support, and respondents to/participants in my research for making my research possible.

References

Boardman F (2019) Human Genome Editing and the Identity Politics of Genetic Disability. *Journal of Community Genetics* 11(2): 125–127. doi:10.1007/s12687-019-00437-4.
Briggs L (2017) *How All Politics Became Reproductive Politics: From Welfare Reform to Foreclosure to Trump*. Oakland, CA: University of California Press.
Cavaliere G (2018) Genome Editing and Assisted Reproduction: Curing Embryos, Society or Prospective Parents? *Medicine, Health Care, & Philosophy* 21(2): 215–225. doi:10.1007/s11019-017-9793-y.

Coller BS (2019) Ethics of Human Genome Editing. *Annual Review of Medicine* 70(1): 289–305. doi:10.1146/annurev-med-112717-094629.

Cyranoski D (2019) Russian Biologist Plans More CRISPR-Edited Babies. *Nature* 570(7760): 145–146. doi:10.1038/d41586-019-01770-x.

Daley GQ, Lovell-Badge R and Steffann J (2019) After the Storm—A Responsible Path for Genome Editing. *New England Journal of Medicine* 380(10): 897–899. doi:10.1056/NEJMp1900504.

Doudna JA (2020) The Promise and Challenge of Therapeutic Genome Editing. *Nature* 578(7794): 229–236. doi:10.1038/s41586-020-1978-5.

Duster T (2003) *Backdoor to Eugenics*, 2nd ed. London: Routledge. www.amazon.co.uk/Backdoor-Eugenics-Troy-Duster/dp/0415946743 (accessed February 8, 2020).

Fauser BCJM and Devroey P (2003) Reproductive Biology and IVF: Ovarian Stimulation and Luteal Phase Consequences. *Trends in Endocrinology & Metabolism* 14(5): 236–242. doi:10.1016/S1043-2760(03)00075-4.

Franklin S (1997) *Embodied Progress: A Cultural Account of Assisted Conception*. First ed. London: Routledge.

Franklin S and Roberts C (2006) *Born and Made: An Ethnography of Preimplantation Genetic Diagnosis*. Princeton, NJ: Princeton University Press.

Heslop D and MacIntyre C (2019) Germ Line Genome Editing and the Emerging Struggle for Supremacy in the Chemical, Biological and Radiological (CBR) Balance of Power. *Global Biosecurity* 1(1): 1. University of New South Wales: 169–173. doi:10.31646/gbio.18.

HFEA (2018) *IVF—What Is In Vitro Fertilisation?* www.hfea.gov.uk/treatments/explore-all-treatments/in-vitro-fertilisation-ivf/ (accessed 15 January 2020).

Inhorn (2015) *Cosmopolitan Conceptions: IVF Sojourns in Global Dubai*. United States: Duke University Press.

Ipsos MORI (2019) *A Public Dialogue on Genomic Medicine: Time for a New Social Contract?* April. London: Genomics England. www.genomicsengland.co.uk/public-dialogue-report-published/.

Jinek M, Chylinski K, Fonfara I, et al. (2012) A Programmable Dual-RNA–Guided DNA Endonuclease in Adaptive Bacterial Immunity. *Science* 337(6096): 816–821. doi:10.1126/science.1225829.

Kaur A (2019) *Understandings of Genetic Editing and Its Potential Uses within Human Reproduction Survey Report*. Cambridge: University of Cambridge Press. www.amarpreetkaur.co.uk/img/Final-Survey-Report.pdf.

Kaur A (2020) Could Seeking Human Germline Genome Editing Force Journeys of Transnational Care? *Multidisciplinary Journal of Gender Studies* 9(2): 184–209. doi:10.17583/generos.2020.5077.

Kaur A and Border P (2020) *Human Germline Genome Editing*. POSTnote 611, January. Parliamentary Office of Science and Technology.

Keller EF (2015) The Postgenomic Genome. In: Richardson SS and Stevens H (eds) *Postgenomics: Perspectives on Biology after the Genome*. Durham: Duke University Press, pp. 9–31.

Kerr A (2004) *Genetics and Society: A Sociology of Disease*. London: Routledge.

Lander ES, Baylis F, Zhang F, et al. (2019) Adopt a Moratorium on Heritable Genome Editing. *Nature* 567(7747): 165–168. doi:10.1038/d41586-019-00726-5.

Lippman A (1991) Prenatal Genetic Testing and Screening: Constructing Needs and Reinforcing Inequities. *American Journal of Law & Medicine* 17(1–2): 15–50.

Lovell-Badge R (2019) CRISPR Babies: A View from the Centre of the Storm. *Development* 146(3). doi:10.1242/dev.175778.

Morrison M and de Saille S (2019) CRISPR in Context: Towards a Socially Responsible Debate on Embryo Editing. *Palgrave Communications* 5(1): 1–9. doi:10.1057/s41599-019-0319-5.

NHS (2017a) *IVF—Availability.* www.nhs.uk/conditions/ivf/availability/ (accessed April 15, 2020).

NHS (2017b) *IVF—Risks.* www.nhs.uk/conditions/ivf/risks/ (accessed January 15, 2020).

Nuffield Council on Bioethics (2018) *Genome Editing and Human Reproduction.* https://nuffieldbioethics.org/publications/genome-editing-and-human-reproduction (accessed January 15, 2020).

Ormond KE, Mortlock DP, Scholes DT, et al. (2017) Human Germline Genome Editing. *The American Journal of Human Genetics* 101(2): 167–176. doi:10.1016/j.ajhg.2017.06.012.

Regalado A (2019) He Jiankui Faces Three Years in Prison for CRISPR Babies. *MIT's Technology Review*, 30 December. www.technologyreview.com/2019/12/30/131061/he-jiankui-sentenced-to-three-years-in-prison-for-crispr-babies/ (accessed April 11, 2020).

Rose N (2006) *The Politics of Life Itself: Biomedicine, Power, and Subjectivity in the Twenty-First Century.* Princeton, NJ: Princeton University Press.

The Royal Society (2019) *New International Commission Launched on Clinical Use of Heritable Human Genome Editing.* https://royalsociety.org/news/2019/05/international-commission-on-heritable-human-genome-editing/ (accessed January 15, 2020).

Sarojini N, Marwah V and Shenoi A (2011) Globalisation of Birth Markets: A Case Study of Assisted Reproductive Technologies in India. *Globalization & Health* 7(1): 27. doi:10.1186/1744-8603-7-27.

Stock G (2002) *Redesigning Humans, Our Inevitable Genetic Future.* 1st Mariner Books Ed edition. Boston: Houghton Mifflin.

van Mil A, Hopkins H and Kinsella S (2017) Potential Uses for Genetic Technologies: Dialogue and Engagement Research Conducted on Behalf of the Royal Society Findings Report. 137.

Wipperman A and Campos M (2016) *Genome Editing Technologies: The Patient Perspective.* London: Genetic Alliance UK. www.geneticalliance.org.uk/media/2623/nerri_finalreport15112016.pdf. November..

World Health Organization (2019) *WHO Launches Global Registry on Human Genome Editing.* www.who.int/news-room/detail/29-08-2019-who-launches-global-registry-on-human-genome-editing (accessed January 15, 2020).

Yotova R (2017) *The Regulation of Genome Editing and Human Reproduction Under International Law, EU Law and Comparative Law.* Nuffield Council on Bioethics.

8

EVALUATING ECTOGENESIS VIA THE METAPHYSICS OF PREGNANCY

Suki Finn and Sasha Isaac

What Is Ectogenesis?

"Ectogenesis" derives from *ecto* meaning "outer," and *genesis* meaning "origin." A Google search defines it as "(chiefly in science fiction) the development of embryos in artificial conditions outside the uterus" (Anon n.d. in *Oxford Dictionaries* 2019). The term *ectogenesis* was coined in 1923 by a British scientist named J. B. S. Haldane in his 1923 essay entitled *Daedalus, or Science and the Future*. The concept was then utilized by Aldous Huxley, a friend of Haldane, in his 1932 novel *Brave New World*. Already by the 1980s, developments in science had started to bring such ideas to life. Between 1982 and 1983, in Bologna and New York City, the first attempts were made to perform fetal implantation outside of the human body (Bulletti et al. 1986). Since then, many other related experiments have taken place (see Klass 1996; Bryner et al. 2014). Most recently, in a *Nature* report from 2017, Alan Flake (from the Children's Hospital of Philadelphia) revealed the development of technology that gestated fetal lambs for 4 weeks inside something that looks akin to a plastic bag with tubes going through and coming out of it (Partridge et al. 2017).

It is notable that the term "ectogenesis" is not used in these scientific studies. Rather, the technology is often referred to as a "device" or a "system." We ask, then, what is meant by "ectogenesis" and how does our understanding of it relate to the fictional concept and to scientific reality?

A preliminary distinction to draw here is between *full* and *partial* ectogenesis: full ectogenesis sees the whole process of pregnancy occurring outside the uterus; partial ectogenesis sees only part of the process of pregnancy occurring outside the uterus. Researchers have yet to provide an example of full human ectogenesis, but there are familiar practices of partial ectogenesis: in-vitro fertilization (IVF) and the use of incubators, tubes, and wires for preterm babies, for instance. Yet the term "ectogenesis" was not intended to capture such technologies and so further work is required to uniquely define the process in question. The recent work of Kingma and Finn (2020) aims to assist in this endeavor.[1]

Kingma and Finn importantly distinguish between technology that preserves *neonatal* physiology outside of the uterus once the baby has been born, which they call "ectogenesis," and technology that preserves *fetal* physiology outside of the uterus where the fetus continues to gestate, which they call "ectogestation." Kingma and Finn show that the more common (and far less controversial) technologies such as IVF and incubation are ectogenetic, whereas the new technology from the 2017 *Nature* report is ectogestative. While the term "artificial wombs" is commonly used to describe ectogestative technologies, in reality such technologies more closely resemble artificial amniotic sacs and artificial placentas. This is because it is not simply the environment of the womb that is being replicated (as "artificial womb" would imply) but also the other organs involved in gestation such as the amniotic sac and the placenta.

In order to avoid the misleading language of "artificial wombs," we endorse the terminology of Kingma and Finn, and use it to challenge the "liberative" prospects of *full* ectogenesis. We shall set aside the question of ectogestation, referring to it only as a helpful contrast. We shall also set aside questions regarding partial ectogenesis, in line with the intuition that it is not such partial forms that attract controversy or promise women's liberation. Acknowledging that full ectogenetic technologies do not currently exist, however, it is helpful to try to picture full ectogenesis as the expansion of its partial forms (with IVF at the start and incubation at the end), where the processes meet in the middle to replicate a full pregnancy.[2] It is this, often idealized, full ectogenesis that we will problematize herein due to its relation to a potentially harmful cultural concept of pregnancy—the Fetal Container Model (see below).

We will begin our analysis by considering philosophical arguments in favor of full ectogenesis more closely, with regard to surveying its potential therapeutic benefits and the social benefits articulated by such feminists as Shulamith Firestone. These considerations are largely ethical and based on hypothetical reasoning, were full ectogenesis to become an available technology. We will then consider criticisms of this stance, providing reasons to doubt its efficacy for women's liberation. Such reasons will again derive from philosophical inquiry, by looking to counter-examples of the supposed benefits and providing

---

1 See also Cannold (1995:56) for an articulation of the partial/full ectogenetic distinction.
2 The current state of science is such that ectogenesis is only available to cover the very first and very last part of a pregnancy—or rather, more accurately, ectogenesis either pre-dates the pregnancy or follows the pregnancy, but cannot replace all pregnant stages. As Kingma and Finn (2020:362) write: "Partial ectogenesis presently exists at both ends of the gestational period: (early) embryos can spend time in a petri-dish in the first few days of development; neonates can spend months in an incubator at the other. It may, and frequently is, glibly assumed that it is only a matter of time before improvements at both ends 'meet in the middle'—so to speak."

intuition-based ethical evaluations. Next, we attempt to re-diagnose the problem of women's oppression: perhaps it is not biological difference that gives rise to such oppressive conditions, but rather the devaluation of pregnancy itself that makes reproduction seem an oppressive practice to some. We will argue for this on the basis of a conceptual analysis of pregnancy, which largely involves analyzing the language used to describe pregnancy and the concepts that underpin it. Our methodology requires the use of tools from the metaphysics of pregnancy, where we look to metaphysics as the abstract study of reality to elucidate the entities involved in a pregnancy and how they are related to one another. We advocate for a non-essentialist view of sex, gender, and sexism, by instead problematizing full ectogenesis through the use of two particular concepts—Containment and Parthood. We conclude that a change in the concepts surrounding pregnancy and gestation is needed to address the problem of women's oppression.

Our argument is two-fold: (1) drawing on metaphysical views of pregnancy and their connections to cultural models of pregnancy, we show that one current conception of pregnancy—the Fetal Container Model—may be harmful; (2) we show that the hypothetical technology understood as full ectogenesis potentially rests upon and perpetuates that harmful (and maybe impossible) conceptualization of pregnancy. We thus conclude that full ectogenesis should not be relied upon to help deliver women's liberation from the trials and tribulations of pregnancy (which we note would also involve "liberating" them from its wonders and joys as well).

The Potential Value of Ectogenesis

There are a multitude of women who want to become pregnant and enjoy giving birth, and who gain enormous self-actualization from doing so. Nevertheless, the process is not without its complications. We need not reiterate the significant side effects of preterm birth,[3] nor of the pregnancy and birthing process itself,[4] to appreciate the potential therapeutic value of full ectogenesis as an alternative or additional option to pregnancy. With the ability to transfer and/or develop fetuses using some sort of reproductive technology, care of preterm neonates and those vulnerable to risky pregnancies could be significantly improved. Any tension between preserving the health of the pregnant person and protecting the life of the fetus would thus be reduced, if not eliminated. Furthermore, those unable or unwilling to undergo pregnancy for any number of reasons, yet wish to have

---

3 Outcomes for babies born preterm depend on multiple factors including appropriate gestational growth at birth, gestational age, conditions surrounding the birth, the culture in which the birth takes place, the place of birth, and so on. Despite current interventions to aid preterm babies, they exist in what is known as the "gray zone" of viability, when survival is sometimes uncertain. See Seri and Evans (2008) for the risks of this gray zone.
4 See Smajdor (2007:340) for data on the risks of pregnancy and birth.

children, may also utilize the technology, adding significantly to its potential social value.

Again, some feminists have instead located the primary value of full ectogenesis in its potential to liberate women (see, for examples, Smajdor 2012; Kendal 2015; MacKay 2020; Cavaliere 2020). Most notably, Shulamith Firestone (1974) argued that the source of women's oppression results from what she described as an uneven distribution of reproductive labor. After declaring the processes of pregnancy and birth "barbaric" (p. 198), she concluded that full ectogenesis (although she did not call it by this name) was a necessary, though not sufficient, part of the solution. This particular argument in favor of full ectogenesis notes that an unfair division of reproductive labor exists, and that full ectogenesis could remedy the situation by eliminating this difference in reproductive ability, thereby removing the condition that had purportedly ensured women's oppression.[5]

However, we question the technology's ability to genuinely address the potential oppressiveness of reproduction. For instance, full ectogenesis could only ensure a fair redistribution of reproductive labor if reproductive work were limitable to the process of pregnancy. Yet, post-birth, it seems to (still) be women who are (largely) expected to feed the newborn, raise and nurture the child, and so on. But this argument is not intended as an exclusionary criterion to dismiss from the debate other people and groups who can and do partake in reproductive work. We do not align with naturalist arguments that problematize such technologies for deviating from "natural" reproductive processes, thereby excluding—whether intentionally or not—such marginalized groups as trans people, people who cannot or do not wish to reproduce, or those unable to conceive, to name only a few, from this important discussion.

Yet still, it remains unclear what full ectogenesis would do to address the social conditions that we believe give rise to the potential oppressiveness of reproduction in the first place. Given these conditions, should fetuses be gestated ectogenetically, it seems likely that women would still be considered responsible for being their primary caretakers.

This brings us to our primary objection against idealizing full ectogenesis as a feminist tool: the technology, rather than alleviating or mitigating the potential devaluation of reproductive work, perhaps instead would perpetuate it. It cannot be ignored that as a society we tend to outsource work we do not value. For example, just as cleaning, once delegated to the housemaid, has now become at least partially the responsibility of machines like the Roomba (the robot vacuum cleaner), so too might we find that full ectogenesis passes the burden of pregnancy down the ranks: from the intended mother to the surrogate mother

---

5 Of course, this requires more than just the elimination of pregnancy, but a complete restructuring of society and women's place within it. See Firestone (1974:10) for a description of this restructuring.

and eventually to technology. Krstić similarly distinguishes opposing feminist responses to ectogenesis based on their conceptual differences of pregnancy as such:

> The attitude of feminist authors…depends upon their interpretation of *ectogenesis* as an instrument of patriarchal oppression, or as a means of empowerment. This interpretation itself depends upon the evaluation of the female body and its specificity—the function of biological reproduction—as a source of strength or weakness in the context of individual or collective female achievement; and upon the evaluation of biological and social motherhood in that same context, as a coercion or a potential for agency. (Krstić 2015:50; italics in original)

Like Krstić, we aim to show how an evaluation of ectogenesis depends upon an evaluation of the metaphysics of pregnancy. We also argue that the problem of women's oppression has potentially been misdiagnosed by feminists like Firestone, leading to the false identification of full ectogenesis as an essential part of the solution. As the problematics of such accounts make clear, we argue that it is the possible devaluation of reproductive work, which can include not only gestation but also household tasks like doing children's laundry, etc., that potentially renders the process oppressive in the first place. Pregnancy, or, per Firestone, the sexual difference between males and females, is to us not necessarily the cause of women's oppression (recognizing that many conditions ultimately underpin this oppression). Rather, it is a certain cultural *concept* of pregnancy currently in circulation—but not necessarily held by all—that is doing much of the oppressive work. As such, a conceptual change away from that specific concept may be more promising in aiding the liberation of women from oppression, rather than this physical change. Pregnancy should not be devalued, and we problematize full ectogenesis because of its potential to devalue pregnancy on the grounds of a certain cultural concept that serves to oppress women.

The specific cultural concept of pregnancy to which we refer is known as the Fetal Container Model, and, as we will show here, the relative ease with which this model lends itself to the devaluation of reproductive work may potentially hinder the liberation effort. As we aim to demonstrate, full ectogenesis shares a problematic relationship with this model. The solution, then, is not to eradicate the process of pregnancy, but rather to change how we think of it. Though Firestone advocates eliminating sexism via challenging "its roots in the biological division of the sexes" (1974:12), we might now reconceive of those sex differences in a way that will not give rise to sexism. That is to say: *we need not eliminate sex difference to eliminate sexism*. And we need not idealize the prospect of full ectogenesis as a step towards eradicating sexism. As we will show in the remainder of this analysis, not only is it unnecessary to do so, but its conceptual entanglements with the Fetal Container Model may prove harmful to the social cause of women's liberation.

The Metaphysics of Pregnancy

Consider the following metaphysical question about pregnancy: Is the fetus a part of, or contained by, the gestator?[6]

Since certain assisted reproductive technologies (ARTs) are meant to emulate the role of gestator during pregnancy, the answer to this question will necessarily impact how we conceive of ectogenesis itself. Understanding the roles of gestating persons will therefore clarify the role their artificial replacement is intended to satisfy. We recognize that the metaphysics of pregnancy will not fully capture that role, as it considers only the mereological (the relation of part to whole) and topological (the connections between entities) relationships between fetus and gestator. This is not necessarily a problem for our account, though, for what we intend to show is that even in a limited, incomplete account of the role of gestating, full ectogenesis—which would obviously rapidly intensify our current process of birthing techno-sapiens—likely distorts or fails to fulfill such a role. There is, of course, much more to understanding pregnancy than the mereology and topology of the entities involved, as women and mothers are not simply their physiologies. In this chapter, we place a narrow focus on the metaphysical mereo-topological relationship between gestator and fetus, yet we recognize the need for a cognitive, emotional, cultural, and perhaps even spiritual account that is sensitive to the biopsychosocial multiplicity and complexity of pregnancy to get a fuller picture.

We will now consider two perspectives of the metaphysical relationship between fetus and gestator, naming them the Parthood view and the Containment view, which underwrite the cultural models of pregnancy named the Parthood Model and the Fetal Container Model.

Parthood: The idea that the fetus is a part of the gestator is held by Kingma (2019:162), who clarifies this position by stating that "one can start by treating talk of [fetuses] being parts of [gestators] as parallel to talk of, say, kidneys being parts of dogs." So, the gestator is the whole, and this gestator may have many parts like limbs and organs, where the fetus is one of (albeit a potentially very special one of) those parts, linked to and interdependent with its gestator. It is important to note that this view does not specify what sort of thing the fetus is; it only states how it is mereologically related to the gestator—namely, as a part of a larger whole. This metaphysical and holistic understanding of the fetal-gestator relationship provides a conceptual basis for the cultural Parthood Model, which we see manifest in our society when we use language about the pregnant "bump" (which is seen as a part of the gestator's body), and slogans like "my body, my choice." All birth activists hold this Parthood view, often using

---

6 This is the language used and the way the debate is set up by Kingma (2019). We follow the terminology of "gestator" or "pregnant person" and "fetus" (as opposed to mother and baby) in order to avoid gendered and social connotations and to stay neutral on whether the fetus meets certain metaphysical and scientific conditions on being regarded as a baby.

the term "MotherBaby" to index the oneness of the mother with the child in her womb (see for example Lalonde et al. 2019).

Containment: In this view, the gestator surrounds and contains the fetus inside of their body. Unlike in the Parthood view, the fetus and gestator are mereologically separate entities. Smith and Brogaard (2003:74) provide the analogy of the fetus being inside the gestator in the same way as "a tub of yogurt is inside your refrigerator." Again, this view does not state what sort of thing the fetus is; it only says that the fetus is inside the gestator without also being a part of them. This metaphysical understanding of the fetal-gestator relationship provides a conceptual basis for the Fetal Container Model, whereby gestators are depicted as "containing" the fetus that they gestate inside their cavity-like wombs.

Kingma argues that the Fetal Container Model is the dominant way in which we conceive of pregnancy in Western culture. The frequency with which we hear of "buns in the oven" provides some support for this claim, but also telling are the efforts to depict: (1) the physical continuity between the fetus and the subsequent baby (using imagery of fetuses as practically fully formed babies rather than what is more appropriate for their gestational stage of development); and (2) the physical *dis*continuity between fetus and gestator (using imagery of the fetus as freely floating inside a bubble-like womb rather than the complex intertwinement within the gestator's body).

There are many harms that appear to be caused or perpetuated by this model. For example: how it may devalue gestation (so long as the gestative work is being done, any container will do); and, per Smith and Brogaard's yogurt-fridge analogy, which portrays pregnancy as a case of *mere* containment (as the contents of a fridge are not considered *part* of it), the dehumanizing effects of being likened to (and treated as) something fungible—exchangeable or replaceable, like a container (or appliance!). Baron captures the concern in her article on surrogacy:

> This Foetal Container model is used in conjunction with social ideals of motherhood to pressure expectant mothers to monitor and modify their behavior and lifestyles, and to emphasise women's responsibility for foetal outcomes; it is used in conjunction with the language of the market to encourage women to view themselves as tools for the development of someone else's child. Different moral frameworks and concepts use the foetal container model to justify different outcomes in these contexts: to nurture the foetus but not mourn miscarriage, or to nurture the foetus but not mourn giving up the child; to claim that the rights of the foetus outweigh the rights of the gestating woman, or to claim that the rights of the commissioning parents outweigh the rights of the gestating woman. The foetal container model of pregnancy does not necessarily entail women's diminished subjectivity; however, in the patriarchal context in which this model has developed, it can pave the way for the reduction of pregnant women to mere containers. (Baron 2018:12)

Note that Baron is suggesting that the metaphysical Containment view is morally neutral and tarnished only by its harmful usage as the Fetal Container Model in a patriarchal context. So, as Baron describes, while the metaphysical Container view may itself be morally neutral, its cultural manifestation as the Fetal Container Model has evidently developed and been used in a patriarchal context with significant harm. In this way, the Fetal Container Model seems to lend itself more to the devaluation of gestation by minimizing the role of the gestator than does the Parthood Model, which places the gestator at the center of the pregnancy process. This does not prove that the Fetal Container Model is *necessarily* morally dubious, but only contingently and instrumentally so.

Some may remain unconvinced by the relationship between the metaphysics and the ethics sketched out thus far. In this case, it is worth pointing out that further to its moral dubiousness, the Containment view looks to be *factually* dubious as well. By conceiving of gestators as containers for fetuses, the Containment view portrays pregnancy as involving two mereologically unrelated entities. But with reference to the connections between fetus and gestator, Kingma (2019:628) reminds us of the biological realities of pregnancy: the umbilical cord, which connects the fetus to the placenta, which itself grows into the uterine wall, connecting the fetus to the gestator; the fetus and the gestator sharing one external boundary, challenging the claim that the two are somehow separate; and, reinforcing this, the lack of any separating cavity between the fetus and the gestator (as would be expected were we dealing with two entities that were not a part of the other).

But while we have aimed to problematize a Containment view of pregnancy, we have yet to demonstrate why this should lead full ectogenesis to a similar fate. In the next section, we will argue that full ectogenesis likely cannot be conceived of without depending on a Fetal Container Model, and because of this inextricability, we ought to be suspicious of any notions about its potential to help liberate women. Furthermore, if the relationship between fetus and gestator involves more than containment, then one might think that the technologies that replicate it should do so too, or else they might give a false (and potentially harmful) picture of what pregnancy involves.

Re-Evaluating Ectogenesis

How does full ectogenesis rely on and perpetuate a Fetal Container Model? Most obviously, the very term "ectogenesis" seems to at least imply it: ecto-genesis literally means originating *outside*, where the contrast would be originating *inside* the body. This inner-outer dichotomy is reminiscent of the language of birth according to the Fetal Container Model being a "mere change of environment" (Smith and Brogaard 2003:65) from inside to outside the gestator's container-like body. Smith and Brogaard (ibid.) go on to state, "birth is the mere passage of an entity from one environment to another (it is analogous to an astronaut leaving her spaceship)." As such, being inside or outside the spaceship/womb implies a topological (containment), and not a mereological (parthood), relationship between the fetus and gestator.

However, were we to adopt the Parthood view, then the prospect of disrupting the part-whole relationship between fetus and gestator (or replicating their interconnectedness) using ectogenetic technology seems far less plausible or desirable. The technology described earlier in this chapter as ecto*gestation* works better in replicating that interconnectedness, whereas ecto*genesis* works better to replicate containment. How pregnancy is perceived plausibly limits what technologies are desirable to pursue. Likewise, the very idea that technology could replace some or all stages of pregnancy depends on our concept of pregnancy. This point is similarly made by Aristarkhova (2005:51):

> Mechanization of the maternal body in philosophy and the life sciences has both derived from and served the devaluation of its participation in genesis and the birth process, as well as the disconnection of the fetus from the uterus. Ectogenesis is a workable concept only if one assumes that the embryo and the mother are two separate and therefore separable entities.

The presupposition of the Fetal Container Model can also be seen in the following quote from Gosden, writing on the wonder of ectogenesis:

> Nothing is more awesome than the emergence in these early weeks of a recognizable human form from a tiny, undifferentiated mass. Such unique events might be expected to need a special environment, but the uterus is just a clever incubator. (Gosden 2000:183–184)

If the uterus is "just a clever incubator," then containment-like technologies such as ectogenesis can succeed in fulfilling their designated roles—liberating women from pregnancy and birth and aiding in our current transformations into technosapiens. And if, as has been observed, there is a strong tendency to conceive of (and treat) gestators as containers or incubators for fetuses, then viewing ARTs in the same way requires no leap of the imagination. Ectogenetic technologies (like incubators) align more closely with the Fetal Container Model, deploying its key tenets to sustain its plausibility.

Were we to accept that the only necessary part of pregnancy is the uterus, where it represents the "clever incubator" and where incubation is ectogenetic technology, full ectogenesis may become a desirable technology. Yet the first premise is simply untrue—the uterus is *not* the only necessary part of pregnancy. Nevertheless, it would be too quick to conclude that ectogenesis therefore necessarily entails or endorses the Fetal Container Model, as ectogenesis might simply be viewed as an alternative to pregnancy, an option that likely only the privileged could choose. Yet it still follows that any technology employing and perpetuating key tenets of an evidently problematic model may unwittingly lead to normalizing and perhaps perpetuating these very same problems (e.g., the devaluation of gestative work and a dismissal of the relationship between fetus and gestator).

On the other hand, the very possibility of full ectogenesis may be taken as evidence that perhaps there *never* existed a parthood relationship between a fetus and its gestator; that it may be precisely *because* there is no parthood relationship in general between fetus and gestator that ARTs like the partial ectogenesis of IVF and incubation "work." Thus, we could move in the direction of learning *about* pregnancy *from* the technology that we create to replicate it.

By the same line of reasoning, however, it might be argued that the very reason full ectogenesis is not currently a reality is *because* pregnancy involves more than containment. It might be that full ectogenesis remains inconceivable because the notion of a mere-containment-like pregnancy is simply inconceivable to us now.

But methodological problems loom. It must be clarified whether the reality of such technologies is evidence for the truth of a metaphysical model of pregnancy, or whether the relationship between fetus and gestator differs depending on the ART (or lack thereof) in play. In other words, it remains to be seen whether ARTs *distort* the relationship between fetus and gestator, or rather whether these technologies *illuminate* what the relationship is like, regardless of such technological factors.

If we proceed with the assumption that there is no parthood relationship between the fetus and the technology that supports it—for example, there being no parthood relationship between fetus and ectogenetic container—then we must select between two options: (1) Would full ectogenesis destroy a parthood relationship that is otherwise present between fetus and gestator? Or (2) would full ectogenesis show us that there was never any parthood relationship between fetus and gestator? In other words, does the environment alter the metaphysical relationship between fetus and whatever/whomever is gestating? And if it does, then we must ask whether it is a welcomed alteration. In this chapter, we hope to have given some preliminary analysis regarding why this might not be the case.

Concluding that ectogenesis may share some relationship with a problematic model of pregnancy does not amount to calling the technology itself *necessarily* problematic, nor for a moratorium or pre-emptive ban on the research and development of any associated technologies. However, when a technology is either founded on or potentially perpetuates a certain representation of women, and when that representation has been used elsewhere to denigrate and mistreat women, good practice dictates that we question the extent to which its ability to alleviate a biological constraint is truly serving the feminist cause overall—especially if it is unable to address the harmful attitudes that make this constraint oppressive in the first place.

Furthermore, it remains unclear whether ethical evaluations of full ectogenesis generally carry over to partial ectogenesis (like IVF and incubation) and vice versa. If partial ectogenesis is to be acceptable when full ectogenesis is not, then some account is necessary to articulate why the reasons for rejecting full ectogenesis do not apply to its partial forms. This may be done by determining just how "partial" ectogenesis must be for it to be deemed acceptable. Or, for those who wish to hold on to the intuition that partial ectogenesis in the forms of IVF and incubation is unproblematic, but full ectogenesis *is* problematic, our approach offers another method for doing so.

Recognizing that pregnancy involves more than containment (and, of course, more than a metaphysical relationship), we might challenge the potential of reproductive technologies designed only to contain rather than to gestate. Note that there is a distinction between containment and *mere* containment that ought to be respected—without any parthood relationship between fetus and gestator, we see pregnancy described as *mere* containment, whereas for as long as there is *some* parthood relationship present, we see pregnancy as *involving* containment without being *defined* by containment. Our criticism of full ectogenesis relates to its reliance on and potential perpetuation of a fetal containment view of pregnancy *as a whole*—a reductionism that partial ectogenesis does not fall foul to in virtue of it being partial. If there is more to gestation than incubation, then the process requires more than ectogenesis to replicate it, and we should shift our conceptions of pregnancy accordingly.

Conclusion: A Conceptual Overhaul

We have argued that we ought to doubt the potential of full ectogenesis as a tool for women's liberation for the very reason that the technology might undermine progress towards such a result. To arrive at this conclusion, we began by considering the arguments in favor of ectogenesis, both from the therapeutic perspective and from a social perspective. Recall that feminists such as Firestone argued that the source of women's oppression stemmed from the biological difference in reproductive ability between the sexes. Full ectogenesis, as an attempt at neutralizing the process of reproduction, was subsequently identified as part of the solution to this problem. We, and others, have revealed the limitations in such an approach to the liberation effort, including the fact that it is not clear that ectogenesis is capable of gender-neutralizing the reproductive process, nor that biological difference really is the source of women's oppression.

Addressing this last point, we have attempted to re-diagnose the problem of women's oppression by suggesting that it is in fact the potential cultural devaluation of pregnancy that can render reproduction an oppressive process. Here we utilized tools and views from the metaphysics of pregnancy. In considering the metaphysical relationship between the fetus and gestator, we can see how and why it might be that full ectogenesis becomes problematic for feminism. As a technology conceptually entangled with the problematic Fetal Container Model of pregnancy, we conclude that full ectogenesis remains inherently limited in securing women's liberation. We further argue that pregnancy or sexual difference is not the cause of oppression; rather, it is our potential concept of pregnancy that can cause oppression. Perhaps, then, it is a *conceptual* overhaul that we require—specifically, the overhaul of the Fetal Containment Model, which is the cultural concept that lends itself to the devaluation of pregnancy—prior to a technological one.

Acknowledgments

Special thanks to Jordan MacKenzie and members of the Bioethics Center at New York University, and to Elselijn Kingma and members of the "Better Understanding the Metaphysics of Pregnancy" project at the University of Southampton, for their very helpful comments on earlier drafts of this paper. Also many thanks to the audience of the Reproductive Ethics Conference in association with Albany Medical College where we presented ideas from this chapter. This chapter was completed during a project that received funding from the European Research Council (ERC) under the European Union's Horizon 2020 research and innovation program, under grant agreement #679586.

References

Anon. (n.d.) Ectogenesis. In: *Oxford Dictionaries*. Retrieved in January 2019 from: https://en.oxforddictionaries.com/definition/ectogenesis.

Aristarkhova, I. (2005) Ectogenesis and Mother as Machine. *Body and Society* 11(3):43–59.

Baron, T. (2018) Nobody Puts Baby in the Container: The Foetal Container Model at Work in Medicine and Commercial Surrogacy. *Journal of Applied Philosophy* 36(3):491–505. https://doi.org/10.1111/japp.12336.

Bryner, B., Gray, B., Perkins, E., Davis, R., Hoffman, H., Barks, J., Owens, G., Bocks, M., Rojas-Peña, A., Hirschl, R., Bartlett, R., Mychaliska, G. (2014) An Extracorporeal Artificial Placenta Supports Extremely Premature Lambs for 1 Week. *Journal of Pediatric Surgery* 50(1):44–49.

Bulletti, C., Jasonni, V.M., Lubicz, S., Flamigni, C., Gurpide, E. (1986) Extracorporeal Perfusion of the Human Uterus. *American Journal of Obstetrics and Gynecology* 154(3):683–688.

Cannold, L. (1995) Women, Ectogenesis and Ethical Theory. *Journal of Applied Philosophy* 12(1):55–64.

Cavaliere, G. (2020) Gestation, Equality and Freedom: Ectogenesis as a Political Perspective. *Journal of Medical Ethics* 46(2):76–82.

Firestone, S. (1974) *The Dialectic of Sex*. London: Verso.

Gosden, R. (2000) *Designing Babies: The Brave New World of Reproductive Technology*. New York: Freeman and Co.

Kendal, E. (2015) *Equal Opportunity and the Case for State Sponsored Ectogenesis*. London: Palgrave Pivot.

Kingma, E. (2019) Were You a Part of Your Mother? The Metaphysics of Pregnancy. *Mind* 128(511):609–646.

Kingma, E., Finn, S. (2020) Neonatal Incubator or Artificial Womb? Distinguishing Ectogestation and Ectogenesis Using the Metaphysics of Pregnancy. *Bioethics* 34(4):354–363. https://doi.org/10.1111/bioe.12717.

Klass, P. (1996) The Artificial Womb Is Born. *The New York Times Magazine*. Retrieved in March 2019 from: www.nytimes.com/1996/09/29/magazine/the-artificial-womb -is-born.html.

Krstić, I. (2015) Extracorporeal Pregnancy as a Feminist Issue. *Journal of Art and Media Studies* 8:45–50. https://fmkjournals.fmk.edu.rs/index.php/AM/article/download /104/pdf.

Lalonde, A., Herschderfer, K., Pascali-Bonaro, D., Hanson, C., Fuchtner, C., Visser, G.H.A. (2019) The International Childbirth Initiative: 12 Steps to Safe and Respectful Motherbaby–Family Maternity Care. *International Journal of Gynecology and Obstetrics* 146(1):65–73.

MacKay, K. (2020) The "Tyranny of Reproduction": Could Ectogenesis Further Women's Liberation? *Bioethics* 34(4):346–353.

Partridge, E., Davey, M., Hornick, M. et al. (2017) An Extra-Uterine System to Physiologically Support the Extreme Premature Lamb. *Nature Communications* 8:15112.

Seri, I., Evans, J. (2008) Limits of Viability: Definition of the Gray Zone. *Journal of Perinatology: Official Journal of the California Perinatal Association* 28(1):4–8.

Smajdor, A. (2007) The Moral Imperative for Ectogenesis. *Cambridge Quarterly of Healthcare Ethics: CQ: The International Journal of Healthcare Ethics Committees* 16(03):336–345.

Smajdor, A. (2012) In Defense of Ectogenesis. *Cambridge Quarterly of Healthcare Ethics: CQ: The International Journal of Healthcare Ethics Committees* 21(1):90–103.

Smith, B., Brogaard, B. (2003) 16 Days: The Ontology of Fetal Development. *Journal of Medicine and Philosophy* 28:45–78.

9

ELECTIVE CESAREAN BIRTHS IN THE US AND THE GLOBAL CESAREAN EPIDEMIC:

Causes, Solutions, and Futuristic Implications

Emaline Reyes

Introduction: Understanding Cesareans

> *Humans have just gone off the deep end, making things "unnatural" as much as they can—for convenience sake amongst other things.* (Respondent #3)

> *If everyone got c-sections, what would happen to humans?* (Respondent #4)

Global rates of cesarean births (CBs) have increased dramatically over past decades. Cesareans have become normalized in affluent and industrialized nations as well as in a number of low-to-middle-resource countries, especially in private hospitals. "Medical" reasons why CBs are presumed to have increased include: improved accessibility to the procedure; improved safety and efficiency; widespread use of continuous electronic fetal monitoring, which shows every fetal heart rate deceleration (most of which are normal), often leading to unnecessary "emergency" CBs (Alfiveric et al. 2017); increased medical need due to declining population health and increased chronic health issues; higher average age of first-time mothers and associated "risks" (e.g., diabetes), previous infertility and use of assisted reproductive technology (which can result in multiparity and preterm delivery); and management of "high risk" pregnancies resulting from disease or chronic health conditions (Lee and Kirkman 2008). They may also be performed in the absence of medical necessity because they are preferable to patients and/or practitioners. Reasons why physicians may prefer CB have been found to be: scheduling convenience (Fischetti and Armstrong 2017); financial incentives (Potter et al. 2001); insurance coverage (Stafford 1990); and legal protection (Donohoe 1996). The literature on non-medically-indicated cesareans shows that doctors may use their authority and power to convince women to plan a CB in advance when that benefits the obstetrician (see Potter et al. 2001).

Practitioner preference and patient preference may overlap. Reasons why women may prefer CB include: perceived superiority and health benefits of the procedure; planning and convenience; and influence of peers (Penna and Arulkumaran 2003). Some women (13%) planning or in the early stages of pregnancy prefer CBs and plan them in advance, largely due to fear of childbirth (Reyes and Rosenberg 2018, 2019). Fear is one of the primary motivators for women who elect CB (Fisher et al. 2006; Serçekuş et al. 2009; Hildingsson 2014; Stoll et al. 2014; Rondung et al. 2016). Women in many countries live in a culture of fearmongering that instills insecurities concerning their physical capabilities and judgment as well as their future birth experiences. The lack of information surrounding birth, or *misinformation*, can create uncertainty and fear. The sources of information that are dominant in our societies—TV, movies, social media—often depict birth (more specifically, vaginal delivery) as frightening, dangerous, traumatic, or even deadly (Morris and McInerney 2010). These sources glorify medicalization and depict surgical interventions as clean, calm, efficient, superior, and advanced (Kitzinger and Kitzinger 2001). The fear-provoking birth narratives that are perpetuated, coupled with the Western notion that biomedicine is far superior to any other form of healing, could contribute to women's preference for CB, or willingness to acquiesce to surgical delivery when recommended by a doctor in the absence of clear medical necessity. This is concerning as, though cesareans can be lifesaving, and more are needed in many countries (Gibbons et al. 2010), they carry more risks than vaginal delivery, decrease beneficial health outcomes, and jeopardize lives when used inappropriately and/or in excess.

Countries with exceedingly high CB rates have seen an increase in mortality and morbidity, for example in Brazil (Williamson and Matsuoka 2019). In Greece, which has an extremely high CB rate of 65%–70%, while mortality rates remain stable, morbidity rates have increased, and maternal mental health has suffered (Georges and Daellenbach 2019). Other countries with high rates of CB include: Turkey (53%; Santas and Santas 2018), China (80% to 100% in private hospitals; Cheung and Pan 2021), many Latin American countries (35% overall; Betran et al. 2009), and the US (32%; Martin et al. 2017). Global policy changes could improve maternal-infant health outcomes—as seen in the countries with CB rates that fall not so far from the WHO recommendation of CB rates no higher than 15% (Gibbons et al. 2010), or 19% on the upper end (Molina et al. 2015; see below).

Hypothesis and Objectives

The surrounding birth environment can impact and influence women's pregnancy and birth experiences (Reyes and Rosenberg 2019). But how is this sociocultural, rather than physical, environment established? In this chapter I argue that social pressures and media depictions intimately shape how women see birth and their own bodies. This fear can serve to further increase CBs, in particular those that are maternally elected. In addition to understanding why women elect CB and what informs their decisions, this chapter explores what could happen to the future of birth if CB becomes the default mode of birth and how we can prevent this from happening.

Methodology

Between September 2017 and February 2018, 368 US women between the ages of 18–30 who had never given birth before but planned to do so in the near future (5–10 years) responded to a quantitative Qualtrics survey that I conducted. Participants could be in the early stages of pregnancy, so long as they had not yet spoken to a doctor about their birth plans and options. I also completed an in-depth literature review, and conducted 6 in-person interviews. I recruited participants via text, email, and social media platforms such as Facebook and Instagram. Recruitment emails were sent to universities throughout the US and were encouraged to be shared widely. My study was approved by the University of Delaware Institutional Review Board.

Results: Reasons for Elective CB in the US

While a majority of women preferred vaginal delivery (86.9%), some preferred CB (13.1%) (Reyes and Rosenberg 2018, 2019). Women who preferred CB reported more fear than those who preferred vaginal delivery (ibid.). The preferred CB group received more of their information on birth from TV/movies (14.6% compared to 7.9%) and less of their information from books/articles (9.8% compared to 20.3%). They were also slightly more likely to have received their information from someone who had never given birth before (2.4% compared to 1.4%) and to report that they had never seen a birth in any form before (10.7% compared to 6.9%). The most common rationale for preferring and planning CB was that it was considered to be "less painful or risky" than vaginal delivery (41.9%).

Women who prefer cesareans often depend on medical management and trust in authority figures such as doctors, rather than in the self and the body. The media, and society in general, do not encourage confidence in women and their own physiologic capabilities.

The 6 women who agreed to be interviewed discussed the media as a source of information on pregnancy and birth, the presence of frightening birth narratives in the media, and the ways in which their imagined "typical" vaginal delivery and CB experiences differed as a result of these depictions. While vaginal birth was described as "painful" and "messy," cesarean birth was described as "calm" and "sterile." The "screaming lady" as often depicted in the media was a common theme. *All* respondents, even those wanting vaginal delivery, preferred the hospital as their birth location and doctors as their attendants (Reyes and Rosenberg 2018), potentially reflecting the abundance of media depictions of doctor-attended hospital births and sparse depictions of midwife-attended births. All interview participants noted the efficiency and convenience of CB, emphasizing the lifesaving (and "miraculous") nature of the surgery. Two of my interlocutors argued that CB was safest/safer than vaginal delivery, reflecting the survey results that 9.9% of women who preferred vaginal delivery thought it to be "safe for neither" mother nor infant. This perception could also result from media depictions, as well as US culture's glorification of medicalization (see Davis-Floyd 2003). In discussing media portrayals of vaginal delivery, Respondent #6 explicitly stated that the media make birth look like a fearful process in its depictions:

> I probably have a little fear and anxiety...because of, I want to say, the media. But like you see TV shows and they're in such pain and everything and it's this whole big—I'm thinking of the show "Friends" right now... It's like this whole big thing centered around it. Not that it's not a big deal, but I think that the media has kind of like amped it up a lot and that's kind of fearful to me because of that. Like you get a baby but there's all of this that comes with it.

Another source of media-derived information that provoked fear was the "horror story." Interview participants discussed the real life (rather than fictional) birth stories that were sensationalized by the news media. These stories, passed on from person to person, differed from the narratives relayed by female family members who had given birth themselves. These "horror stories" were almost folktales, or *cautionary* tales. They served as cultural rather than personal narratives, perpetuating the myth that birth is always traumatizing and potentially deadly, whereas stories from those who had given birth characterized birth as difficult and painful, but not as a "horror." Respondent #5 discussed the impact of stories and storytelling (from both friends and family):

> I have some fear and anxiety, just because hearing about women's experiences with childbirth. It doesn't sound like the most "pleasant" affair. Also, the stories you hear about women dying from childbirth or complications and things like that. Sounds horrible. So, I guess it's just like the pain and complications too.

Though Respondent #5 did not know anyone personally who had died, hearing these stories secondhand impacted her. Respondent #6 also described the stories she often heard (excluding the story of her own delivery that her mother told her) as "horror stories":

> A little anecdote—my hairdresser had a baby two years ago and before she gave birth (it was her first kid) she was talking about how she was really nervous and stuff. But then she thought about it (kind of what I told you) like "oh women have been doing this a long time," and then she thought,

"you know I have a few friends who really didn't think they could handle it but then they did." So, it's kind of like that actually made me feel a little bit better about it. And then I guess on the other end, why it (the fear) is medium, would just be because you've been told horror stories about how it hurts so badly and all this stuff.

While the personal anecdotes from those who had experienced birth served to comfort the interlocutors, the "horror stories" of the dangers of birth instilled fear in them. Those who prefer CB rely more heavily on these stories. Both fictitious media depictions of treacherous deliveries and anomalous news stories of the most risk-filled births intimately shaped how women thought of *all births*. Similar studies confirm the finding that media depictions of dramatic births serve to cultivate the culture of fear surrounding birth in our society (Leachman 2017), impacting women's birth preferences and planning (Morris and McInerney 2010).

Discussion: The Impacts of Cesarean Birth

Studies clearly show that fear is a primary motivator for elective CB (Fisher et al. 2006; Serçekuş et al. 2009; Hildingsson 2014; Stoll et al. 2014; Rondung et al. 2016; Reyes and Rosenberg 2018, 2019). Physicians' fear of birth may contribute to their own preference for performing CB (Gamble et al. 2007; Weaver et al. 2007). Patient fear may even lead to emergency CB as well (Ryding et al. 1998; Laursen et al. 2008). In this way, fear contributes to the increase of *all* CB, from elective to emergency. But why does it matter if CB rates rise?

Immediate Risks of Cesarean Births and Poor Long-Term Health Outcomes

Cesarean section is a major surgery, and as such should only be used when absolutely necessary. Delivering by cesarean can jeopardize the health and wellbeing of a mother and her child, both in regards to short-term risks and long-term health outcomes. According to Collard et al. (2008), for mothers, CB (both emergency and elective) can lead to: increased morbidity and mortality, infection and pain, poor birth experience, delayed infant contact and bonding, longer hospital stay and recovery, and future complications in subsequent births. Many of these factors can lead to poor maternal mental health outcomes and jeopardized psychosocial wellbeing (Lobel and Deluca 2007). For infants, CB can result in increased morbidity, specifically: respiratory problems, accidental surgery cuts and injuries, and difficulty initiating breastfeeding and bonding (Collard et al. 2008).

Intergenerational and Epigenetic Effects

These factors can also shape child development. Emerging evidence demonstrates the epigenetic impacts of surgical delivery, signaling potential intergenerational consequences (Dominguez-Bello et al. 2010; Cho and Norman 2013). CB results in minimal microbial contact with the birth canal (especially when procedures are pre-planned and labor is not attempted), which is needed to build a strong immune system in infants to protect against disease and allergies (Dominguez-Bello et al. 2010). A weakened immune system and compromised microbiome could lead to increased risk of digestive issues, allergies, asthma, chronic diseases, and autoimmune disorders; many of these conditions as well as the microbiome itself can be inherited (Dominguez-Bellow et al. 2010). Does a future of high CB rates mean a future of altered microbiomes, immunological struggles, and chronic health issues for children? In addition to these physiological implications, there are psychological implications, as CB can alter behavioral response and immunological gene expression due to an adverse birth stress response in delivery (Cho and Norman 2013).

Futuristic Implications of Normalizing Cesareans

In addition to negative physiologic and psychological impacts, normalizing CB also alters our society's attitudes towards reproduction, birth, and women's bodies (Wendland 2007). We need to consider if birth as a ritual, ceremony, tradition, cultural experience, and rite of passage (Davis-Floyd 2003) will be altered if CB becomes the default mode of birth for all; and we will need to learn more about how to help women form attachments with their infants following birth, initiate and encourage breastfeeding, remember their birth experiences with satisfaction, and feel confident in their own bodies. How will we as a society *and* as individuals change? How will we change biologically *and* culturally?

In regards to human biology and evolution, Mitteroecker et al. (2017) hypothesize that the potential for CB may be genetically inherited and that daughters who are delivered surgically may end up delivering surgically themselves, thus further increasing CB rates over time. In considering human emotions and affection, Odent (2004) speculates that over-performing CB will lead to a society of people who have difficulty connecting with others, bonding, and forming meaningful relationships. While I am skeptical of both claims, they are thought-provoking. My primary concerns lie in how society and culture will be changed. The medicalization of birth has led to the supremacy of white, masculine knowledge and has displaced the knowledge of BIPOC (Black, Indigenous, and People of Color) communities (Fraser 1995; Davis-Floyd and Sargent 1997; Davis 2019). If CB becomes the default, we could lose all non-medical traditions and cultural knowledge surrounding birth. Midwives, both traditional and professional, may cease to exist, and childbirth education will be rendered obsolete, as childbearers will simply plan their cesareans. Obstetricians will be trained to solely perform surgical deliveries, as they currently are for breech deliveries in many countries (Daviss and Bisits 2021). Breastfeeding and mother-baby bonding will become more of a challenge, unless immediately facilitated. We must imagine what a future dominated by cesarean birth will look like, as it is possible that such a future may come to pass. And while most of this is now just speculation, we can look to the countries with the highest CB rates to see how they have already been impacted.

Cesareans in Global Perspective

Countries with High CB Rates

For years Brazil was considered to be the "cesarean capital of the world." In 2012, Brazil had a 52% overall CB rate, resulting from the 45% CB rate in the public sphere and the 88% CB rate in the private sphere (Leal et al. 2012), compared to the WHO target CB rate of 10–15% (Gibbons et al. 2010) or the slightly higher recommendation of 19%, on the upper end (Molina et al. 2015). While many countries have similar rates to Brazil, and some have even surpassed it, studying the Brazilian healthcare system remains essential to understanding medicalization in birth and CB culture. In Brazil, a majority of CBs have not been as "elective" (on the part of the patients) as they seemed (Potter et al. 2001; Williamson and Matsuoka 2019). *Practitioner preference* has been a much more prevalent driving force of surgical deliveries, and those women who elected CB in the absence of medical necessity did so due to practitioner "recommendation," or rather, coercion (ibid.). Insecurity and fear surrounding the birth process and/ or fear of poor treatment from obstetricians, most common amongst women of the lower classes and of Afro-Brazilian ancestry, contribute to women's willingness to elect or agree to CB (ibid.). Cesareans are associated with the upper class, and therefore with "superior" treatment and care; furthermore, Black and Indigenous women in Brazil are more afraid of the medical interventions and abuses that characterize medicalized vaginal delivery than of CB itself (ibid.). For many Brazilian women, this has led to low levels of satisfaction with their birth experiences and perinatal care, as well as poor maternal and infant mortality and morbidity. The assumption that medicalization and intervention should automatically improve outcomes is not validated here. Rather, we see abusive interventions and unnecessary surgeries jeopardizing psychological and physical health (Sadler et al. 2016). In Brazil, these issues exist within the larger cultural context of racism, classism, and misogyny.

In recent years, the "true" "cesarean capital of the world" could be considered Greece (Georges and Daellenbach 2019). The vast majority of women there are delivering via cesarean, and almost all deliveries in the private sector are surgical. In the public sector, CB rates are 60%–70%. The private sector rate is unknown, but it is, reasonably, believed to be even higher (Georges and Daellenbach 2019). In Greece, even vaginal delivery could still be considered "operative delivery" as it is characterized by episiotomies and forceps or vacuum extraction (ibid.). Nevertheless, many women in Greece begin their pregnancies preferring and planning vaginal delivery or "natural birth" (ibid.). Yet "normal," physiologic delivery is near impossible to achieve in the "Alpha" and "Beta" wards for wealthier childbearers where obstetricians are the primary attendants, but not in the "Gamma" wards for the poor, where midwives prevail (ibid.).

General Recommendations for Reducing CB Rates and Improving the CB Experience

Changing Cesarean Birth Practices

Odent (2004) provides recommendations for when and how to perform cesareans so that they are not "overused" or "misused" and to maximize health outcomes of women and children. As Odent describes, emergency CB can be extremely dangerous and traumatic. Elective or pre-planned cesareans are also problematic, in that they lead to an increase in preterm births (as due dates are often wrong and elective CB is often scheduled too early in the fetus's development) and the infant is denied the benefits of hormonally initiating and undergoing the first stage of labor (Odent 2004). Yet after an infant is born by cesarean, practitioners can take steps to maximize health outcomes: exposing the newborn to the vaginal microbiome, thereby supporting the baby to internalize diverse gut bacteria and thus to develop a strong immune system, allowing and supporting immediate skin-to-skin contact with the mother after her cesarean birth, and encouraging breastfeeding initiation (Rosenberg and Trevathan 2018). Using these recommendations, obstetricians can more responsibly perform CB for those who need it and can decrease risks during the delivery itself, as well as improve postpartum care and long-term health outcomes.

Adjusting Environment and Discourse

In addition to changing medical practices, we need to re-evaluate the socio-cultural birth environment. How birth is discussed and what information is presented leaves a lasting impact on viewers and consumers of media. As the media is a major influence for contemporary women, changing the tone and focus of these platforms can help to properly inform women and to provide comfort rather than create (or exacerbate) fear. Luce et al. (2017) recommend that midwives engage with the media as the medical community does so that they can educate women and demonstrate a wider range of care options available, and can inform women of the pros and cons of these varying options. Similarly, Weatherspoon et al. (2015) and Daniels et al. (2015) provide recommendations for childbirth educators in regards to connecting to and properly communicating with young pregnant women using social media platforms, so as to provide them with the most accurate information available and make sure that they feel prepared for birth and that their childbirth decisions are well-informed, as does the website of Childbirth Connection. Early studies have already begun to assess what women need from the media and how to best support them, using focus groups that discuss the convenience and accessibility of the media in health care (Lupton 2016).

Shifting the focus of the discourse surrounding birth using the media is a way to combat years of fearmongering. However, negative sources of information still run rampant, and in order to reduce women's likelihood of requesting or agreeing to CB and to improve their birth experiences and outcomes, their fears must be reduced. Both changing the cultural conversations surrounding birth and providing psychological care and support are crucial to cultivating confidence and positive mindsets in women, and by extension positive attitudes towards birth.

Countries with "On-Target" Rates

In addition to these general practice changes, we can look to the countries with on-target CB rates for inspiration in regards to birth practices and social outlooks on/attitudes towards reproduction. While most countries are either well above or below the recommended CB rate range (10%–15% or 19%), there are a number of countries that fall within this recommended range, that have done so *intentionally* and have benefited from positive maternal-infant health outcomes and overall population health. These include Iceland, Belgium, Finland, Norway, and Sweden (Gibbons et al. 2010). Other countries with reasonable CB rates, competent care, and excellent outcomes include the Netherlands (Jordan 1993; De Vries 2009; Cheyney et al. 2019) and Japan (Williamson and Matsuoka 2019). Each country has its own unique set of circumstances and its own particular beliefs about birth. Jordan (1993) noted that Sweden was one of the first countries to almost entirely embrace clinical or hospital birth and to do away with home birth. Nevertheless, Swedish midwives and obstetricians offer competent care and keep their CB rates within a reasonable range, even decreasing the rates in recent years, approximating the target range (Högberg 2004; Mesterton et al. 2017). The Netherlands has remained one of the last high-resource nations in the world to keep their homebirth rates high—at a current 13%—their CB rates reasonably low, at around 16%, and their birth experiences relatively unmedicalized (Cheyney et al. 2019). The Netherlands also has a state-organized healthcare system, well-educated and autonomous community midwives fully integrated into the maternity care system, a system for postpartum care and for well-child visits, political support for midwifery and for births at home and in birth centers, and easy access to specialist care. They invest their money in the long-term social, emotional, and physical well-being of their citizens rather than in medical technology or pharmaceuticals (ibid.). Scandinavian countries, including Sweden, also have universal health care, more births supervised by midwives and attended by doulas, and overall political support for women's reproductive rights and health (Högberg 2004; Mesterton et al. 2017). These countries have some of the lowest perinatal mortality rates as well as some of the best maternal outcomes and patient satisfaction. Should the US choose to reduce the current CB rate of 32% and to administer care as many of these countries have—which would entail much greater numbers of midwife-attended births in all settings—we could expect to see similar benefits.

As well as modeling maternity care on these systems, we should be cognizant of the larger socio-cultural contexts in which this care takes place. Countries with healthcare equity, evenly distributed resources, recommended CB rates, and healthy women and children invest in their families and in their communities. They are not just focused on the moment of birth, but rather everything leading up to and following it: a life-long approach. Social determinants of health and (uneven) administration of care impact CB rates and distribution. As we saw in Brazil, and can see in the US, cesareans are classed and racialized (Davis 2019). Insurance, monetary incentives, and competing healthcare systems only serve to further this stratification and exacerbate inequalities. It is not enough to solely limit the number of cesareans—we must make sure that they are only being performed when absolutely necessary, are not discriminatory, and are not being used inappropriately, but that they *are* accessible to those who need them. Revolutionizing birth means re-modeling our care as well as our culture—most especially the culture of obstetrics and the training of obstetricians.

Concluding Remarks: Birthing Techno-Sapiens

As the chapters in this book demonstrate, we are well on our way to becoming techno-sapiens. The media influence our birth perspectives and planning, and technology is heavily relied on in order to bring us into this world, far too often culminating in the surgical removal of the infant. Technology has led the way to seeming miracles, such as those described in other chapters in this volume, including helping those to conceive who would otherwise be unable, saving the lives of women and children in birth who would otherwise die, and providing nourishment to infants who would otherwise starve. Yet over-dependence on technology, and the normalization of its implementation, have serious implications, not only in regards to our physiology and psychology, but also to the fabric of our society. This medicalization is often used to control the bodies of women and minorities and to reinforce pre-existing power structures and stratifications (Jordan 1993; Davis-Floyd and Sargent 1997; Davis 2019). We will always be co-dependent with our technologies; however, we can choose to use them wisely. While technology can be used to control bodies ("the cyborg as oppressor"), it can also be used to liberate them ("the cyborg as liberator"—see Introduction).

For example, during COVID-19, the telehealth used to administer care, both by midwives and obstetricians, transferred agency, power, and control back to the patients. Pregnant women were put in charge of their pregnancies, taking measurements, recording vitals, and monitoring physical conditions, all the while reporting back to healthcare workers and guiding the virtual "appointment" (Davis-Floyd, Gutschow, and Schwartz 2020). This technology allows mothers to be autonomous in their pregnancies in a way that is rarely observed in Western medical systems. *Living in a world of technological advancement does not mean living in a world devoid of patient rights and reproductive justice.* Clearly, techno-sapiens can be as replete with holistic possibilities as they are with the vast potentials of technology, both in birth and in life.

Acknowledgments

Many thanks to Karen Rosenberg, who oversaw this research, and to the women who participated in my study and were willing to share their thoughts and feelings on childbirth.

References

Alfirevic Z, Gyte GML, Cuthbert A, Devane D. 2017. Continuous Cardiotocography as a Form of Electronic Fetal Monitoring for Fetal Assessment During Labour. *Cochrane Database of Systematic Reviews* 2. Art. No.: CD006066. DOI: 10.1002/14651858. CD006066.pub3

Betrán AP, Gulmezoglu AM, Robson M et al. 2009. WHO Global Survey on Maternal and Perinatal Health in Latin America: Classifying Caesarean Sections. *Reproductive Health* 6(1):18.

Cheung NF, Pan A. 2021. Changing Childbirth in China: Reclaiming Midwives and Family Care. In: *Birthing Models on the Human Rights Frontier: Speaking Truth to Power*, eds. Daviss BA, R Davis-Floyd. London: Routledge, in press.

Cheyney M, Goodarzi B, Wiegers T, Davis-Floyd R, Vedam S. 2019. Giving Birth in the United States and the Netherlands: Midwifery Care as Integrated Option or Contested Privilege? In: *Birth in Eight Cultures*, eds. Davis-Floyd R. Cheyney M Long Grove, IL: Waveland Press, 165–202.

Cho CE, Norman M. 2013. Cesarean Section and Development of the Immune System in the Offspring. *American Journal of Obstetrics and Gynecology* 208(4):249–254.

Collard TD, Diallo H, Habinsky A, Hentschell C, Vezeau TM. 2008. Elective Cesarean Section: Why Women Choose It and What Nurses Need to Know. *Nursing for Women's Health* 12(6):480–488.

Daniels M, Wedler JA. 2015. Enhancing Childbirth Education through Technology. *International Journal of Childbirth Education* 30(3).

Davis DA. 2019. Obstetric Racism: The Racial Politics of Pregnancy, Labor, and Birthing. *Medical Anthropology* 38(7):560–573.

Davis-Floyd RE. 2003. *Birth as an American Rite of Passage*, 2nd ed. Berkeley: University of California Press.

Davis-Floyd RE, Gutschow K, Schwartz DA. 2020. Pregnancy, Birth and the COVID-19 Pandemic in the United States. *Medical Anthropology* 39(5):413–427. doi:10.1080/0 1459740.2020.1761804.

Davis-Floyd RE, Sargent CF. 1997. *Childbirth and Authoritative Knowledge: Cross-Cultural Perspectives*. Berkeley: University of California Press.

Daviss BA, Bisits A. 2021. Bringing Back Breech: Dismantling Hierarchies and Re-Skilling Practitioners. In: *Birthing Models on the Human Rights Frontier: Speaking Truth to Power*, eds. Daviss BA, R Davis-Floyd. London: Routledge, Chapter 5, in press.

De Vries R. 2009. The Dutch Obstetrical System: Vanguard of the Future in Maternity Care. In: *Birth Models That Work*, eds. Davis-Floyd R, L Barclay, BA Daviss, J Tritten. Berkeley: University of California Press, 31–54.

Dominguez-Bello MG, Costello EK, Contreras M, Magris M, Hidalgo G, Fierer N, Knight R. 2010. Delivery Mode Shapes the Acquisition and Structure of the Initial

Microbiota Across Multiple Body Habitats in Newborns. *Proceedings of the National Academy of Sciences of the United States of America* 107(26):11971–11975.

Donohoe MM. 1996. Our Epidemic of Unnecessary Cesarean Sections: The Role of the Law in Creating It, the Role of the Law in Stopping It. *Wisconsin Women's Law Journal* 11:197.

Fischetti M, Armstrong Z. 2017. The Baby Spike. *Scientific American* 317(1):76.

Fisher C, Hauck Y, Fenwick J. 2006. How Social Context Impacts on Women's Fears of Childbirth: A Western Australian Example. *Social Science and Medicine* 63(1):64–75.

Fraser G. 1995. Modern Bodies, Modern Minds: Midwifery and Reproductive Change in an African American Community. In: *Conceiving the New World Order: The Global Politics of Reproduction*, eds. Ginsburg F, Rapp R. Berkeley: University of California Press, 42–58.

Gamble J, Creedy DK, McCourt C, Weaver J, Beake S. 2007. A Critique of the Literature on Women's Request for Cesarean Section. *Birth* 34(4):331–340.

Georges E, Daellenbach R. 2019. Divergent Meanings and Practices of Childbirth in Greece and New Zealand. In: *Birth in Eight Cultures*, eds. Davis-Floyd R, Cheyney M Long. Grove, IL: Waveland Press, 89–128.

Gibbons L, Belizán JM, Lauer JA, Betrán AP, Merialdi M, Althabe F. 2010. The Global Numbers and Costs of Additionally Needed and Unnecessary Caesarean Sections Performed per Year: Overuse as a Barrier to Universal Coverage. *World Health Report* 30(1):1–31.

Hildingsson I. 2014. Swedish Couples' Attitudes Towards Birth, Childbirth Fear and Birth Preferences and Relation to Mode of Birth—A Longitudinal Cohort Study. *Sexual and Reproductive Healthcare: Official Journal of the Swedish Association of Midwives* 5(2):75–80.

Högberg U. 2004. The Decline in Maternal Mortality in Sweden: The Role of Community Midwifery. *American Journal of Public Health* 94(8):1312–1320.

Jordan B, Davis-Floyd R. 1993. The Crosscultural Comparison of Birthing Systems: Toward A Biosocial Analysis. In: *Birth in Four Cultures: A Crosscultural Investigation of Childbirth in Yucatan, Holland, Sweden, and the United States*. Prospect Heights, IL: Waveland Press, 45–90.

Kitzinger S, Kitzinger J. 2001. Sheila Kitzinger's and Jenny Kitzinger's Letter from Europe: Childbirth and Breastfeeding in the British Media. *Birth* 28(1):60–61.

Laursen M, Hedegaard M, Johansen C, Danish National Birth Cohort. 2008. Fear of Childbirth: Predictors and Temporal Changes Among Nulliparous Women in the Danish National Birth Cohort. *BJOG: An International Journal of Obstetrics and Gynaecology* 115(3):354–360.

Leachman A. 2017. How Media Promote Fear Around Childbirth. In: *Midwifery, Childbirth and the Media*. Switzerland: Springer Nature, 61–77.

Leal MC, da Silva AAM, Dias MAB, da Gama SGN, Rattner D, Moreira ME, Bittencourt SDA. 2012. Birth in Brazil: National Survey into Labour and Birth. *Reproductive Health* 9(1):1–8.

Lee ASM, Kirkman M. 2008. Disciplinary Discourses: Rates of Cesarean Section Explained by Medicine, Midwifery, and Feminism. *Health Care for Women International* 29(5):448–467.

Lobel M, DeLuca RS. 2007. Psychosocial Sequelae of Cesarean Delivery: Review and Analysis of Their Causes and Implications. *Social Science and Medicine* 64(11):2272–2284.

Luce A, Hundley V, van Teijlingen E, Ridden S, Edlund S. 2017. Midwives' Engagement with the Media. In: *Midwifery, Childbirth and the Media*. Switzerland: Springer Nature, 97–110.

Lupton D. 2016. The Use and Value of Digital Media for Information About Pregnancy and Early Motherhood: A Focus Group Study. *BMC Pregnancy and Childbirth* 16(1):1–10.

Martin JA, Hamilton BE, Osterman MJK, Driscoll AK, Mathews TJ. 2017. Births: Final Data for 2015. *National Vital Statistics Reports: From the Centers for Disease Control and Prevention, National Center for Health Statistics, National Vital Statistics System* 66(1):1.

Mesterton J, Ladfors L, Ekenberg Abreu A, Lindgren P, Saltvedt S, Weichselbraun M, Amer-Wåhlin I. 2017. Case Mix Adjusted Variation in Cesarean Section Rate in Sweden. *Acta Obstetricia et Gynecologica Scandinavica* 96(5):597–606.

Mitteroecker P, Windhager S, Pavlicev M. 2017. Cliff-Edge Model Predicts Intergenerational Predisposition to Dystocia and Caesarean Delivery. *Proceedings of the National Academy of Sciences of the United States of America* 114(44):11669–11672.

Molina G, Weiser TG, Lipsitz SR et al. 2015. Relationship Between Cesarean Delivery Rate and Maternal and Neonatal Mortality. *JAMA* 314(21):2263–2270.

Morris T, McInerney K. 2010. Media Representations of Pregnancy and Childbirth: An Analysis of Reality Television Programs in the United States. *Birth* 37(2):134–140.

Odent M. 2004. *The Caesarean*. London: Free Assn Books.

Penna L, Arulkumaran S. 2003. Cesarean Section for Non-Medical Reasons. *International Journal of Gynecology and Obstetrics* 82(3):399–409.

Potter JE, Berquó E, Perpétuo IH, Leal OF, Hopkins K, Souza MR, de Carvalho Formiga MC. 2001. Unwanted Caesarean Sections Among Public and Private Patients in Brazil: Prospective Study. *British Medical Journal* 323(7322):1155–1158.

Reyes E, Rosenberg K. 2018. *Maternal Motives Behind Elective Cesarean Sections*. Dissertation, University of Delaware.

Reyes E, Rosenberg K. 2019. Maternal Motives Behind Elective Cesarean Sections. *American Journal of Human Biology: The Official Journal of the Human Biology Council* 31(2):e23226.

Rondung E, Thomtén J, Sundin Ö. 2016. Psychological Perspectives on Fear of Childbirth. *Journal of Anxiety Disorders* 44:80–91.

Rosenberg K, Trevathan W. 2018. Evolutionary Perspectives on Cesarean Section. *Evolution, Medicine, and Public Health* 1(1):67–81.

Ryding E, Wijma B, Wijma K, Rydhström H. 1998. Fear of Childbirth During Pregnancy May Increase the Risk of Emergency Cesarean Section. *Acta Obstetricia et Gynecologica Scandinavica* 77(5):542–547.

Sadler M, Santos MJDS, Ruiz-Berdún D et al. 2016. Moving Beyond Disrespect and Abuse: Addressing the Structural Dimensions of Obstetric Violence. *Reproductive Health Matters* 24(47):47–55.

Santas G, Santas F. 2018. Trends of Caesarean Section Rates in Turkey. *Journal of Obstetrics and Gynaecology: The Journal of the Institute of Obstetrics and Gynaecology* 38(5):658–662.

Serçekuş P, Okumuş H. 2009. Fears Associated with Childbirth Among Nulliparous Women in Turkey. *Midwifery* 25(2):155–162.

Stafford RS. 1990. Cesarean Section Use and Source of Payment: An Analysis of California Hospital Discharge Abstracts. *American Journal of Public Health* 80(3):313–315.

Stoll K, Hall W, Janssen P, Carty E. 2014. Why Are Young Canadians Afraid of Birth? A Survey Study of Childbirth Fear and Birth Preferences Among Canadian University Students. *Midwifery* 30(2):220–226.

Weatherspoon D, Weatherspoon C, Ristau C. 2015. Speaking Their Language: Integrating Social Media into Childbirth Education Practice. *International Journal of Childbirth Education* 30(3):21–24.

Weaver JJ, Statham H, Richards M. 2007. Are There "Unnecessary" Cesarean Sections? Perceptions of Women and Obstetricians About Cesarean Sections for Nonclinical Indications. *Birth* 34(1):32–41.

Wendland CL. 2007. The Vanishing Mother: Cesarean Section and "Evidence-Based Obstetrics." *Medical Anthropology Quarterly* 21(2):218–233.

Williamson KE, Matsuoka E. 2019. Comparing Childbirth in Brazil and Japan: Social Hierarchies, Cultural Values, and the Meaning of Place. In: *Birth in Eight Cultures*, eds. Davis-Floyd R, M Cheyney. Long Grove, IL: Waveland Press, 89–128.

10

CANCEROUS CONTRACEPTIVES AND THE INCUBATION OF MONSTERS:

Quechua Reproductive Etiology and Producing *Necro-Techno-Sapiens*

Rebecca Irons

Introducing *Necro-Techno-Sapiens*

Biomedical pharmaceuticals, and specifically hormonal contraceptives, are often framed as tools to help women gain control over their lives through planning future offspring and being granted the ability to pursue life projects free of child-rearing concerns. However, not all perceive such reproductive technology as beneficial. For the Quechua of the Peruvian Andes, this technology may instead be the bringer of death, through causing cancerous tumors and the production of what I am calling *necro-techno-sapiens*.

While the cyborgs of contemporary imagination may have the presence of metal and machines as key features, this was not necessarily so in the original conception of the cyborg. Clynes and Kline (1960), who coined the term in reference to the future astronauts of space travel, did not solely envisage a human merged with mechanics, but an enhanced human organism achieved through the careful administration of pharmaceuticals (74). Rather than having the human rely on external machinery, they perceived cyborgs as humans enhanced biologically through injected drugs that would allow them to stay awake for extended periods, avoid radiation damage, and control metabolic function, among other things designed to facilitate survival in outer space (74–75). For the cyborg, first came the alteration of human biology with pills and potions; machinery came later. With this in mind, cyborgs and techno-sapiens may not only be produced through mechanical or electronic devices, but also through pharmaceutical interventions.

In reproduction, hormonal contraceptives are one such pharmaceutical that could potentially be framed as "biohacking" (Malantino 2017) by "enhancing" humans and rendering them cyborgian by suppressing "unwanted" menstruation and its associated bodily troubles. As suggested by Dumit and Davis–Floyd

(1998:8), among other views, the cyborg can be seen as a "mutilator of natural processes" (see Introduction), and certainly using hormones to interfere with menstrual cycles is one expression of this "mutilation." However, as Malantino notes, "biohacking" in this way remains the purview of "a small handful of entitled, enfranchised subjects" while other, racialized subjects are denied the same agency in their dealings with these new technologies, including "forms of birth control with minimal deleterious side-effects" (2017:189), with the poor sometimes becoming "the guinea pigs of the cyborgification of…reproduction" (Dumit and Davis-Floyd 1998:2).

At first glance, it may seem out of place to focus on hormonal contraceptives—pharmaceuticals that *stop* the conception of babies—in a volume about the *production* of techno-sapiens. However, a type of techno-sapiens *can* be produced through hormonal contraceptives, according to the Quechua etiology of hormones and how they work on the reproductive body—a *necro-techno-sapiens*. In this instance, one needs to remove their biomedical hat when approaching hormonal contraceptives as drugs that suppress ovulation with the intention of avoiding fertilization, and see them Quechually: as a potion that makes your menstruation stop all of a sudden, as happens during pregnancy, but that results in the production of no living child. Where does this blood go? Two things can happen: it can form a cancerous tumor, or it can distort the development of a "fetus" into a monstrous form, as will be addressed in this chapter. These "monsters" that can have human teeth, hair, skin, and fat, but no tangible life— biomedically called "teratoma tumors"—are a "dead life" produced by artificial hormones. However, with their human tissues, their *sapiens-substances*, they are nonetheless a remnant of life. In this sense, sex hormones hold the ability to produce necro-techno-sapiens—technologically culpable dead [human] life. As Haraway once stated, cyborg modes of reproduction represent a "promise of monsters" (quoted in Dumit and Davis-Floyd 1998:13). Thanks to biomedical pharmaceuticals, in the Andes that promise is made good.

This chapter is based on ethnographic research undertaken over one year in a rural Quechua community in the province of Ayacucho, in the Peruvian Andes. My research investigated Indigenous women's relationships to biomedical contraception, sexual and reproductive health care, and wider interactions with the national family planning program and state health workers. All names are anonymized and all translations are mine.

To properly contextualize the experiences and beliefs presented in this chapter, it is necessary to briefly touch upon the fraught relationship between Indigenous Quechua and the Peruvian state—particularly as this relationship applies to reproductive health care—to understand why the Quechua might perceive mal-intent on the part of biomedicine aside from Indigenous etiologies.

In the period 1996–2000, an estimated 300,000+ Indigenous women underwent enforced sterilization in Peru (Ewig 2010) as part of the national family planning program; many women did not give their consent, nor understand the permanence of the procedure. As the state denies culpability, instead blaming individual health workers, justice has still not been granted for those who were sterilized. Understandably, Quechua women have been wary of state family planning ever since. Nevertheless, maternal care in Peru has continued to be medicalized, with home births and traditional midwives officially banned in 2005. Although this ban was introduced as an "intercultural birthing model," whereby Indigenous women could use some elements of Quechua cultural birth (such as upright birthing positions and the use of sheep's wool to coddle the newborn), they are obligated to give birth using biomedical facilities and university-trained *obstetras* (professional direct-entry midwives not trained as nurses). While this policy has been successful in reducing maternal mortality, it has been argued that this intercultural birth model is a way of luring Indigenous women into biomedical facilities and thereby influencing their subjectivities (Guerra Reyes 2019). In the case of family planning and contraceptives, women are also obligated to accept hormonal contraceptives in some instances—for example as a condition of returning home after giving birth, and to receive government welfare checks (Irons 2020). However, many Quechua women *do* want to practice family planning; despite prejudiced perceptions that Andean women are hyper-fertile, they mostly desire small families—they just wish to avoid the myriad conditions and perceived health complications that come with some forms of family planning.

Peruvian sociologist Anibal Quijano (2000) suggested that there is a power relationship of dominance present in situations of such disjuncture between the "official" view of the body and Indigenous etiologies. Ultimately, it is the postcolonial state's medical preference—biomedicine—that is imposed upon the Quechua through the obligation to birth in hospitals, and even the kind of contraceptives on offer (e.g., hormonal rather than behavioral). This is because of a "coloniality of power" (ibid.), whereby the Peruvian government continues to impose dominance over colonized people in the form of obligations and imposition of discourse and lifeways.

It is against this backdrop that Quechua women experience hormonal contraceptives, with the three-month injection Depo-Provera being one of the principal methods used in the rural Andes. Crucially, Indigenous understandings of the mechanisms of action differ from the biomedical model. For Quechua women, the effects produced on the body by sex hormones are potentially *cancerous*. In some cases, tumors are more than "cancer"—they are evidence of a distorted life that the biomedical pharmaceuticals have manipulated—an "estranged recognition" (Comaroff and Comaroff 2002) of fetal life. This kind of disrupted fetus, which, thanks to technological intervention of hormonal contraceptives, is "dead" but nevertheless held the promise of life, is an example of a necro-techno-sapiens.

Cancerous Contraceptives

In a quiet room of a rural hospital in Ayacucho, Eusebia, a 30-year-old Quechua woman who was using the contraceptive injection, confided that "sometimes we women get worried when there's no blood coming down…you should see blood every month." We were deep in a discussion about reasons why some women have problems with the hormonal contraceptives on offer in the hospital, and why people may feel that those methods could cause you harm. Eusebia had two children and desired another later on, but had decided to discontinue use of the injection as she was dubious as to what it was "really doing" inside of her, and what effects this could have on her future ability to bear children. Her concerns rotated specifically around the perceived accumulation of blood that she believed happened over the duration of the injection's three months—during which she did not see her menstruation at all. Explaining the dangerous effects of the contraceptives, Eusebia expressed concerns: "They say that it forms a tumor, it forms cancer. The blood accumulates inside of you and it forms a small ball (*bolita*), like a tumor."

Like many others, she had heard it rumored that hormonal contraceptives were giving women cancer due to accumulated menstrual blood, that instead of being released monthly as it should, was "stuck" inside the uterus and festering into a cancerous tumor. For the Quechua, absence of blood and menstrual suppression was not desired. Instead, this idea was replaced by the more fearsome notion of undesirable "blood accumulation." Eusebia was not the only one who felt this way, as the comments of other women suggested:

> With the [contraceptive] injection there was no blood, but when I stopped using it a lot of blood came, why would that be? Was it because of blood accumulation? (Paucar, 27)

> When I used the [contraceptive] injection, my blood didn't come for many months, and later it came out like clots (*coagulaciones*). Here they say that it's cancer, it's *tumorcitos* (little tumors). (Fermentina, 38)

> I didn't see my blood with the [contraceptive] injection, *¿a donde va esa sangre?* Where does that blood go? It stays inside you! (Samaira, 22)

> Because my menstruation did not come [when I used contraceptives], I thought that the blood was inside, *sancochada* (parboiling). Inside it became like gelatin! (Eulogia, 48)

Many women expressed concern about the lack of menstruation for up to 3 months, as this is well beyond the timeframe of a "missed period" and can indicate serious consequences; women wondered if the blood had accumulated inside and was "stuck" up there, rotting and fermenting. As these quotes indicate, this trapped blood is thought to coagulate inside the uterus ("belly") and develop into a cancerous tumor.

Blood is an extremely important substance in the Andes, a "dominant symbol" of "vitality" (Bastien 2003:173), and some consider blood a finite resource. Loss of blood can result in physical weakness, and for this reason pregnancy is considered a "temporary death" in which the woman is physically vulnerable (La Riva Gonzales 2017). However, it is not only blood loss that poses a problem; accumulation of blood is also problematic, as "body flows are of primary concern for wellbeing...impeded flow of essential substances (blood, bile, phlegm, urine, semen, feces, sweat, fat, air, water) are causes for bodily disorders" (Hammer 2001:244). When a woman does not menstruate, this flow of blood is thought to be accumulating inside instead of being expelled monthly, which would be the healthy cycle of blood. In biomedical understanding, the uterine lining will build up and thicken during a menstrual cycle in preparation for pregnancy. If an egg is not fertilized during this cycle, the lining will slough off as menstruation. The contraceptive injection can cause this uterine lining to cease building; hence the lack of menstrual blood, as it has not been produced in the first place. However, clearly this is not the dominant etiology in Quechua understandings of the reproductive body. Hammer (2001:245–246) succinctly describes Quechua women's views of menstrual regulation flows:

> Women...become distressed about irregular and delayed menstrual periods. When menstruation fails to begin in a given month, women worry that the blood is stuck inside the abdomen...women say that this blood becomes 'like a baby'...while embryos are formed essentially of blood, lumps of cold blood or other growths that appear in the abdomen unrelated to male insemination are signs of danger to the woman's well-being. Women use the borrowed Western terms, tumor and cancer, to describe severe, often terminal cases of menstrual malfunction identified with the growth of masses in the belly.

Hammer's interlocutors also used "cancer" as an explanation for their hindered menstrual flows; however, she sees this as a "borrowed term" rather than respecting Quechua women's embodied knowledge. One could argue that in Ayacucho, women are not "borrowing terms"—they are identifying a Quechua etiology of cancer. When they talk of tumors and cancer, they arguably *mean* biomedical ("Western") cancer. Hammer noted that (cold) blood clots or growths in the abdomen unrelated to male insemination are dangerous (2001:246). However, when contraception enters the equation, it may not be so easy to tell the difference. Women are using hormonal contraception precisely because they are engaging in sexual intercourse, and thus there is a possibility of insemination.

Returning to women's comments, often the 3-month contraceptive injection was perceived as the most dangerous method, and for good reason, as this 3-month time frame and blood coagulation are significant within understandings of reproduction across the Andes. Until 3 months, as mentioned above, it is thought that a fetus is *not* a living entity per se, but a coagulation of blood; a *trozo de sangre* (chunk of flesh) (Morgan 1997:341). La Riva Gonzalez (2017:175) outlines the predominant theory of conception in the Peruvian Andes:

> Conception is a process of "cooking" or "maturation" of the masculine substance (*muhu*), by the menstrual blood, the semen is considered metaphorically like alimentation that "grows," that "cooks" in the woman's body, in her blood.

Over time, this "fetus feeds on the maternal blood (liquid element) and the father gives…the solid part…the association of the female sex with the smooth, liquid element and the masculine sex with the solid element seems to confirm the idea that the body of the fetus does not form at the same time…and *during those first months is purely blood (yawarlla)*" (2017:176) (emphasis added). It is thought that this view is pan-Andean, also found in Aymara, Peru, where the fetus is "plain blood"/ *sangre plena / wila p'alt'a* for the first 4 months (2017:176), and the Ecuadorian Andes, where fetal "fermentation" can take between 1 and 4 months (Morgan 1997).

Thus, the process of blood coagulation resulting in a fetus must be understood as it relates to the process of blood coagulation resulting in a cancerous tumor. Both the development of life (fetus) and death (cancer) begin the exact same way—blood coagulates inside the uterus—however, its destined final product dictates the outcome for the woman.

There is hardly 100% faith in hormonal contraceptives, and the line between blood coagulation that will lead to a healthy, living baby and blood coagulation that will result in a deadly cancerous tumor is thin. After all, the initial process of blood coagulation inside the abdomen is the same in both scenarios. Because most Quechua users are engaging in sexual intercourse and therefore having contact with semen, what could develop is a fetus, were it not for the contraceptives. Yet contraceptive use does not discount the possible formation of a "fetus." However, it is not a (future human) coagulation-entity that is eventually formed when contraception is used, but a cancerous tumor.

It is worth noting that there is some crossover between Quechua reproductive etiology and how the fetus has been portrayed in biomedical textbooks. As Martin points out, the fetus has previously been described as a "tumor" from an immunological point of view (1998:131), due to its nature as a genetically different tissue mass, distinct from the mother, yet growing within her and thriving from her blood source. However, in this North American example, the question is posed as to why this "tumor-fetus" is not attacked by the *mother's* body. For the Quechua, the attack is the other way around, with the tumor potentially harming the woman. Even more interesting is the notion that these tumors can turn into something other than cancer—an abstraction of a fetus-that-might-have-been, were it not for the interference of the reproductive technologies. If hormones are involved and tumors are afoot, here there be monsters.

The Incubation of Monsters

While tumors have been associated with fetuses and reproduction beyond the Andean context, monster myths are found with even more frequency

(Bewell 1988). Indeed, pregnancy is riddled with potential monstrosity, with Frankensteinian imagery a particular feature of Western gestational tales and fears of catastrophic creation, forewarning the perils of overzealous use of technologies such as IVF (Almond 1998), and in this case, contraceptives.

While some perceptions of pregnancy and monsters have been analyzed as projections of latent maternal fears, there are some very real biomedical examples of "monsters" in obstetrics that may fuel such notions. Since the 16th century, medical and popular documentation of "monstrous" pregnancies and deformed fetuses has been widely discussed (Bates 2002), including in specific relation to Indigenous pregnancies in colonial Latin America (Few 2009). Today reproductive abnormalities still hold the power to incense the emotions, whether these are the "strong visceral…revulsion and fascination" (Angel 2013) produced through viewing a teratoma in a pathology museum, or the fear and indignation felt by a Quechua woman whose fetus had perceptibly gone "awry" due to hormonal contraception.

Ovarian teratomas (dermoid cysts) are germ cell tumors that can grow to the size of a grapefruit and are usually benign, though they can cause pain and infertility if left untreated. As these tumors form from a totipotential germ cell, they are able to develop a number of different types of human tissue within, including teeth, wax, fat, bone, eyes, hair, and in rare cases, partly developed limbs and brain tissue (Kim et al. 2011; see Figure 10.1). (The hair within teratomas can be of a different color from the woman's due to germ cell variation, which may contribute to perceptions that these tumors are growths of a separate human such as a fetus or a twin.) Because of this, teratomas are widely perceived as "evil twins," although biomedically this is incorrect. Like the acardiac (the congenital absence of a heart), the presence of sapiens-substance without life has influenced their naming: *teras* is Greek for "monster." Despite their inherently fascinating properties, virtually no anthropological attention has been afforded the teratoma in terms of reproductive health or otherwise, besides musings over whether they might be related to the global myth of the *vagina dentata* ("toothed vagina") (Jackson 1971; Angel 2013). Their lack of attention outside of medical research may be due to their rarity, although they arguably deserve more reflection, as for those in a rural Quechua community, the appearance of a teratoma had very much to do with fetal development and hormonal contraception's interference in it.

While the most commonly perceived corporeal outcome of contraceptive use may be a cancerous tumor as an abstraction of "normal" fetal development, in the following instance the fetal development had taken a very different turn. Although many women reported on the presence in, and belief about, hormones producing cancer, Pilajia had undergone a different experience, although it began in very much the same way. She had, as she described, experienced a sort of tumor-pregnancy.

Pilajia was married with 5 children and had been using the injection as recommended by the hospital to avoid getting pregnant again. In her mid-40s, she had agreed to use contraception to curb her fertility and avoid future offspring.

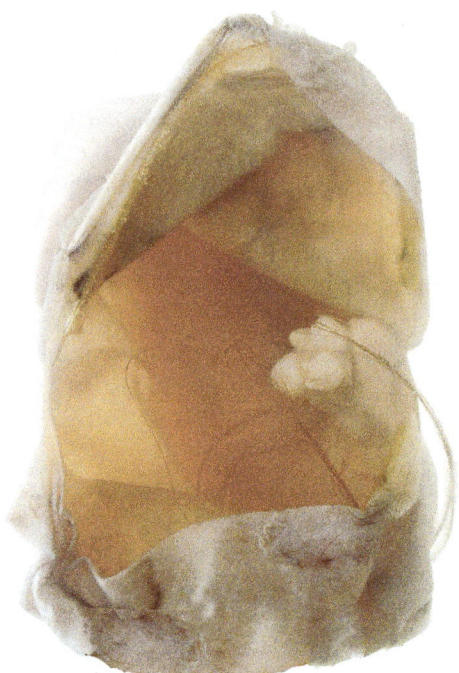

FIGURE 10.1 © UCL Pathology Collections: LDUCPC-UCH-MX.GYN.143.1, Dermoid Cyst/Teratoma Tumor. Used with permission of UCL Pathology Collections.

However, a short while after being injected, she discovered a "ball" developing inside of her. According to Quechua etiology, this would usually be identified as a cancerous tumor; however, Pilajia began to have sharp pains and so had to be referred to the regional hospital in Ayacucho city for observation. The health workers in the rural district had a name for what happened to her—it was a teratoma. However, Pilajia held a different perception of this occurrence:

> The [contraceptive] injection made me grow a *bolita* (small ball) inside, like a *tumorcito* (small tumor), and on top of it, hair started to grow! It seems that when you use the injection it could make hairs start to grow on top of these tumors…but then I said to myself, a *wawa* (baby) must have appeared. Sometimes accumulated blood (*sangre acumulado*) can make tumors appear, but then for me hairs appeared on top, so it was a *wawa*! They told me that I had to have an operation in Ayacucho city, but I asked myself what could have happened to my blood? Hairs started to grow on top, it was like a *wawa*, so they said that had to take it out—because of the injection it was not a baby. But what would it be if not a *wawa*? *Una wawita,* I thought,

but they [the ob/gyn] said that it was not a baby that was growing inside of me, even though it grew hair! So, what would it be I asked myself, *un monstruito*, a little monster, growing inside, from the injection? I was afraid about what it would be.

Pilajia was rightfully confused about what had happened. She said that nobody had explained anything to her, although post-operation she had been shown the mass with hair. (The healthcare workers had diagnosed this as a teratoma via ultrasound, during which they also may have indicated to Pilajia that the mass contained hair.) As hair is a sapiens-substance, it seemed logical that what the hospital had removed had been a fetus, apart from one very significant fact: she had been using the contraceptive injection, which meant that she could not become pregnant in the first place. Certainly, there had been a coagulation of blood, as in the initial process of fetal formation according to Quechua etiology. In many women's perceptions, this coagulation would go on to either become a fetus (if not using contraceptives), or a cancerous tumor (if using contraceptives). In Pilajia's case it became something in-between: a tumor, but with human features such as hair. (It is very rare for women to see one of the "cancerous tumors" they perceive themselves as having.)

Pilajia's upset about this complicated case is understandable, and likely not helped by the seeming lack of information given by medical staff as to what this "little monster" might be, biomedically speaking or otherwise. Whether she had been provided with them or not, Pilajia did not mention biomedical explanations for this something-in-between, so it is important to understand her experience from her perception and not impose a biomedical framework. Therefore, while this occurrence may have been a diagnosable teratoma for health workers, for Pilajia it was much more confusing, according to Quechua reproductive etiology. In hushed tones she wondered if the injection had caused her *wawa* to become deformed into something monstrous that then needed surgical removal. In harking back to historical mistreatment of Indigenous women by state health services, it is not difficult to see why she might be inclined to suspect malintent.

This was not an isolated case, although Pilajia was the only woman interviewed who had personally experienced it. Other women mentioned that they had heard of such stories, that sometimes a contraception-tumor could grow *into* a baby, although there were no reported cases in which any woman had actually given birth to one of these "fetuses," so we do not know what kind of baby had "grown." Indeed, in a relatively small province, these rumors could very well have pertained to Pilajia, although this is difficult to evidence. There was also some confusion as to what "it" was, and stories around these incidences were ambiguous at best. Iraida, a market-seller from a small village, recalled a story about another woman from the regional capital:

Iraida: They say that there was a woman in Ayacucho, and her blood accumulated but it became like a tumor. They said that it had teeth and hair like a *wawa*, but supposedly she had used the [contraceptive] injection, so maybe it couldn't be a *wawa*, but something else growing inside…but with teeth!

RI: Do you know what happened to the woman?

Iraida: They operated on her, I believe…there in Ayacucho they took it out, like when they cut the *wawa* out [cesarean]. But it was dead.

The "it" that had been produced was ambiguous for Iraida. Women had been told that use of the injection meant they would not conceive, but the presence of human tissue such as hair makes the "it" something other than a tumor. The "ball may be an 'it,' but not in the same way that a prior-to-three-month blood-ball is an 'it' that may eventually become a 'someone'" (Morgan 1997). Pilajia's "it," and the "it" that Iraida spoke of could not be a someone, as "it was dead"; "a little monster," produced because the woman was using biomedical technology in the form of the contraceptive injection.

These incidences reveal that, because of pharmaceutical use, some kind of monstrous "it" *could* grow inside Quechua women. One way to understand this literal embodiment of an "other" within the reproductive system itself (the "other" here being biomedicine and its wider associations with a harmful post-colonial state), is through the concept of "estranged recognition" (Comaroff and Comaroff, 2002:795). According to the Comaroffs, "estranged recognition" refers to "invisible predations" that lurk beneath the surface when someone or something that was seemingly once "knowable" becomes "estranged." In their research, they discussed how people become turned into one kind of recognizable monster: the zombie. Once zombified, the person in question is no longer themselves, and their relationship to the community and their kin is forever changed.

For the Quechua, it can be argued that using biomedical contraceptives may also produce "estranged recognition" of a reproductive process that should follow a known etiology but has become disrupted due to the external intervention of hormonal interference. The same process that should lead to a healthy fetus and the reproduction of kin is instead leading to a woman's potential death through cancer, or in the case of Pilajia, a "monstrous" non-pregnancy of human form, but without tangible life; a *dead life*. There is something still recognizable in the grisly matter, or the *trozo de sangre*, as Morgan refers to Andean fetal development (1997). The hair and tissue mass found in Pilajia's body are not surprising in and of themselves, as they reflect the first part of healthy fetal development in Quechua etiology. However, because of the hormones within the injection, she should not have been pregnant in the first place and no *trozo de sangre* should be growing; thus this process is estranged, as it has resulted in an unexpected and unnerving conclusion that warps the normal reproductive process.

As the Comaroffs suggest, monster stories and fears may reflect wider societal concerns about power imbalances in post-colonial societies. Indeed, the presence of monstrous "others" can tell us rather a lot about the wider social processes in which they occur, beyond bodies and health alone. For example, across Africa and Haiti, the zombie monster figure has come to represent the displaced person; the explosion of contemporary culture references to this creature are perceived as a reference to the mounting fears of uncontrolled migration (Stratton 2011). In reproduction, "monstrous births" have long been viewed as signs of contemporaneous events (Bates 2002), as well as being linked to colonial Latin America and discrimination towards Indigenous pregnancies (Few 2009). More recently, the image of the Frankensteinian monster is employed to represent widening concerns over artificial, technological pregnancies such as those generated via IVF (Almond 1998). These fears arise from the "natural" process of pregnancy being taken out of human hands and placed under the strict control of biomedicine and "science."

There are those who may be more accepting of this type of control in the Andean context; for example, Roberts (2012) shows how IVF is increasingly sought by women in Ecuador who wish to control their fertility. However, as with the case of Brazilian women using hormonal contraceptives to control their biology (Sanabria 2016), these forms of "biohacking" (Malatino 2017) are neither enjoyed nor available to all: they are for the white and wealthy. Indigenous women in the Andes have a very different experience of them.

Importantly, a key feature of contemporary monster theories is that of domination and colonization. For example, the zombie-monster can be seen as a product of colonization, as it arose from the power imbalances caused during this time (Lauro and Embry 2008:96); yet it is not content with its solitary existence and must produce "a multiplication of its condition" (Lauro and Embry 2008:100). As colonizers sought to expand their territory, so do monsters seek to reproduce. Touching upon the Quechua etiology of contraception-tumors, cancer can be similarly viewed as a "a phenomenally successful *invader* and *colonizer* in part because it exploits the very features that make us successful as a species or as an organism" (Mukherjee 2011:38) (emphasis added).

The notion of hormonal contraceptives producing something akin to a monstrous dead-life as well as a cancerous tumor could be read as part of the same story—a story of an increasing coloniality of power (Quijano 2000), and of the creeping dominance of the state and its biomedical institutions. The estranged recognition of reproductive processes that results serves to make a wider comment on this situation: although Quechua people want to use biomedicine and reproductive technologies, they are also afraid of the consequences, and indeed, afraid of the technology itself.

Necro-Techno-Sapiens and Reproductive Technologies

Certainly, reproductive technologies and techno-sapiens, produced through an increasing cyborgification of reproduction, may be helpful and sought after. The ability to practice biohacking—interfering with one's biology to gain control over its functions—is desirable for certain individuals in some parts of the world. However, this desire is unequally distributed and differs in its perceptions. Malatino (2017:189) suggests that pharmaceutical inequity has colonial roots, and in the Andes, the negative perceived consequences of dominant reproductive technologies among Indigenous communities can be seen as part of the coloniality of power (Quijano 2000)—which disproportionately favors some while overlooking and obscuring the experiences and reproductive etiologies of previously colonized communities. The fact that Quechua etiology sees hormonal contraceptives as cancer and monster-producing needs to be addressed—not through "educating" them as to the biomedical model's explanation, but by making *behavioral*, instead of only hormonal, contraceptive options available to them and involving them in understanding and selecting those options.

In this chapter, the concept of a *necro-techno-sapiens* has been introduced and applied to a very limited subject of obstetric concern, the monstrous contraceptive-fetus, or teratoma. However, there are arguably far more uses and questions that may evolve from this concept throughout reproduction and cyborg research: what about fertilized but un-implanted embryos awaiting a never-coming moment of IVF stardom—are they necro-techno-sapiens? What about fetuses that are devastatingly miscarried through technological interventions such as amniocentesis or radiography? Would they be necro-techno-sapiens? These questions cannot be answered here, yet they open up wider possibilities for discussion on the darker side of techno-sapiens, and for a focus on what happens when technological intervention into reproduction goes awry.

References

Almond, B. 1998. The Monster Within: Mary Shelley's Frankenstein and a Patient's Fears of Childbirth and Mothering. *International Journal of Psycho-Analysis* 79(4):775–786.

Angel, G. 2013. Pulling Teeth: Ovarian Teratomas & the Myth of Vagina Dentata. *UCL Researchers in Museums Blog*, blogs.ucl.ac.uk/researchers-in-museums.

Bastien, J. 2003. Sucking Blood or Snatching Fat: Chagas Disease in Bolivia. In: *Medical Pluralism in the Andes*, eds. Koss-Chioino, J., Leatherman, T., Greenway, K. New York: Routledge, 113–128.

Bates, A. 2002. *Emblematic Monsters: The Description and Interpretation of Human Birth Defects in Europe, 1500–1700*. MD Thesis. UCL.

Bewell, A. 1988. "An Issue of Monstrous Desire": Frankenstein and Obstetrics. *Yale Journal of Criticism* 2(1):105–128.

Clynes, M., Kline, N. 1960. Cyborgs and Space. *Astronautics* 14(9):26–27.

Comaroff, J., Comaroff, J. 2002. Alien Nation: Zombies, Immigrants, and Millennial Capitalism. *South Atlantic Quarterly* 101(4):779–805.

Dumit, J., Davis-Floyd, R. 1998. Cyborg Babies: Children of the Third Millennium. In: *Cyborg Babies: From Techno-Sex to Techno-Tots*, eds. David-Floyd, R., Dumit, J. London: Routledge, 1–20.

Ewig, C. 2010. *Second-Wave Neoliberalism: Gender, Race, and Health Sector Reform in Peru*. Philadelphia, PA: Pennsylvania University Press.

Few, M. 2009. Atlantic World Monsters: Monstrous Births and the Politics of Pregnancy in Colonial Guatemala. In: *Women, Religion, and the Atlantic World (1600–1800)*, eds. Kostroun, D., Vollendorf, L. Toronto, ON: University of Toronto Press.

Guerra Reyes, L. 2019. *Changing Birth in the Andes: Culture, Policy, and Safe Motherhood in Peru*. Nashville TN: Vanderbilt University Press.

Hammer, P. 2001. Bloodmakers Made of Blood: Quechua Ethnophysiology of Menstruation. In: *Regulating Menstruation: Beliefs, Practices, Interpretations*, eds. Van de Walle, E., Renne, E. Chicago, IL: University of Chicago Press.

Irons, R. 2020. *Planning Quechua Families: Indigenous Subjectivities, Inequalities, and Kinship under the Peruvian National Family Planning Programme*. PhD Thesis. UCL.

Jackson, B. 1971. Vagina Dentata and Cystic Teratoma. *Journal of American Folklore* 84(333):341–342.

Kim, M. et al. 2011. Clinical Characteristics of Ovarian Teratoma: Age-Focused Retrospective Analysis of 580 Cases. *American Journal of Obstetrics and Gynecology* 205(1):32–32.

La Riva González, P. 2017. El Walthana Hampi o la reconstrucción del cuerpo. Concepción del embarazo en los Andes del sur de Perú. In: *Recuperando la vida: Etnografías de sanación en Perú y México*, eds. Torres, V., Anguiano, V. Lima: Ríos Profundos, 90–105.

Lauro, S. Embry, K. 2008. A Zombie Manifesto: The Nonhuman Condition in the Era of Advanced Capitalism. *Boundary 2* 35(1):85–108.

Malatino, H. 2017. Biohacking Gender. *Angelaki* 22(2):179–190.

Martin, E. 1998. The Fetus as Intruder: Mother's Bodies and Medical Metaphors. In: *Cyborg Babies: From Techno-Sex to Techno-Tots*, eds. David-Floyd, R., Dumit, J. New York: Routledge, 125–142.

Morgan, L. 1997. Imagining the Unborn in the Ecuadorian Andes. *Feminist Studies* 23(2):322–350.

Mukherjee, S. 2011. *The Emperor of All Maladies: A Biography of Cancer*. New York: Fourth Estate.

Quijano, A. 2000. Coloniality of Power, Eurocentrism, and Latin America. In: *Nepantla: Views from the South 1.3*, ed. Mignolo, W. Durham, NC: Duke University Press., 223–245.

Roberts, E. 2012. *God's Laboratory: Assisted Reproduction in the Andes*. Berkeley, CA: University of California Press.

Sanabria, E. 2016. *Plastic Bodies: Sex Hormones and Menstrual Suppression in Brazil*. Durham, NC: Duke University Press.

Stratton, J. 2011. Zombie Trouble: Zombie Texts, Bare Life and Displaced People. *European Journal of Cultural Studies* 14(3):265–281.

PART II
Imagining Techno-Holistic Reproductive Futures

11

WATER AS A TECHNOLOGY TO SUPPORT EMBODIED AUTONOMOUS BIRTHING

Kelly Kara and Suzanne Miller

Introduction: Water Immersion as a Health Technology

The World Health Organization states that "a health technology is the application of organized knowledge and skills in the form of devices, medicines, vaccines, procedures, and systems developed to solve a health problem and improve quality of lives" (WHO 2007:106). This definition fits the use of water immersion for labor and birth as a technology backed by a set of professional skills and knowledge that can greatly help with the sensations of labor, assisting in achieving a positive birthing experience and avoiding the current continual increase of interventions in labor and birth. As a counter to the technology of epidural analgesia, which can trigger a cascade of intervention, water immersion in a large tub or small inflatable pool during labor has the potential to instead function as a breakwater to the incoming tide of intervention by providing a sanctuary in which a laboring woman feels safe and private, and where opportunities to perform invasive procedures are reduced.

Water Immersion in Its Current Form

Water immersion has long been used to help with the sensations of labor and birth. Its availability varies across birth settings internationally. There is generally greater availability within midwife-led and primary birthing settings such as freestanding birth centers, and more restricted availability within biomedical facilities. Water immersion is a safe technology for use in labor, with no difference in neonatal outcomes when compared to "land births" and improved maternal outcomes, including heightened maternal satisfaction with the birthing experience (Cluett et al. 2018; Lathrop et al. 2018).

Despite this evidence, water immersion is controversial in some settings, with concern expressed that there is insufficient research to quantify maternal or perinatal benefits (AAP & ACOG 2014; ACOG 2016). The American Academy of Pediatrics (AAP) suggests that water immersion in second stage labor should be considered an "experimental procedure" with no maternal or fetal benefits, and notes concerns about the risk of neonatal infections, NICU admissions, and drowning (ibid.). However systematic reviews and observational studies (see below) have confirmed the safety of water immersion, and their authors, such as Snapp et al. (2020) note that frequently the concerns cited are based upon case reviews and isolated cases rather than quality research and meta-analysis.

Water immersion during labor is highly valued by women for pain management and for the control, comfort, and privacy it provides. When using water immersion, women say they are more in control of their labor process, able to adopt positions that feel right for them, and feel protected from the demands and potential interventions of the institution (Ulfsdottir et al. 2018). While not removing the sensations of labor as epidurals do, women report that the feelings of buoyancy, warmth, and relaxation from the water make these sensations manageable. This buoyancy and ease of movement support the upright positioning that is also key to physiologic birth (Carlsson and Ulfsdottir 2020). Maintaining upright positions such as kneeling and squatting, which optimize the pelvic diameter, is easier in water, and freedom from gravity also provides beneficial effects. The feelings of safety, privacy, and control engendered by water immersion facilitate the essential hormonal interactions of labor and birth that enhance the physiologic process and support confidence, safety, and autonomy for birthing people (Dixon et al. 2013).

Water immersion is associated with a reduction in both the duration of the first stage of labor (Cluett et al. 2018) and in the perception of pain in the second stage (Ulfsdottir et al. 2019). Unlike other birth technologies such as continuous electronic fetal monitoring (CEFM) and epidurals, which disembody childbearers from their experiences of labor and birth, water immersion supports them to be present in their bodies and in the birth space, and to actively work towards birthing their babies.

Too often within birthing, the interventive use of technologies has separated women from their bodily experiences of birth and shifted the power from women and midwives to the dominant biomedical and technocratic management of labor and birth. In many resource-rich countries, it is far more common to use epidurals for management of labor sensations than it is to use water immersion (Seijmonsbergen-Schermers et al. 2020). In the United States currently, 78% of women use epidurals for labor pain management (ibid.), whereas in other countries with strongly established midwifery systems, the epidural rate sits between a fifth and a third of birthing people (New Zealand College of Midwives [NZCOM] 2018). While epidural analgesia is effective pain relief, it is negatively associated with the woman's sense of her own abilities and satisfaction with her birth experience. It is therefore important to consider that this increasing trend may not actually be serving childbearers' needs (Ulfsdottir et al. 2019), and that it is associated with increased use of other interventions—particularly synthetic oxytocin administration due to delayed first and second stage of labor caused by epidurals (Anim-Somuah et al. 2018).

The technocratic restrictions on the availability of water immersion for labor and birth can take the form of institutional policies, accreditation requirements, or waivers that women are required to sign (Newnham et al. 2015). Evidence from Aotearoa New Zealand (now so called to acknowledge the Indigenous name for New Zealand) confirms that the use of water in labor is most common at home (27%) or in midwifery-led birth centers and small community hospitals (34%), and reduces to only 3%–7% in obstetric-led settings (NZCOM 2018). Lack of availability of water immersion is often attributed to restrictive institutional policies and a lack of tubs, but is perhaps more closely related to institutional birth cultures that value biomedical technologies over those that return the autonomy and control of the birth experience to the woman. Within these institutional cultures, it is apparent that the choice of water immersion is open to the influence of personal and professional bias, which contributes to the challenges midwives experience when supporting a woman choosing water immersion. Midwives providing continuity of care are more knowledgeable and supportive of water immersion and facilitate it more often than other birth practitioners (Plint and Davis 2016). In contrast, obstetricians in general believe that water immersion in labor and birth is risky, do not value it, and lack both the education and the confidence to work with women who make this choice (ibid.).

Restricting women's choice to use water immersion—which would grant them more autonomy—within technocratic settings demonstrates the continuing influence of patriarchy in birth. The ongoing biomedical and societal acceptance of the iatrogenic complexity associated with birth interventions demonstrates that feminist critiques of the patriarchal power inherent within biomedical birth settings continue to be valid (McAra-Couper et al. 2010). Women's decreased satisfaction associated with interventions, along with continued restrictions on supportive technologies such as water, suggests that the childbearer's voice is not being adequately valued and respected within maternity care (Downe et al. 2018).

Developments in cardiotocography (electronic fetal monitoring) technologies now mean that CEFM (telemetry) is possible with water immersion. This possibility is slowly influencing changes to water immersion guidelines in Aotearoa New Zealand. But rather than simply a change in the availability of equipment, this will also require a paradigm shift around embracing women's autonomy, the value of the birth experience, and its ongoing impacts on early parenting and family wellbeing.

Water immersion pivots the focus from obstetric risk management practices to respectful midwifery care focused on the woman's needs. Within the growing movement for humanizing birth, an environment that is private, safe, supportive, and that recognizes women's rights and need for holistic care is key (Curtin et al.

2020). Technology should be used appropriately to optimize and improve both birth outcomes *and* the experiences of those giving birth and being born. The experiences of women and babies are not *opposing* priorities but are inseparably entwined in their dyad, so both can be prioritized. We argue for the discontinuation of the current obstetric narrative that suggests that to prioritize the woman's experience is somehow risking her baby's wellbeing. As Davis-Floyd (2003:160) put it, "what is good for the mother is good for the baby"; thus the safety of the baby and the emotional needs of the mother should not be pitted against each other.

Evidence of Negative Side Effects of Technocratic Birthing Environments

The inexorable rise of birth interventions around the world over the last 50 years has not resulted in the expected decrease in adverse outcomes that increased surveillance and control over peoples' birthing bodies were predicated on. Neonatal encephalopathy and cerebral palsy rates have shown only modest decreases as a result of the near-universalization of continuous electronic fetal monitoring (CEFM), yet it is a major global cause of rising cesarean rates, as the excess of information it provides easily leads to detecting normal fetal heart rate decelerations and to assuming a non-existent danger (Alfiveric et al. 2017). Although the available evidence rejects the routine use of CEFM for well women (Gibb and Arulkumaran 2008), common practice reflects a different reality (Maude et al. 2014). As a birth technology, water immersion has the potential to mitigate against this rise in interventions by decreasing the incidence of labor dystocia (slow progress leading to artificial augmentation) and use of epidurals (Ulfsdottir et al. 2019). The short and long-term impacts of synthetic oxytocin and of epidural analgesia are now more fully appreciated, and a growing debate exists within midwifery *and* obstetrics about the harm being caused to parents and babies from these common birth practices (Bisits 2016; Newnham et al. 2017). The "too much too soon" (TMTS) and "too little too late" (TLTL) phenomena common in many countries are not serving the interests of laboring people (Miller et al. 2016). Cheyney and Davis-Floyd (Chapter 1) recommend RARTRW care—"the right amount at the right time in the right way."

The psychological and physical sequelae of women's birth experiences heavily influence their future lives and maternity choices. A negative birth experience may influence a delay or even avoidance of a subsequent pregnancy (Gotvall and Waldenstrom 2002). Post-traumatic stress disorder (PTSD) and tokophobia (fear of birth) are increasingly reported (see Chapter 9), alongside challenges to relationships between the woman and her baby, or the woman and her intimate partner, along with a reduction in her ability to meet the daily needs of her family (see Simpson and Catling 2016). Women who have experienced cesarean births also contend with having a "high risk" label for their future pregnancies, which can affect both the care available to them and their own sense of themselves as capable birthing women (Chalmers 2017).

The childbirth continuum is probably the time in a person's life when they are most often asked to share the parts of their body that relate to their sexuality with people other than their current sexual partner. This can be profoundly challenging for some. From sexual health testing procedures, to transvaginal ultrasound, vaginal examination in labor, and obstetric intervention during birth through to perineal repair and breastfeeding support, the potential for touch by "intimate strangers" is ubiquitous. Water immersion during labor presents an opportunity for increasing privacy and decreasing the imposition of physically and psychologically uncomfortable touch by reducing the need for such interventions and by adding a barrier to/distance from the potential interventionists.

How people feel about *other's* interactions with their bodies strongly shapes their sense of agency and control. Obstetric disrespect, abuse, or violence marring pregnancy and birth can have lifelong effects (Sadler et al. 2016). The actions of maternity care providers can affect peoples' sense of agency and control, with implications for their ongoing sexual and psychological well-being beyond the childbirth continuum. The term "birthrape" (Kitzinger 2006) describes the situation where unconsented procedures occur during birth, perpetrated by healthcare providers. The term itself stirs strong emotional responses. As one mother said "People disagree that [birthrape] is sexual…that's where people end up being heated. But the way I felt was that it was a sexual thing. It deals with your sexual organs." A birth trauma worker summed it up: "The people that should be concerned about naming obstetric violence 'birth rape' should be the perpetrators. Women get to define their experience" (Pencz 2012). Water immersion can be an effective deterrent against birthrape.

Addressing the physical sequelae of cesareans, which water immersion can often prevent, a subsequent pregnancy may be more likely to include placental complications, sub- or infertility, or even stillbirth (see Goer and Romano 2013). Disturbances to the development of the neonatal microbiome are reported (Dahlen et al. 2013; Almgren et al. 2014). Neonatal gut colonization (the microbiome) is in part stimulated by contact with the mother's vaginal micro-organisms during vaginal birth. These organisms are implicated in long-term health, and an increase in the development of asthma, obesity, and gastrointestinal disease (e.g. Kristensen and Henriksen 2016) is noted when these beneficial gut flora are not collected by the fetus during cesarean birth (as also explained in Chapter 9).

Epigenetic research is the new frontier in terms of our understanding of the negative sequelae of common birth interventions. When labor unfolds physiologically, the orchestration of *endogenous* oxytocin (with other hormones) ensures a smooth transition through labor and into early mothering, optimizing maternal-infant interaction and establishing an environment for successful lactation and early neonatal life (Buckley 2015). With the *exogenous* administration of synthetic oxytocin, neuroendocrine mechanisms are triggered because exogenous oxytocin is released directly into the brain, while endogenous oxytocin in the woman's circulation does not cross the blood–brain barrier (Uvnas-Moberg et al. 2019). Epigenetic research is focusing on the implications of disruption to the oxytocin system of both women and neonates arising from exogenous oxytocin use.

More than half of all women in technocratic birth settings are exposed to synthetic oxytocin during induction and augmentation of labor (Miller 2020). "DNA methylation" is the process by which methyl groups are added to a DNA molecule, altering the activity of the DNA sequence (Moore et al. 2013). Disturbances to this process caused by synthetic oxytocin use may result in gene expression disruption by "silencing" gene transcription. This modification of oxytocin receptors may play role in social, behavioral, and emotional disorders (Plothe 2010; Dahlen et al. 2013; Bell et al. 2014). The first contact a maturing hormone receptor has with its target hormone determines the binding capacity of that receptor for life. Flooding the oxytocin receptors within the uterine musculature during birth produces down-regulation of oxytocin receptors (Phaneuf et al. 2000); in a fetus exposed to synthetic oxytocin during birth, this receptor saturation may result in faulty imprinting, with lifelong consequences such as those associated with disturbed maternal-infant attachment and adverse social behaviors (Bell et al. 2014).

The neuroscience community remains uncertain about the extent to which exogenous oxytocin can breach the "leaky" fetal neurovascular unit—the blood/brain barrier (Ek, Dziegielewska et al. 2012; Saunders et al. 2012; Kenkel et al. 2014), but there is more certainty about synthetic oxytocin crossing the placenta (Bell et al. 2014). Several studies have examined links between synthetic oxytocin use and cognitive spectrum disorders such as autism and attention deficit hyperactivity disorder (ADHD), with some reporting increased incidence (Wahl 2004; Weisman et al. 2015) while others deny a link (Guastella et al. 2018). Irrespective of where the scientific consensus ultimately arrives, it is clear that there might be potentially harmful outcomes for women and babies associated with such widespread synthetic oxytocin use, including the associated over-stimulation of the uterus, which can lead to fetal asphyxia (Hayes et al. 2013).

Water immersion in labor is linked with decreased rates of labor dystocia, and therefore can mitigate against the use of exogenous oxytocin. Other benefits include the possible reduction of Group B strep colonization in the baby (Zanetti-Dallenbach et al. 2007), and birth in water does not appear to disturb the development of the neonatal microbiome (Fehevary et al. 2004; Combellick et al. 2018). A minimization of "birthrape" via a reduction in the number of (usually painful and disruptive) vaginal examinations, known to occur when women labor in water, also reduces the likelihood of disturbance to the vaginal micro-organisms from the use of chlorhexidine-based lubricants on the practitioner's gloves (McElroy and Regan 2016).

Our developing understanding of the evidence about both short- and long-term health impacts of common birth interventions makes it essential that all birth attendants prioritize supporting safe physiologic birth and facilitating emotionally satisfying birth experiences. In the future, we envision that it will no longer be acceptable to minimize or dismiss the use of "low" technologies like water immersion that improve the woman's experience in preference to those high technologies that provide practitioners and their medico-legal teams and insurance companies with increased comfort. Given that telemetry (CEFM) can be used in water, it need not be "and/or"—it can be "both/both"—an example of obstetric technologies as "flexible helpers" whose meanings are generated in practice, as described by Skeide in Chapter 15. While water immersion has enormous potential to de-escalate the TMTS cascade of interventions, and despite the concerns associated with many birth interventions, the use of water as a technology for supporting even complex labors holds promise as a way to minimize interventions and interference and improve women's experiences.

Water Immersion in Complex Pregnancy in Aotearoa New Zealand

Our qualitative descriptive study used interviews to explore the experiences of 7 women with complex pregnancies who negotiated to use water immersion for their labors and births within the hospital setting, despite this contravening current water immersion guidelines. These women identified their use of water immersion as a conscious and determined choice that they negotiated as a response to previous negative experiences of hospital birth. Most women in the study had previously birthed within "high-tech/low touch" hospital environments as characterized by Davis-Floyd (2018:34) and shared that they were left dissatisfied and at times traumatized by their birth experiences. They reported that the use of CEFM, IVs, augmentation of labor with synthetic oxytocin, and epidurals had left them feeling separated from their support people, trapped on the birthing bed, and disembodied from the process of birthing their baby. In other words, these women felt their needs were usurped by the requirements of technological surveillance.

In cyborg birth, physiology and technology often compete during the birth process. This phenomenon is perfectly described as the "1-2 Punch" effect of technological mutilation and prosthesis described in the Introduction and in Chapter 1 of this volume, where technology is firstly applied to alter/mutilate a natural process, and is secondly required to prosthetically fix the problems caused by this mutilation.

The women in our study also identified that in their previous births, they had trusted that by following the recommendations of their providers as passive recipients of care, they would receive a safe and satisfying birthing experience. Yet this was rarely the case, and these women were dissatisfied with the care and support that they had received. In contrast, in their most recent births, our interlocutors used water immersion as an active strategy to reduce the possibility of unwarranted intervention into their birthing journeys. These women were informed and knowledgeable about the risks of early intervention in labor and the common cascade of interventions. They also recognized that privacy, safety, and a feeling of control were important to them and felt that water immersion would support these aims. Shani explained:

> If I'm in a bath, I can't really have an epidural, well…then I probably can't go down the line of forceps. I just didn't want anything to get away from me really in terms of intervention. I didn't want any, which I was lucky enough not to need any. But, I was like ok, if we start with water then it starts to make a lot of those early interventions more difficult to do.

As a result of using water immersion for their labors and births, the women in our study were overwhelmingly positive about their labor experiences. They noted that being in the water supported them to feel in control, made the sensations of labor manageable, and generally supported them to labor in ways that worked for their bodies (see Figure 11.1). They described feelings of privacy within their birthing space, in contrast to their previous experiences of feeling exposed and observed throughout. These women had been concerned that their next birth would also involve exposure and the loss of their dignity. They shared that it had been a relief to come to the end of their birthing journey with feelings of safety, privacy, and joy. Being an involved and active participant in their birthing process was valued by these women, as was the feeling of being capable, strong mothers moving forwards into their parenting journey. Renee exclaimed,

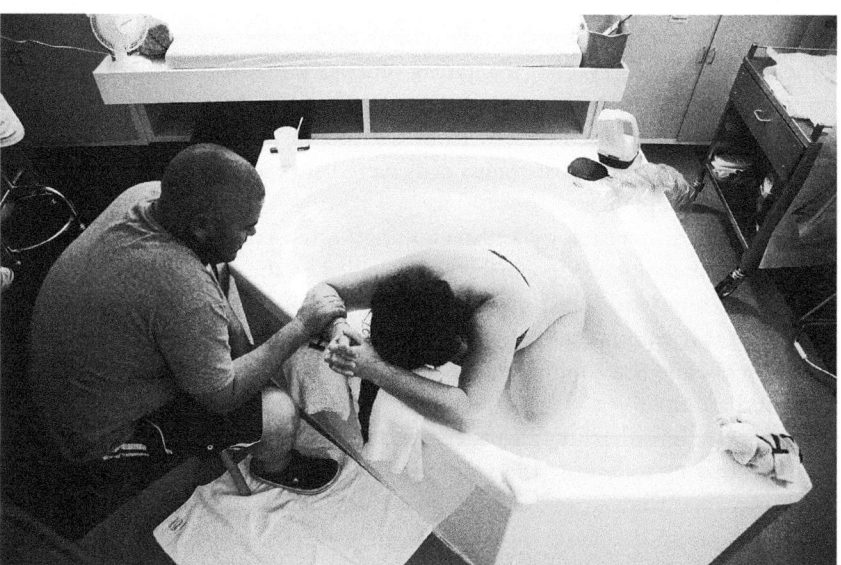

FIGURE 11.1 A water labor in Aotearoa New Zealand. Photo by Sharon Thompson, used with the permission of all involved.

"It was so raw and beautiful and I was on a high from it… There is something so healing about childbirth."

These women identified that continuity of care from a known midwife throughout their pregnancy and birth was vital in supporting their ability to make and negotiate this choice. They viewed this continuity as integral in the development of a shared understanding of previous experiences and birthing priorities with their midwife. Women also noted that their midwife supported their decision making by providing literature, support groups, and advocacy when needed to foster their informed decision making around the use of water immersion.

The "partnership model" of midwifery care (Guilliland and Pairman 1995) is an underpinning philosophy of midwifery practice in Aotearoa New Zealand and was valued by the women in this study. This model, based on shared decision making and a core belief in women's right to be actively involved participants in their maternity care, supported the women to negotiate the choice of water immersion with their midwives, who were then able to advocate for this choice in the hospital despite the institutional challenges to that choice.

Conclusion: The Future as It Needs to Be

As we move towards a future of birth that incorporates this knowledge, it becomes professionally unacceptable to take a one-dimensional view of safety in birth based upon neonatal outcomes. The psychological and physical wellbeing of the mother can no longer be viewed, even sub-consciously, as a "nice-to-have" within an otherwise disempowering birthing process. Therefore, the expectation will be that birth attendants will prioritize wellbeing in all its facets rather than physical outcomes above all others.

Humanistic maternity care, with the use of technology to *enhance* the birthing experience, will be viewed as an essential aspect of the expected skills, professionalism, and ethical responsibility of birth practitioners. The benefits of humanistic care are already known, with both midwives and obstetricians recognizing the value of care that promotes the woman's psychological wellbeing alongside her physical wellbeing (Chalmers 2017; Curtin et al. 2020). There are also professional benefits to providing this kind of care, including increased job satisfaction, increased esteem in their profession and practice, and increased confidence to change practice in humanistic, woman-centered ways.

As it is currently expected that all professionals who work in the birth arena have the skills and knowledge to manage clinical emergencies such as postpartum hemorrhage and neonatal resuscitation, it will become a professional imperative that their skills broaden to reduce medicalization of birth and include physiology-promoting technologies such as water immersion and upright (including all-fours) positions for birth. All birth practitioners must embrace the body of knowledge and essential skill set that includes the ability to support, prioritize, and promote physiologic birthing and holistic birth care that enhances childbearers' and families' wellbeing.

As a part of this commitment, birth technologies that foster emotional satisfaction, safety, women's sense of protagonism, and physiologic birth will be taught in the education curricula of all maternity care professionals. It will no longer be acceptable for any such professional to lack an understanding of supportive birth technologies. Within all birth settings, the ability to facilitate emotionally satisfying experiences where the woman is in a position of power and her autonomy will be prioritized. In hospitals with sufficient resources, this will mean the universal provision of large tubs or small pools within birthing spaces for laboring people to use at *their* desire and discretion.

Rather than water immersion being framed as an "alternative other" within biomedical birth settings, it will be viewed as simply another option that women can choose as part of their usual personal decision making in birth and valued as a breakwater against a tide of unnecessary interventions. Telemetry for fetal monitoring in water will become widely available; its non-invasive use will satisfy legal and other needs for information about fetal status. Birthing women will thus still be surveilled, but that surveillance will be much less intrusive, and interventions, even in high-risk pregnancies, will be fewer due to the physiologic and emotional relaxation and sense of privacy that water immersion can provide.

The cost savings of water immersion that will accompany the associated decrease in interventions such as labor augmentations and epidurals, and the evidence of its safety, will mean that the implementation of change will have no logical barriers. The requirement for signed acknowledgment by women of the limitations of water immersion and accreditation for health professionals will no longer exist, as it will be recognized that rather than being evidence-based, these requirements are merely an explicit demonstration of professional bias. Given the evidence of emotional trauma associated with the TMTS ("too much too soon") cascade of interventions within current technocratic hospital settings, in the future, humanistic maternity care with the use of technologies that enhance the woman's abilities and foster a positive experience of birth will become an ethical and professional responsibility (see Figure 11.2).

This aligns with the futuristic priority of all birth attendants to support women to exit their birth experience with confidence and satisfaction that carry them forward into their parenting journey. The birthing journey will not be seen as isolated from the rest of life, but rather as a launchpad to their early journey as parents and as a family. The recognition that a traumatic birthing experience can negatively influence the course of the early years within the family will provide impetus to health professionals to prioritize the woman as a holistic being who needs to emerge from her birthing experience feeling safe, satisfied, and empowered. When maternity carers support the transformation from *techno*-obstetrics to *eco*-obstetrics, everyone becomes a winner. As we move further along our path of becoming techno-sapiens, we must ensure that this brave new species we are creating is imbued with the human characteristics of compassion, respect, and love.

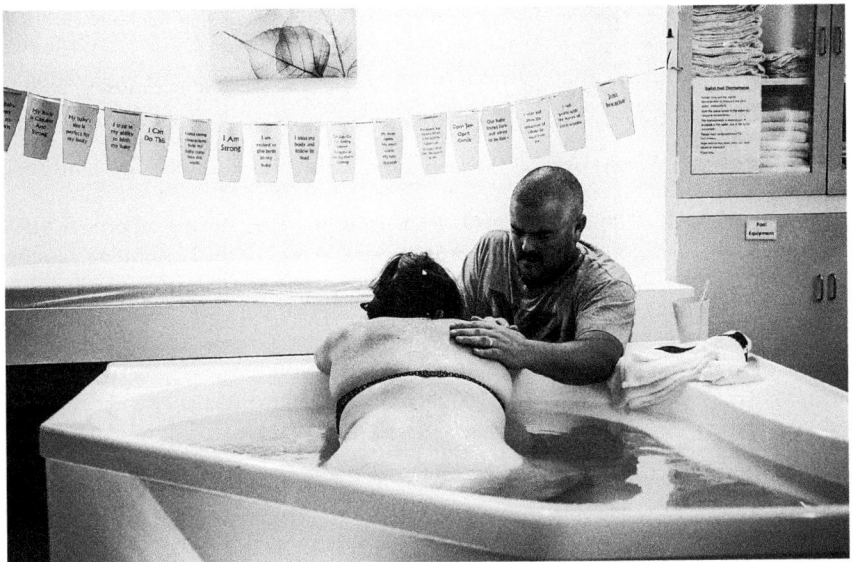

FIGURE 11.2 Photo by Sharon Thompson, used with the permission of all involved.

References

Alfirevic Z, Gyte GML, Cuthbert A, Devane D. 2017. Continuous cardiotocography as a form of electronic fetal monitoring for fetal assessment during labour. *Cochrane Database of Systematic Reviews* 4.

Almgren M, Schlinzig T, Gomez-Cabrero D et al. 2014. Cesarean delivery and hematopoietic stem cell epigenetics in the newborn infant: Implications for future health? *American Journal of Obstetrics and Gynecology* 211(502):e1–8. https://doi.org/10.1016/j.ajog.2014.05.014

American Academy of Pediatrics Committee on Fetus and Newborn, & American College of Obstetricians and Gynecologists Committee on Obstetric Practice, American College of Obstetricians and Gynecologists Committee on Obstetric Practice. 2014. Immersion in water during labor and delivery. *Pediatrics* 133(4):758–761. https://doi.org/10.1542/peds.2013-3794

American College of Obstetricians and Gynecologists & Committee on Obstetric Practice. 2016. Committee opinion no. 679: Immersion in water during labor and delivery. *Obstetrics and Gynecology* 128(5):e231. https://doi.org/10.1097/acog.0000000000001771

Anim-Soumah M, Smythe R, Cyna A, Cuthbert A. 2018. Epidural versus non-epidural or no analgesia for pain management in labour. *Cochrane Database of Systematic Reviews* 2018 (5): Art. No.: CD000331. DOI: 10.1002/14651858.CD000331.pub4.

Bell A, Erikson E, Carter S. 2014. Beyond labor: The role of natural and synthetic oxytocin in the transition to motherhood. *Journal of Midwifery and Women's Health* 59(1):35–42. https://doi.org/10.1111/jmwh.12101

Bisits A. 2016. Risk in obstetrics—Perspectives and reflections. *Midwifery* 38:12–13. https://doi.org/10.1016/j.midw.2016.05.010

Buckley S. 2015. Executive summary of hormonal physiology of childbearing: Evidence and implications for women, babies, and maternity care. *Journal of Perinatal Education* 24(3):145–153. http:/doi.org/10.1891/1058-1243.24.3.145

Carlsson T, Ulfsdottir H. 2020. Waterbirth in low-risk pregnancy: An exploration of women's experiences. *Journal of Advanced Nursing* 76(5):1221–1231. https://doi.org/10.1111/jan.14336

Chalmers B. 2017. *Family-Centred Perinatal Care*. Cambridge: Cambridge University Press.

Cluett ER, Burns E, Cuthbert A. 2018. Immersion in water during labor and birth. *Cochrane Database of Systematic Reviews* 5. https://doi.org/10.1002/14651858.cd000111.pub4

Combellick J, Shin H, Shin D, Cai Y, Hagan H, Lacher C, Lin D McCauley K, Lynch S, Dominguez-Bello MG. 2018. Differences in the fetal microbiota of neonates born at home or in the hospital. *Scientific Reports* 8:15660 DOI:10.1038/s41598-018-33995-7

Curtin M, Savage E, Leahy-Warren P. 2020. Humanisation in pregnancy and childbirth: A concept analysis. *Journal of Clinical Nursing* 29(9–10):1744–1757. https://doi.org/10.1111/jocn.15152

Dahlen H, Kennedy H, Anderson C et al. 2013. The EPIIC hypothesis: Intrapartum effects on the neonatal epigenome and consequent health outcomes. *Medical Hypotheses* 80(5):656–662. https://doi.org/10.1016/j.mehy.2013.01.017

Davis-Floyd R. 2003. *Birth as an American Rite of Passage*. Berkeley: University of California Press.

Davis-Floyd R. 2018. *Ways of Knowing about Birth: Mothers, Midwives, Medicine, and Birth Activism*. Long Grove, IL: Waveland Press.

Dixon L, Skinner J, Foureur M. 2013. The emotional and hormonal pathways of labor and birth: Integrating mind, body and behavior. *New Zealand College of Midwives Journal* 48:15–23. https://doi.org/10.12784/nzcomjnl48.2013.3.15-23

Downe S, Finlayson K, Oladapo O, Bonet M, Gülmezoglu AM. 2018. What matters to women during childbirth: A systematic qualitative review. *PLOS ONE* 13(4):e0194906. https://doi.org/10.1371/journal.pone.0194906

Ek C, Dziegielewska K, Habgood M, Saunders N. 2012. Barriers in the developing brain and neurotoxicology. *Neurotoxicology* 33(3):586–604. http://doi.org/10.1016/j.neuro.2011.12.009

Fehevary P, Lauinger-Lorsch E, Hof H, Melchert F, Bauer L, Zieger W. 2004. Water birth: Microbial colonisation of the newborn, neonatal and maternal infection rate in comparison to conventional bed deliveries. *Archives of Gynecology and Obstetrics* 270:6–9. DOI: 10.1007/s00404-002-0467-4

Gibb and Arulkumaran. 2008. *Fetal Monitoring in Practice*. Elsevier.

Goer H, Roman A. 2013. *Optimal Care in Childbirth*. London: Pinter and Martin Ltd.

Gottvall K, Waldenstrom U. 2002. Does a traumatic birth experience have an impact on future reproduction? *BJOG: An International Journal of Obstetrics and Gynaecology* 109(3):254–260. https://doi.org/10.1097/00006254-200209000-00004

Guastella A, Cooper M, White C, White M, Pennell C, Whitehouse A. 2018. Does perinatal exposure to exogenous oxytocin influence child behavioural problems and autistic-like behaviours to 20 years of age? *Journal of Child Psychology and Psychiatry, and Allied Disciplines* 59(12):1323–1332. https://doi.org/10.1111/jcpp.12924

Guilliland K, Pairman S. 1995/1. *The Midwifery Partnership: A Model for Practice*. Wellington: Department of Nursing and Midwifery, Victoria University of Wellington.

Hayes B, McGarvey C, Mulvany S, Kennedy J, Geary MD, Matthews T, King M. 2013. A case-control study of hypoxic-ischemic encephalopathy in newborn infants at >36 weeks gestation. *American Journal of Obstetrics and Gynecology* 209(29):e1–19. http://doi .org/10.1016/j.ajog.2013.03.023

Kenkel W, Yee J, Carter S. 2014. Is oxytocin a maternal–foetal signalling molecule at birth? Implications for development. *Journal of Neuroendocrinology* 26(10):739–749. https://doi.org/10.1111/jne.12186

Kitzinger S. 2006. Birth as rape: There must be an end to "just in case" obstetrics. *British Journal of Midwifery* 14(9):544–545. https://doi.org/10.12968/bjom.2006.14 .9.21799

Kristensen K, Henriksen L. 2016. Cesarean section and disease associated with immune function. *Journal of Allergy and Clinical Immunology* 137(2):587–590. https://doi.org/10 .1016/j.jaci.2015.07.040

Lathrop A, Bonsack CF, Haas DM. 2018. Women's experiences with water birth: A matched groups prospective study. *Birth* 45(4):416–423. https://doi.org/10.1111/birt .12362

Maude R, Skinner J, Foureur M. 2014. Intelligent Structured Intermittent Auscultation (ISIA): Evaluation of a decision-making framework for fetal heart monitoring of low-risk women. *BMC Pregnancy and Childbirth* 14(1):184–197. DOI: 10.1186/1471-2393-14-184

McAra-Couper J, Jones M, Smythe E. 2010. Rising rates of intervention in childbirth. *British Journal of Midwifery* 18(3):160–169. https://doi.org/10.12968/bjom.2010.18.3. 46917

McElroy K, Rean M. 2016. Vaginal microbiota and lubricant use during labor: Implications for nursing, research, practice and policy. *SAGE Open Nursing* 2:1–8. DOI: 10.1177/237796081 6662286

Miller S. 2020. *"Moving Things Forward": Birthing Suite Culture and Labour Augmentation for Healthy First-Time Mothers* (Unpublished PhD thesis). Wellington: Victoria University of Wellington.

Miller S, Abalos E, Chamillard M et al. 2016. Beyond too little, too late and too much, too soon: A pathway towards evidence-based, respectful maternity care worldwide. *Lancet* 388(10056):2176–2192. https://doi.org/10.1016/s0140-6736(16)31 472-6

Moore l, Le T, Fan G. 2013. DNA methylation and its basic function. *Neuropsychopharmacology: Official Publication of the American College of Neuropsychopharmacology* 38(1): 23–38. https://doi.org/10.1038/npp.2012.112

Newnham EC, McKellar LV, Pincombe JI. 2015. Documenting risk: A comparison of policy and information pamphlets for using epidural or water in labor. *Women and Birth: Journal of the Australian College of Midwives* 28(3):221–227. https://doi.org/10.1 016/j.wombi.2015.01.012

Newnham EC, McKellar LV, Pincombe JI. 2017. Paradox of the institution: Findings from a hospital labor ward ethnography. *BMC Pregnancy and Childbirth* 17(1):2. https ://doi.org/10.1186/s12884-016-1193-4

New Zealand College of Midwives (NZCOM). 2018. *MMPO Report on New Zealand's MMPO Midwives: Care Activities and Outcomes.* Christchurch: NZCOM

Pencz B. 2012. *Unhappy Birthdays, Part 2. The Politics of "Birth Rape" and Mothers with PTSD.* www.vancouverobserver.com/blogs/feminista/2012/05/08/unhappy-birt hdays-part-2-politics-birth-rape-and-mothers-ptsd

Phaneuf S, Rodríguez Liñares B, TambyRaja [stet]R, MacKenzie IZ, López Bernal A. 2000. Loss of myometrial oxytocin receptors during oxytocin-induced and oxytocin-augmented labor. *Journal of Reproduction and Fertility* 120(1):91–97. https://doi.org/10 .1530/reprod/120.1.91

Plint E, Davis D. 2016. Sink or swim: Water immersion for labour and birth in a tertiary maternity unit in Australia. *International Journal of Childbirth* 6(40):206–222. DOI 10.1891/2156-5287.6.4.206

Plothe C. 2010. The perinatal application of synthetic oxytocin and its possible influence on the human psyche and the etiology of autism. *Journal of Prenatal and Perinatal Psychology and Health* 25(2):89–105.

Sadler M, Mário JD, Santos S, Ruiz-Berdún D, Skoko E, Gillen P, Clausen JA. 2016. Moving beyond disrespect and abuse: Addressing the structural dimensions of obstetric violence. *Reproductive Health Matters* 24(47):47–55.

Saunders N, Liddelow S, Dziegielewska K. 2012. Barrier mechanisms in the developing brain. *Frontiers in Pharmacology* 3(46):1–18. https://doi.org/10.3389/fphar.2012.00046

Seijmonsbergen-Schermers AE, van den Akker T, Rydahl E et al. 2020. Variations in use of childbirth interventions in 13 high-income countries: A multinational cross-sectional study. *PLOS Medicine* 17(5):e1003103. https://doi.org/10.1371/journal.pmed.1003103

Simpson M, Catling C. 2016. Understanding psychological traumatic birth experiences: A literature review. *Women and Birth: Journal of the Australian College of Midwives* 29(3):203–207. http://doi.org/10.1016/j.wombi.2015.10.009

Snapp C, Stapleton SR, Wright J, Niemczyk NA, Jolles D. 2020. The experience of land and water birth within the American Association of Birth Centers Perinatal Data Registry, 2012–2017. *The Journal of Perinatal and Neonatal Nursing* 34(1):16–26. https://doi.org/10.1097/JPN.0000000000000450

Ulfsdottir H, Saltvedt S, Ekborn M, Georgsson S. 2018. Like an empowering micro-home: A qualitative study of women's experience of giving birth in water. *Midwifery* 67:26–31. https://doi.org/10.1016/j.midw.2018.09.004

Ulfsdottir H, Saltvedt S, Georgsson S. 2019. Women's experiences of waterbirth compared with conventional uncomplicated births. *Midwifery* 79:102547. https://doi.org/10.1016/j.midw.2019.102547

Uvnäs-Moberg K, Ekström-Bergström A, Berg M et al. 2019. Maternal plasma levels of oxytocin during physiological childbirth—A systematic review with implications for uterine contractions and central actions of oxytocin. *BMC Pregnancy and Childbirth* 19(1):285. https://doi.org/10.1186/s12884-019-2365-9

Wahl R. 2004. Could oxytocin administration during labor contribute to autism and related behavioral disorders?—A look at the literature. *Medical Hypotheses* 63(3):456–460. https://doi.org/10.1016/j.mehy.2004.03.008

Weisman O, Agerbo E, Carter C et al. 2015. Oxytocin-augmented labor and risk for autism in males. *Behavioural Brain Research* 284:207–212. https://doi.org/10.1016/j.bbr.2015.02.028

World Health Organization. 2007. *World Health Assembly WHA60.29 Health Technologies.* www.who.int/healthsystems/WHA60_29.pdf

Zanetti-Dallenbach R, Lapaire O, Holzgreve W, Hosli I. 2007. Neonatal colonization-rate with Group B Streptococcus is lower in neonates born underwater than after conventional vaginal delivery. *Geburtsh Frauenheilk* 67(10):1114–1119.

12

THE BIRTH OF A NEW HUMAN BEING:

The Utopian Project of the Late Soviet Waterbirth Movement and Its Inheritors

Anna Ozhiganova

Introduction: Igor Charkovsky and the Aquaculture Project

In the spring of 2018, people on the beach of the popular Egyptian resort Dahab accidentally witnessed an amazing event—the birth of a child into the Red Sea—which became famous thanks to the photos published in *Cosmopolitan* magazine (2018). A pregnant woman entered the sea, and soon her husband and an elderly man carried ashore a newborn and a placenta with an attached umbilical cord. The elderly man was later recognized as Igor Charkovsky, the creator of the Russian waterbirth method called "Aquaculture." In recent years, he has been living permanently in Israel and from time to time has come to Egypt at the request of his followers to attend births and train babies to swim.

Igor Charkovsky and His "Aquaculture" Project: A Brief History

In order to understand what happened in 2018 on that Egyptian beach, we need to return to Moscow in the early 1960s. In 1962–1964, Charkovsky, then a student at the Institute of Physical Culture and Sports, started swimming with his daughter, who was born premature. He trained his daughter to swim at home in an ordinary bathtub from the first days of her life, and when she reached 7 months of age, in the *Moskva* Pool (Moscow Pool) (for a time the world's largest open air swimming pool), where he worked as a lifeguard. The little girl spent many hours in water, where she ate, slept, dove for toys, and watched filmstrips projected onto the pool wall. Ten years later, in 1974, an article called "Amphibian Girl" dedicated to these workouts, which demonstrated the success of aquatic rehabilitation of premature babies, was published in the newspaper *Soviet Sport*, in the section "Swimming before Walking." Charkovsky's words about water birth were also quoted there:

> Birth on the land is unfavorable for newborns because they are immediately exposed to the powerful effects of gravity. You can get rid of this enemy only in two environments—in space and in water. There's no need to talk about space yet, but water is nearby. (Quoted in Schenkman 1974:36)

In subsequent years, several more articles about the ideas and experiments of Igor Charkovsky, who had already become a research fellow in the laboratory of the All-Union Scientific Research Institute of Physical Culture and Sports (VNIIFK), were published in various Russian popular magazines. The then-Director of VNIIIFK, Professor I. Ratov, supported these studies of "the perspectives to influence human evolution" (Korop 1972a:47). Charkovsky conducted experiments with land insects and animals—flies, cockroaches, hens, mice, and cats—and found that the fear of water could be overcome through training, which was especially effective for animal newborns. He also discovered that if the newborns were transferred to *aquatic* mothers (for example, chickens to ducks, kittens to nutria), they began to lead an aquatic lifestyle and acquired various advantages: large size, great strength and endurance, and high life expectancy (Korop 1972a:44). Then he claimed that a fetus was an aquatic animal because it was swimming in the amniotic fluid, and proposed to conduct an experiment with a childbirth into the sea near a flock of dolphins:

> Maybe dolphin milk, which is especially high in fat and designed for an aquatic lifestyle, is suitable for a baby. The instinct will make our newborn hold on tightly to the dolphin, and the oncoming water-air flow will turn on thousands of "micro reflectors" on the baby's sensitive body, so the baby will automatically take the most optimal pose with the lowest possible resistance to the aquatic environment. (Quoted in Korop 1972b:47)

Many Soviet people were inspired by these ideas, despite the fact that they sounded like science fiction, and no babies were actually breastfed by dolphins. Tatyana Sargunas recalls how she heard Charkovsky speak for the first time in 1982, saying "Today, psychics from Australia called me and said that the dolphins gave their permission for ocean childbirth" (Interview 1). Tatyana and her husband Alexei Sargunas became active followers of Charkovsky: they gave birth to 3 children at home in water, founded a childbirth preparation center, and helped many couples with their home births.

A professional midwife, Irina Martynova, met Charkovsky in 1978 and immediately started preparing the experiment about which he had long dreamed—a water birth. They organized a home mini-maternity hospital where two aquariums were installed: the large one was supposed to serve for labor and the smaller one for birth. The main idea was that a baby should be born into the water and remain underwater while the umbilical cord was still pulsating, providing the newborn with oxygen-rich blood. In the fall of 1979, a group of five pregnant women-volunteers was formed, and the first delivery into the water happened

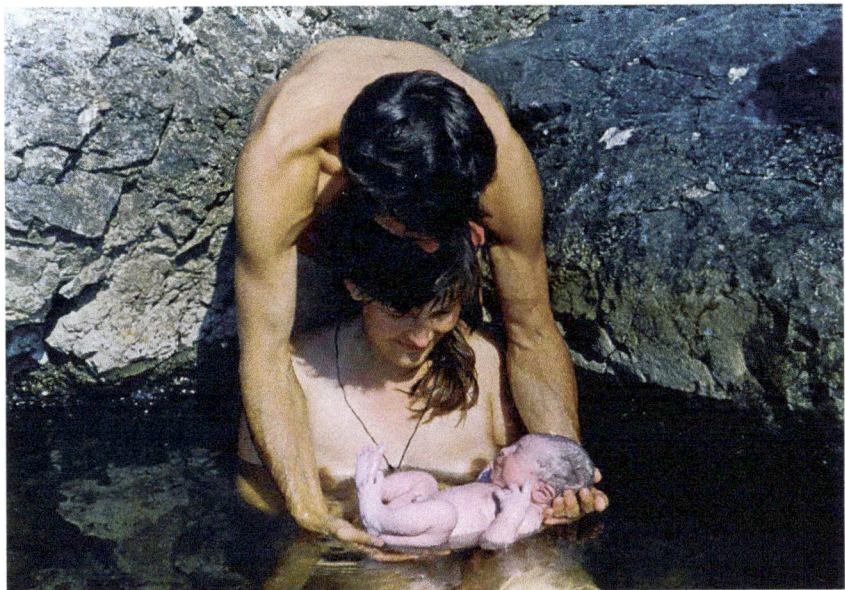

FIGURE 12.1   The birth of Eya Bagriansky. Black Sea, Crimea, Sudak, Alchak mountain, July 22, 1986. © Vladimir Bagriansky. Used with permission.

in the spring of 1980 under the supervision of Charkovsky and Martynova. Although water birth remained a very rare event for the next several years, Martynova (2017) claimed that there, "the secret revolution in obstetrics began."

In 1986, the first ocean birth took place in Crimea: a girl, named Eya, was born to the Bagryansky family (see Figure 12.1). This event happened without Charkovsky's participation; Tatyana Sargunas helped the mother in childbirth, and Alexey Sargunas shot this event with an amateur movie camera. These shots were subsequently included in the film "Igor Charkovsky—An Impossible Dream" (1989). Vladimir Bagryansky (2011) described the sea birth of his daughter as "the spiritual revival of nature and transition from the old to the new life."

In 1988, Charkovsky's follower Marina Dadasheva assisted in a water birth in a maternity hospital in the Siberian city of Tomsk (Interview 2). Although official permission was obtained for this demonstration and the delivery was successful, this event did not affect obstetric practice. Water birth appeared in the practice of maternity hospitals only in the second half of the 1990s as a new "Western" trend.

The "Aquaculture" Project as a Human Enhancement Utopia

In her dissertation about the "Aquaculture" method, Belousova (2012:84) notes that it is possible to trace the origins of Charkovsky's ideas back to the lineage of "Russian cosmists"—philosophers of cosmic evolution: Nikolay Fedorov,

Konstantin Tsiolkovsky, and Vladimir Vernadsky. She also connects Charkovsky with Soviet science fiction, particularly with the novel *Amphibian Man* (1928) by Alexander Belyaev, which was very popular among Soviet readers. John Lilly's book *Man and Dolphin*, which was published in Russian in 1965, likely also served as a source of inspiration for Charkovsky. Additionally, many of his ideas resemble quotes from the book *Homo Delphinus: The Dolphin Within Man* (published in Russian in 1987) by the famous French diver Jacques Mayol, known for his mystical approach to dolphins. Charkovsky himself did not write anything; his method was implemented in practice. Yet the ideas of Aquaculture certainly correspond to the utopian cognitive style that Karl Mannheim (1979:173) defined as "transcendent": incongruous with the state of reality within which it occurs and at the same time "breaks the bond of the existing order."

Some critics of Charkovsky claim that he did not come up with anything new, and even claimed that he borrowed the idea of water birth from the French obstetrician Michel Odent, who had put baths and pools into obstetric practice in the 1970s in Pithiviers, France. Some students of Charkovsky, on the contrary, argue that it was the "Russian method of home waterbirth" that later spread around the world. In fact, these methods were initially completely different. Odent (1984) suggested using water only for pain relief during contractions and even recommended that women in labor get out of the pool to give birth to facilitate the "fetus ejection reflex." Water technology was fully integrated into his approach, which was focused on the physiologic and emotional needs of women. In contrast, the emphasis of the Aquaculture method was on the child, insisting that being born in water would provide great advantages. Thus, Aquaculture was a human enhancement project.

The current discussion in bioethics has concluded that human enhancement—the attempt to improve human cognitive, emotional, and physical capacities through technological means—has been part of the human condition right from the beginning (Kourany 2014:981). People often dream of overcoming their body and mind limitations, expanding their abilities, and living longer, healthier, and more productive lives. However, the emergence of new classes of enhancements—pharmacological, cybernetic, genetic, and nanotechnological—is often perceived as a threat to humankind. Critics have said that these technologies "not only introduce unnatural structures, but they do so in order to produce unnatural results—characteristics or abilities that go beyond the normal or species-typical function" (Kourany 2014:984). So, such new and increasingly possible enhancements, unlike the old ones provided by education, training, and healthy lifestyle, are considered *unnatural* and part of the creation of humans as cyborgs.

However, is it possible to make a clear distinction between human enhancement via nurture and learning and its radical transformations or transmutations? What could be the principles of such a distinction: the difference in aims or in means such as technologies? When we talk about childbirth technology, we usually mean the intervention of biomedical technologies into the normal physiologic process. However, could the idea of natural, demedicalized childbirth form a kind of technology, the goal of which is the radical transformation of a human being? Charkovsky believed that with the help of a special technology—the use of water in tubs or in bodies of water like lakes or oceans, it is possible to give birth to a special human being—a baby-dolphin, a mutant with a dual nature: sapiens and animal. Could we call water birth "natural" if it aims for the emergence of post-humans—creatures with enhanced or supernatural abilities? What is the role of the mother in these experiments: does she possess subjectivity, or is she objectified, with her task being only to provide the necessary conditions for the birth of a new (post-) human being? Donna Haraway (2016:11) showed that the idea of human mutants, creatures with human-animal origins, elides the dichotomy of human/non-human and prepares the emergence of cyborgs: "The cyborg appears in myth precisely where the boundary between human and animal is transgressed." We may also wonder: what kind of a human being is "disassembled and reassembled" in the Aquaculture project, and is that human already a kind of cyborg?

Considering the history of the Russian homebirth movement, I rely on my field research, which I started in 2015 and have continued to the present. My field materials include over 70 interviews with homebirth midwives and women who gave birth outside hospitals. In this chapter, I quote only 7 of them—including the first followers of Charkovsky (Tatyana Sargunas, Vladimir Bagrianski, Marina Dadasheva, and Margarita Razenkova) and well-known homebirth midwives (Natalia Kotlar, Julia Postnova, and Svetlana Akimova), who were already students of Sargunas and Dadasheva (see the *List of Interviews* below).

Supermoms: Giving Birth to a New Kind of Human Being

"Aqua-Mothers": Techniques of Conduct and Counter-Conduct

Special preparation for childbirth was an important part of the Aquaculture method. Charkovsky believed that aqua training—swimming and diving—would help women to overcome their "instinctive fear of water." At the same time, these workouts were aimed at the prenatal preparation of infants: "If a mom during pregnancy practices how to hold her breath, then she gives birth to a trained baby" (Sargunas and Sargunas 1985:8). Charkovsky even advised pregnant women to dive and suck a nipple with milk or juice underwater so that the baby could learn what to do after birth. After experiments with animals, Charkovsky believed that a mother, as a land creature, could not give birth to an aquatic child; therefore, he urged women to meditate and imagine themselves as dolphins:

> If during swimming, a mother imagines herself as a dolphin, she thereby transfers the dolphin information flow to the child. If a mother deprives the child of communication with dolphins and closes the connection within herself, then she automatically encloses the child in her own pathology. (Sargunas and Sargunas 1985:9)

The importance of water birth in the Aquaculture concept was crucial. For many years in Russia, home birth meant water birth and water birth meant home birth. Only in the mid-2000s did Russian homebirth midwives (who practice illegally in Russia) begin to move away from the imperative to give birth only in the water and attend births on land as well. For Charkovsky, water birth was "soft" and "natural" specifically for the child, because that child "naturally" moved from the amniotic fluid to the aquatic environment. Charkovsky also insisted to give birth not in a comfortable water temperature of 35°–36° Celsius, but in cold water: "We usually prepare a woman to give birth in the sea, and a baby is able to be in the water of 20°–18°" (meeting with I. B. Charkovsky 1985:13).

Immediately after the birth, a woman should be ready for intensive workouts with her baby. Charkovsky was indignant that mothers often refused to breast-feed their children underwater:

> Women do not understand anything and do not want to understand, they behave like females, and work on ancient instincts that came from animals, they themselves do not know why they cannot understand simple things. Therefore, a man must prepare everything [to feed a child from a bottle]). (Sargunas and Sargunas 1985:11)

Thus, for the patriarchal Charkovsky, as well as for technocratic obstetrics, only a child as the "end product" mattered and the "mother was a secondary by-product" (Davis-Floyd and Dumit 1998:5): she has to follow instructions and ensure the birth of a water baby. But unlike technocratic obstetrics, which treats the woman's body as a defective machine (Davis-Floyd 2001), Charkovsky considered that the maternal "biological program" (or instincts) was improper and prevented her from raising her child in the right way, so it was necessary to use a special technology or to seek help from dolphins.

When some women who were followers of the Aquaculture method became lay midwives and childbirth instructors, they changed Charkovsky's approach to the activities of expectant mothers. Proper preparation was considered as key to success, because women had to be ready for unassisted childbirth: there were few homebirth midwives in Russia in the 1980s and 1990s and they had little or no formal training. The childbirth preparation courses took several months and included serious physical, informational, and psychological training. Svetlana Akimova, who later became a homebirth midwife, recalled her studies during her first pregnancy in the course taught by Tatyana Sargunas: "We were preparing like Special Forces: had a dry fasting [fasting without water] for 42 hours once a week, did gymnastics every day, doused ourselves with cold water, and swam in the ice hole" (Interview 6).

Not only women, but also their husbands, began to perceive childbirth as a family affair: some of them assisted at births and trained their babies, and some became active members of the homebirth movement, male midwives, and aqua coaches. One of these active fathers explained why that was so important for him:

> We perceived this birth in three ways (besides, of course, the fact of the birth of our child): as our small contribution to the formation of a new attitude to childbirth, mother and baby; as our contribution to the propagation and struggle for the official recognition of water birth; as a protest against the existing obstetric system. (Anonymous, "The Story of One Birth" 1985:20)

Thus, the "Aquaculture" method showed the parents the way out of the control and supervision of the state institutions and directed their protest or *counter-con-duct* as a specific "revolt of conduct" (Foucault 2007; Dean 2009) to transforming or strengthening the body and mind, and giving birth to new "free" children.

Babies-Dolphins and Charkovsky's "New Physiology"

Babies-Dolphins: Nature and Technology

According to Aquaculture, workouts with babies should begin immediately after birth. In the first hours, it is necessary to do baby yoga, a kind of neonatal manual therapy. Then parents need to do a special set of exercises with a child, called "dynamic gymnastics," and a series of hundreds of rhythmic dives into water (see Figure 12.2)

Charkovsky constantly created various devices or "trainers": the frame on which the child was attached in a certain position, the mount for nipples to feed a child underwater, and others. M. Dadasheva told me how Charkovsky had once made an imitation of a placenta for a child who was born in a hospital and doctors immediately cut the umbilical cord:

> Charkovsky took a bottle, put water into it, attached a hose and began to dive the child with this device into the water. The child immediately turned on, at the energy level [got extra energy]. I saw how the state of the child was changing, how the eyes of the parents were changing, because the child was starting to turn on [become more active]. He began to crawl after this training, imitating the placenta [formed by the device]. Before, he had a decreased tone and, obviously, anemia due to early cutting of the umbilical cord. (Interview 2)

There was an idea that the "placenta was an additional organ of the baby," a "second heart"; therefore, the umbilical cord was usually only cut a few hours or even days after the birth. Dadasheva explains that the image of the placenta was preserved in the child's "subtle plane," so the device "completed" this experience and provided the necessary "energy balance." Thus, a temporary artificial organ, provided with para-scientific explanations, was created and used as a superstructure for the child's body to recreate its imaginary integrity.

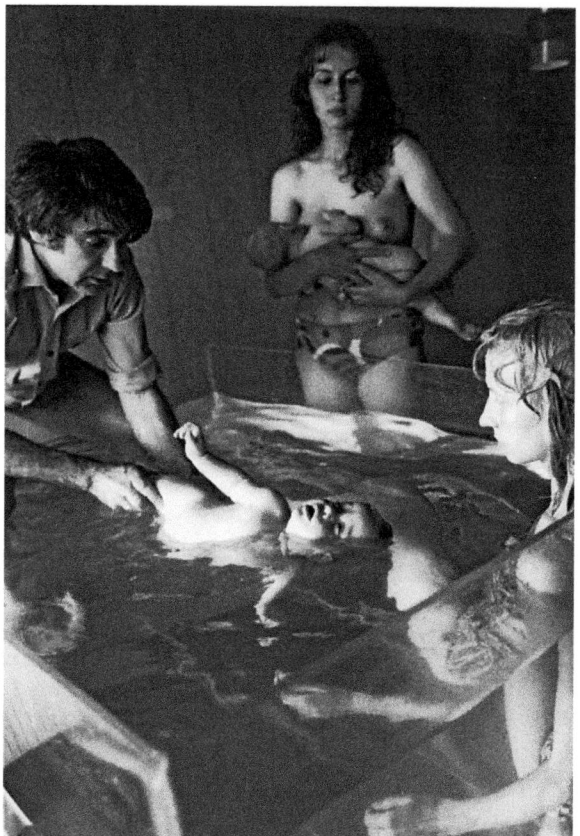

FIGURE 12.2 Igor Charkovsky and his followers performing water trainings with infants. Moscow, 1980s. Photo by Alexei Sargunas. © Natalya Kotlar. Used with permission.

In the concept of Aquaculture, the most effective way to develop the aquatic abilities of a newborn was to get into contact with dolphins, because only they were able to create a favorable environment:

> When we contact with dolphins, almost all the fears associated with water are removed; it seems as if they take us into their flock, and we get information about the life of the Ocean. (Sargunas and Sargunas 1985:11)

Dolphins are attributed such qualities as sentience, high intelligence, kindness, friendliness, high morality, ability to see internally, and even connection with the cosmos. Charkovsky and his followers believed that dolphins came to help humans in difficult situations; for example, they could attend human births and save drowning children. According to Charkovsky, newborns understood the dolphins' language better than their mothers, because babies were also aquatic creatures. Thus, "technology" in the form of various artificial devices and "nature" represented by dolphins could be used equally to achieve the main goal of the Aquaculture project—human enhancement.

In the film "Igor Charkovsky—An Impossible Dream" (1989), Alexey Sargunas explained that there were three directions in the Aquaculture method: a "clinic" was for healing, a "sports school" was valuable for developing the capabilities of the body, and a "spiritual school" or "ashram" was needed to extend extrasensory abilities. Tatyana Sargunas told me that there was one more direction, which they called *kolkhoz* as a joke. (The word "kolhoz" (a contraction of the Russian words for "collective ownership"—a form of a state collective farm in the Soviet Union) was used as a humorous colloquial expression to denote a friendly, cheerful group of people):

> This is the bulk of people who do not have any special problems, they just want to live peacefully and happily, without any special undertakings. We chose "kolkhoz" for ourselves because we wanted a harmonious and comprehensive development. (Interview 1)

The most devoted followers of Aquaculture usually say that Charkovsky's method is the most effective in healing and claim that they witnessed the miraculous healings of little patients whom official medicine could not help. They usually do not mention the potentially negative effects of these workouts, although it is known that several children actually died during the process. Charkovsky follower and former aqua-coach Margarita Razenkova admitted:

> Some parents held the children under water so that they turned blue. I even wrote about this: with such activities, not all children will live to the Age of Aquarius, you just drown them. (Interview 3)

The main idea of this therapy was that the child's organism needs to be stressed to increase its resistance to diseases. Natalia Kotlar told me a story she heard from her teacher:

> Charkovsky said that he loved babies like a fox loved a hare. The rabbit lives a short life, because he sits in a cage and does not move much, and a hare is constantly forced to run away from the fox, so he lives a long time. When he saw hopeless children, he said: I will now start the wheels of this idle machine, since it won't start with a key, I'll start this car from a hill, the wheels will spin and the engine will start. (Interview 4)

This story provides analogies from the world of nature as well as from the world of technology. The need for training is explained by examples from the animal world; at the same time, the child's body is compared to a machine that needs repair.

A striking event that was supposed to demonstrate the success of Charkovsky's "sports school" took place in 1992 when Vasya Razenkov, who was born in water and trained in accordance with the Aquaculture method, at the age of 1 year and 9 months swam in the school pool 33 kilometers for 15 hours non-stop. This event was captured in photographs and videos and included in the Russian analog of the *Guinness Book of World Records* (Divo 1993:36). According to his mother and aqua-coach Margarita, part of this time Vasya was listening to music on special waterproof earphones, periodically eating liquid food from a plastic nipple, and most of the time he was just sleeping. According to Charkovsky, babies trained according to his system were able to swim while sleeping, like dolphins. Margarita does not connect the success of this demonstration with any supernatural abilities of her son: "It was just the result of training. If I had trained another child, he would have swum the same way" (Interview 3). At the same time, Vladimir Bagryansky described this event as one of many Charkovsky's "hoaxes," literally as a "performance with deception," ultimately alienating many people from him and his ideas (Interview 7).

Charkovsky claimed that children born in water demonstrated outpaced growth: they began to sit on their own at 2 months, walk at 3 months, etc., but he considered these achievements only as signs of a higher form of consciousness. Water birth and postnatal baby training were believed to enhance supernatural abilities: clairvoyance, telepathy, the ability to communicate with animals, birds and insects, flowers, and trees. These children were attributed an exceptionally high sensitivity to everything that happens around them; therefore, they were also called "sensitives."

Natalia Kotlar, a follower of Charkovsky and a homebirth midwife, went to Goa in 2007 to give birth to her 5th child in the Indian Ocean (see Figure 12.3). She perceived this childbirth as an event of incredible spiritual unity with nature, which was personified by dolphins:

> The dolphin swam quite close. And hung, looking at my belly without stopping. At the same time, I felt my baby moving inside me toward the exit. Our daughter floated into the water, opened her eyes and, oh, what a miracle! smiled in response to our happy laugh. Alpha [the name Natalia and her husband gave to one of the dolphins]) swam very close, and with her nose very carefully pushed the child to the surface of the water. Her large blue eyes, as if from time immemorial, radiated a powerful stream of wisdom. (Kotlar 2008:102)

The coming of the "messiah children"—children with extraordinary abilities who should change the world—was a constant theme of Charkovsky's dreams: "These children will be able to stop the arms race. Therefore, the creation of such a New Race is extremely important" (Sargunas and Sargunas 1985:7).

On a practical level, Charkovsky's ideas inspired the then-Chairman of the USSR Swimming Federation, Zakhary Fisov, and thanks to his efforts, the state

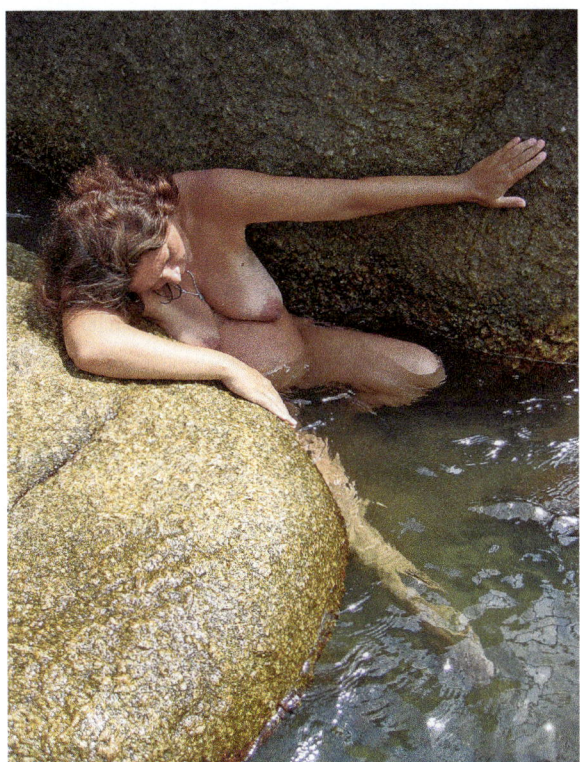

FIGURE 12.3   The birth of Anna Sargunas, while her mother was in touch with dolphins. One is just barely visible in this photo—the gray blur in front of the mother. India, Goa, May 8, 2007. Photo by Alexei Sargunas. © Natalya Kotlar. Used with permission.

program for teaching infants to swim in bathtubs at children's clinics started in 1980. The practice of water birth appeared in some maternity hospitals in the 1990s thanks to the efforts of Charkovsky's followers and the enthusiasm of some doctors, but very briefly, as an experiment. In the 2000s, some home-birth midwives, former Charkovsky followers, received a formal education and began to work in the maternity hospitals, and to a certain extent contributed to the humanization of obstetric practice, at least in such cities as Moscow and St. Petersburg (Ozhiganova 2015).

The Machinery of Utopia: The "New Physiology" of Childbirth and Infancy

Charkovsky argued that the Aquaculture method was based on a thorough knowledge of physiology. Firstly, he believed that, when born on land, the newborn experienced a "gravitational shock," which significantly limited his or her abilities. According to Charkovsky, brain volume, and consequently intellectual potential, increased in the weightlessness induced in water; therefore it was so important to give birth in water and "prolong the state of weightlessness as much as possible" by water training: "You can give birth to a child who will surpass Leonardo da Vinci by its potential" (Sargunas 1985:9).

Secondly, Charkovsky talked about the benefits of hypoxia, which occurred when a child was dipped underwater—this was probably the most fantastical part of his teaching. He believed that a newborn, like a dolphin, had a reflex that blocked the respiratory tract underwater, and that this reflex could be preserved if a child is constantly dipped underwater. Moreover, he argued that diving caused blood vessels to spasm and oxygen to feed only the brain, which therefore grew quickly. Charkovsky insisted on feeding children underwater; he said, "It has been shown in animals that diving without food leads to much less success, about 30%, and with food you can reach 100%." It turns out that he believed in the possibility of anaerobic respiration, thanks to which the child receives oxygen through the ingestion of food, "just like the fetus received oxygen through the placenta" (Sargunas and Sargunas 1985:9).

These ideas, rather strange from a scientific point of view, have unexpected parallels in the works of a famous Russian physiologist, academician Ilya Arshavsky (1903–1996). Arshavsky formulated the concept of the physiological immaturity of newborns, called its "signs" (decreased muscle tone, weak reflexes, and others), and proposed compensation methods: cold strengthening, physical activity, and most importantly, swimming and diving. Like Charkovsky, he also claimed that a short-term oxygen deficiency, which arose during diving, was the "trigger" that stimulated the body (Arshavsky 1982:195). Arshavsky was well acquainted with Charkovsky and wrote many positive reviews of his aquatic activities with babies: he spoke about the benefits of water weightlessness and confirmed that according to his observations, "amphibian babies" were stronger and more developed than ordinary children. He also noted the benefits of prenatal training, citing the results of his experiments with animals: if the fetus received nutrients and oxygen in excess, then it had no incentive to develop and would begin to lag behind, while, in contrast, the lack of nutrients and oxygen stimulated its rapid development and growth.

Thus, Arshavsky worked on creating a kind of "new physiology," in which was inherent a firm belief in the huge but hidden reserves that infants have for their development. Infant strengthening was the main instrument for the mobilization of these reserves. This approach was simultaneously *natural*, or physiological, since it appealed to the image of harsh nature, which trained its creatures living on the brink of survival, and *technological* since the concept of *strengthening* was equated to metal hardening. "New physiology" represented utopian transcendental knowledge, incongruous with conventional scientific knowledge, and thus provided the theoretical basis of the Aquaculture project.

Conclusions: Aquaculture and Techno-Sapiens

The utopian project of Aquaculture arose in the so-called "era of stagnation" in the Soviet Union, when the inability to influence Communist social reality combined with the idea of the omnipotence of man and his power over nature. "Aquaculture" can be placed in line with such projects of Soviet modernism as space exploration and the (proposed) rotation of Siberian rivers: it was also aimed at exploration of a different kind of space—the world's oceans. For Charkovsky and his followers, this proximity was evident: "It's an interesting coincidence that the first flights into space, into space weightlessness, and the first birth into water, into water weightlessness took place in our country (Sargunas 1985:6).

At the same time, in the late Soviet Union and during the 1990s, Charkovsky's project belonged to the numerous esoteric or para-scientific teachings that shared a faith in hidden human potential and the ability to master it through special technologies. In the peculiar anthology of Russian spiritual teachings, compiled by Russian transpersonal psychologists, one entry was devoted to the Aquaculture project: "Charkovsky's research shed light on the unexplored human possibilities and has opened practical ways to improve the nervous system and brain of a newborn person" (Kozlov and Maykov 2007:1146). Thus, the Aquaculture and "new physiology" identified by Arshavsky and Charkovsky became two of the many examples of ambiguous collaboration of scientific and para-scientific knowledge that were rich in late Soviet and post-Soviet history.

The Russian project of home water birth and active development of infants has undergone significant transformations, along with the political and social changes and crises that the whole country has experienced. Firstly, it shifted from the Soviet utopia of creating a new human being to the spiritual search of the 1990s, and then to the commercialization and professionalization of homebirth midwifery, which began in 2000 and is currently ongoing. Such phenomena as "conscious parenthood" and "spiritual midwifery" in their Russian versions are closely related to the Aquaculture project. Nowadays, participants in the Russian homebirth movement often critically evaluate the personality and methods of Charkovsky. As Alexander Naumov (2001:230), a homebirth male midwife, stated: "We need to clear the idea of waterbirth from all the fog and myths that are associated with the name of Charkovsky."

Not only did the methods change, but also the very purpose of the Aquaculture project. Charkovsky dreamed of the birth of a new (post)human being—a baby-dolphin, who was supposed to be more perfect than today's people, yet his followers just wanted their children to grow up healthy and harmoniously developed. Some of these children have chosen creative professions as adults, some have become health specialists; according to their parents, they retained excellent health and love of swimming, but none claim to possess superhuman abilities.

However, it is important to understand that the essence of the Aquaculture project was *titanism*—a utopian idea of the extreme plasticity of human nature, and the possibility of its radical transformation to achieve the ideal human. Charkovsky considered today's people to be a kind of cyborgs, or "biorobots," controlled by certain programs: they could be "switched on" or "switched off," "start" or "stop," "connect" or "disconnect," redo or "reprogram" one way or another. The goal of the project was the production of an enhanced model of what we could now, as a result of this book, call "techno-sapiens." Paradoxically, it was believed that the new (post-) human being would be not only a more perfect version of *sapiens*, but also more *natural*, despite the fact that this new being had to be assembled by a special demedicalized water-birth technology, complex prenatal preparation, and postnatal training. So, the Aquaculture project could be considered as a variant of the "cyborg myth about transgressed boundaries, potent fusions, and dangerous possibilities" (Haraway 2016:14). The baby-dolphin was simultaneously a product of technology and nature—a mutant and cyborg who demonstrated the relativity of the categories of *natural* and *artificial*, *traditional* and *new* modes of human enhancement, a chimera in which "myth and tool mutually constitute each other" (Haraway 2016:33).

List of Interviewees

Interview 1. Tatyana Sargunas, a homebirth midwife, head of the birth preparation center "Aqua." Moscow, 2018.

Interview 2. Marina Dadasheva, a homebirth midwife, head of a birth preparation center. Moscow, 2020.

Interview 3. Razenkova Margarita, a former aqua couch. Moscow, 2020.

Interview 4. Natalya Kotlar, a homebirth midwife, head of the birth preparation center "Our Stork." Moscow, 2020.

Interview 5. Postnova Julia, a homebirth midwife, head of the birth preparation center "Jewel." Moscow, 2018.

Interview 6. Akimova Svetlana, a midwife, head of the birth preparation center "Magic Baby." Moscow, 2019.

Interview 7. Vladimir Bagriansky. Moscow–Poissy (France), 2020 (via Skype).

References

Anonymous 1985. The story of one birth. *Aqua* 2:18–24. (In Russian).

Arshavsky IA 1982. *Physiological Mechanisms of Individual Development*. Moscow: Nauka. (In Russian).

Bagryansky V 2011. *The Lessons of I. B. Charkovsky: Ethical Conflicts as the Essence of All the Problems of Russia (2)*. Annunciation of Aphrodite. Personal Blog at Facebook.

Belousova E 2012. *Waterbirth and Russian-American Exchange: From the Iron Curtain to Facebook*. Doctoral Dissertation. Houston, TX: Rice University. https://scholarship.rice.edu/bitstream/handle/1911/64601/BELOUSOVA-THESIS.pdf?sequence=1&isAllowed=y.

Davis-Floyd R 2001. The technocratic, humanistic, and holistic paradigms of childbirth. *International Journal of Gynecology & Obstetrics* 75:S5–S23.

Davis-Floyd R, Dumit J, eds. 1998. *Cyborg Babies: From Techno-Sex to Techno-Tots.* New York: Routledge.

Dean M 2009. *Governmentality: Power and Rule in Modern Society,* 2nd edition. London: Sage.

Divo 1993. *Russian Book of Records and Achievements,* ed. V Ponomareva. Moscow: Russkaja kniga. www.vixri.com/d/Russkaja%20kniga%20rekordov%20i%20dosti zhenij.pdf. (In Russian).

Foucault M 2007. *Security, Territory, Population: Lectures at the College de France (1977–1978),* ed. M Senellart. New York: Picador.

Haraway DJ 2016. *A Cyborg Manifesto: Science, Technology, and Socialist-Feminism in the Late Twentieth Century.* Minneapolis, MN: University of Minnesota Press.

Igor Charkovsky or Impossible Dream (Film) 1989. *France USSR. Igor Tcharkovsky ou le reve Impossible, Co-Prod.* JC Patrice, S Simonenko: Les Films Auramax, Paris–Gosteleradio, URSS.

Korop P 1972a. Escape from gravity? *Technique for Youth* 3:42–46. (In Russian).

Korop P 1972b. The path leading to the ocean. *Technique for Youth* 12:44–47. (In Russian).

Kotlar N 2008. *Anna is Grace. The Story of one Reincarnation. Diary of Events of the Spring of 2007.* Moscow. http://alexnatali.com/uploads/pdf/Kotlar_block_web.pdf. (In Russian).

Kourany JA 2014. Human enhancement: Making the debate more productive. *Erkenntnis* 79(S5):981–998.

Kozlov V, Maykov V 2007. *Transpersonal Project: Psychology, Anthropology, Spiritual Traditions,* Vol. II. Moscow: Yaroslavl State University. (In Russian).

Mannheim K 1979. *Ideology and Utopia: An Introduction to the Sociology of Knowledge.* London: Routledge.

Martynova IA 2017. *Born of One's Own Will: Chronicle of Midwifery,* 2nd edition. St. Petersburg: Publisher Yablokov S.Yu. (In Russian).

Meeting of I.B. Charkovsky with Esther Myers in Moscow. *Aqua* 2:14–18.

Naumov AB 2001. *Home Water Birth. The Current State of the Problem.* Moscow: Sovremennik. (In Russian).

Odent M 1984. *Birth Reborn.* New York: Pantheon.

Ozhiganova A 2015. Official (biomedical) obstetrics and alternative (home) midwifery: Formalized and informal interaction practices. *Journal of Economic Sociology* 20(5):28–52. (in Russian).

Russian Woman Gave Birth to a Child on Vacation in Egypt in the Red Sea 2018. *Cosmopolitan,* 14 March. www.cosmo.ru/lifestyle/news/14-03-2018/rossiyanka-rodil a-rebenka-na-otdyhe-v-egipte-v-krasnom-more/#part0.

Sargunas A 1985. History and general ideas of the "babies- dolphins" program (1985). *Aqua* 2:5–12. (In Russian).

Sargunas A, Sargunas T 1985. Five conversations with I.B. Charkovsky. *Aqua* 1:4–18. (In Russian).

Schenkman S 1974. Amphibian girl. *Physical Education & Sports* 11:36–37. (In Russian).

13

SAFETY, CO-REGULATION, AND POLYVAGAL THEORY:

The Autonomic Nervous System as the Missing Link in Childbirth Outcomes and Experiences

Sarah Melancon

Introduction: Pam's Stalled Labor and Lucia's Solution

Pam had been in labor in a hospital for half the day when Lucia was called in as a backup midwife. The two had never met before. Lucia describes her experience:

> Pam has been stuck at five centimeters' dilation for several hours; the contractions are painful, and she is writhing and moaning [in a high-pitched tone], "Oh God, Oh God, Oh Godddd…"
>
> I sit quietly behind Pam, [wrapping my arms and legs around her] and synchronize my breathing with hers. "Oh good," I breathe softly into her ear, in rhythm with her. "Oh Good. Oh good. Oh gooooood." She picks it up. "Oh goooooood," her voice dips with mine into the lowest abdominal registers, good primal rhythmic toning.
>
> Later Pam tells me that her bag of waters was artificially ruptured against her will when she was six centimeters dilated with her first child. She was plunged into agonizing contractions and then had to take them on her back…in the hospital. Pam's body remembered, although her conscious mind didn't; her body tensed and balked at the possibility of a repeat performance in this labor. "Oh goooood" broke the hold of the past and allowed Pam to relax, unencumbered, into the present. (Roncalli 2011:183–185)

What exactly happened here? Such stories are common among midwives, though less so in hospital settings, for important reasons. This chapter will explore Pam's experience using the lens of the autonomic nervous system and Stephen Porges' Polyvagal Theory (2011). Here I ask, what if the midwife had instead been an obstetrician? Labor would likely have been augmented with pitocin to forcibly strengthen her contractions, with an epidural for increased pain. If labor continued, Pam faced increased risk of instrumental (vacuum or forceps) delivery. If she remained "stuck," Pam's birth would have ended in a cesarean. This "cascade of interventions" is part of the reason why the United States has a 32% cesarean rate (Martin et al. 2017).

While interventions can be life-saving, Pam's needs were simpler, and much more human. Pam needed social connection and attuned support, which begs the question: How many mothers on the operating room table just needed to feel a sense of safety and close connection? On the whole, research demonstrates the importance of supporting women's innate birthing capabilities for optimal birth outcomes, breastfeeding, attachment, and maternal satisfaction (Buckley 2015).

This chapter attempts to fill a gap in our understanding of childbirth experiences, outcomes, and their subsequent impacts, centering our human needs for intimate safety and autonomic co-regulation in the birth of our next generation. I will first review Polyvagal Theory and the autonomic regulation of childbirth. Next I will cover the role of the vagus nerve, the optimal autonomic state for birth, and autonomic contributors to birth trauma. Finally, I will return to Pam's story and offer an interpretation of her experience from the perspective of Polyvagal Theory, concluding with reflections on the cyborgification of birth and a reminder to center factors from our evolutionary past (see Chapter 1) for safe, sane, and humane birth as we move toward the future.

Polyvagal Theory and the Autonomic Nervous System

Polyvagal Theory, created by Stephen Porges (2011), is an evolutionarily informed approach to understanding human behavior via the autonomic nervous system, which is divided into 3 subsystems: social engagement, mobilization, and immobilization. Human beings are inherently social creatures; this sociality is reflected in our biology. Our social engagement system is generally characterized by a sense of safety via positive social interaction and feelings of calm, relaxation, and well-being, induced by eye contact, warm facial expressions, and vocal rhythms. The social engagement system includes cranial nerves V, VII, IX, and XI, which control the face and head, and the ventral branch of cranial nerve X—the vagus nerve. The vagus nerve has two separate branches; hence the name "polyvagal." These nerves supply the heart, lungs, digestive tract, liver, pancreas (Porges 2011), uterus, and cervix (Komisaruk and Sansone 2003). The ventral branch of the vagus nerve is responsible for the heart-face connection, linking neural regulation of the heart to regulation of the face and head muscles, enabling mammals to engage in social life (Porges 2011).

When sensing threat, humans have two defensive states—mobilization and immobilization. Fear activates the *mobilization system* and flight-or-fight mechanisms in the sympathetic nervous system, operating like a gas pedal, involving increased heart rate, hypervigilance, panic, and emotional overwhelm (Porges 2011)—a state of "hyperarousal" (Ogden et al. 2006). The *immobilization system*—often known as the "freeze" response, as in "fight, flight, or freeze"—involves the dorsal branch of the vagus nerve, activated under extreme danger—an evolutionary mechanism from early vertebrates who "play dead" when facing a predator. Analogous to a brake pedal, immobilization includes low oxygen levels, weak muscle tone, reduced heart rate and blood pressure, fainting, dissociation, defecation (diarrhea), and in extreme cases, death (Porges 2011; 2017)—a state of "hypoarousal." Immobilization includes a sense of collapse and feelings of hopelessness, helplessness, numbness, and depersonalization. Behaviorally, immobilization can involve total submission and passive compliance (Ogden et al. 2006).

What determines the state of the autonomic nervous system? Through a process called "neuroception," neural circuits evaluate sensory information from the immediate environment for risk or threat, without conscious awareness. When perceiving safety, the social engagement system is activated and defensive systems are inhibited. When a potential threat is detected, often the mobilization system will become activated in preparation for flight, then fight. A "freeze" response occurs when both the sympathetic (gas pedal) and immobilization (brake) systems are activated simultaneously. When a threat is perceived as life-threatening or terrifying, and flight or fight is not an option, sympathetic activation withdraws. The immobilization system then leads to "behavioral shutdown and frequently, dissociation" (Porges 2011, 2018).

Research on the autonomic nervous system is possible through measurements such as heart rate variability (HRV). HRV is the variation in time between heartbeats, and serves as a measure of the autonomic nervous system. While numerous indicators for HRV exist, HRV is particularly important for the purposes of this chapter in providing an index of vagal tone (Laborde et al. 2017). "Vagal tone" refers to the activity of the ventral vagal branch parasympathetic system. Generally, higher tone reflects a healthier state. Vagal tone can be compromised by stress, poor attachment, and trauma (Porges 2011). Research on HRV, pregnancy, and birth is limited but appears to be growing, and provides important insight into autonomic aspects of reproduction (see Mizuno et al. 2017; Kozar et al. 2018).

The Autonomic Regulation of Childbirth

Past research has claimed that birth is solely regulated by the sympathetic nervous system and spinal nerves (Enderli 2017). However, according to Polyvagal Theory, reproductive behaviors including sex, childbirth, and nursing involve the parasympathetic dorsal vagal immobilization system—the primitive defensive system that has been "modified to serve intimate social needs" in mammals, termed *immobilization without fear* (Porges 2011:14). While "immobilization" sounds paradoxical, as healthy birthing entails a great deal of movement, Porges' terminology stems from research into mammalian mating behavior, wherein females of many species enter a crouching posture (called "lordosis") for reproduction, wherein the body is physically immobilized (ibid.).

Despite utilizing the same neural circuits, immobilization without fear is a fundamentally different state than immobilization when fear is present. The social engagement and immobilization systems are coupled in sexual intimacy. Safe intimate experiences, Porges suggests, act as a "neural exercise optimizing the ability of the social engagement system to regulate the dorsal vagal pathway" (2018:63). For women, this may serve as a "preparatory neural exercise...[to] optimize the reproductive behaviors and processes, including facilitating childbirth" (2018:63).

In *Childbirth Without Fear* (2006 [1942]), Grantly Dick-Read posited fear as the root of labor pain: fear creates tension, which the body interprets as pain. Pain increases fear, prompting a desire to escape, thus increasing tension and pain. Fear activates the sympathetic nervous system, creating excess tension in the uterus. The uterus has three layers of muscle fibers: (1) outer longitudinal, expulsive fibers that contract and shorten to empty the uterus, "innervated" by (supplied by nerves from) the parasympathetic nervous system and local nerves; (2) middle figure-8-shaped fibers, innervated by the sympathetic nervous system; and (3) inner layer fibers circling around the lower half and neck of the uterus; innervated by the sympathetic nervous system, these inner layer fibers can contract to inhibit uterine expulsion. These fibers are meant to work in harmony: longitudinal fibers contract to expel the baby, and circular fibers relax (Dick-Read 1942). The cervix is also innervated by both sympathetic and parasympathetic nerves, and importantly, the vagus nerve innervates both the uterus and cervix. In rats, the vagus nerve plays a role in cervical ripening (Komisaruk and Sansone 2003; Reyes-Lagos et al. 2019).

Thus, in Dick-Read's fear-tension-pain cycle, removing fear—the source of sympathetic activation—is the solution to pain. Some sympathetic activity, however, may be necessary for the labor process. This "healthy stress" increases contractions, aids attachment, and helps mother and infant adapt during and after labor. Labor pain itself creates a stress response, stimulating the sympathetic nervous system with large increases of epinephrine (adrenaline). The "fetal ejection reflex," rarely observed in hospitals, is a surge of epinephrine-norepinephrine creating several extremely strong, involuntary contractions to "eject" the baby (Buckley 2015). After the healthy stress of birth, skin-to-skin and early breastfeeding stimulate the vagus nerve and social engagement system to calm infants and help them to integrate the experience (Olza-Fernandez et al. 2014). However, excess sympathetic activity can slow or stall labor, allowing the mother time to escape threat and move to safety before continuing the birth process. These hormonal and autonomic responses can increase stress, fear, and pain, and complications and length of labor (Buckley 2015).

Painless—and Pleasurable?—Childbirth

Dick-Read (2006 [1942]) believed that with proper education and preparation, childbirth could be both painless and joyful. Unfortunately, his approach was often unable to overcome the impact of the medicalized institutional environment. Many women who read his book, or who were taught his approach, intended to have a "natural birth," yet "failed." When intervention is accepted as normal (Newnhan et al. 2016), "by virtue of being in the hospital in the first place, most women never stand a chance of achieving 'natural' birth" (Davis-Floyd 2003:176).

Some women's experiences lend credence to Dick-Read's claims. An obvious minority, some mothers describe their births as painless, and others as ecstatic, pleasurable, euphoric, sexual, or orgasmic (Davis and Pascali-Bonaro 2010). Pain and pleasure may co-exist, or pleasure may counteract some or all of the pain. Some purposefully stimulate their clitoris or nipples, or ask their partners to do so, utilizing sexual pleasure as a pain-relieving and oxytocin-stimulating technique in "the best-kept secret" about birth (ibid.; Bolaza 2020). As stress increases, endorphins, epinephrine-norepinephrine, and cortisol are released to bring the body into balance. High levels of these hormones can create euphoria, excitement, and pleasure (Buckley 2010). While difficult to study, it would be helpful to understand what is happening autonomically during pleasurable or orgasmic birth experiences to help more women enjoy their births.

Safety, the Vagus Nerve, and Optimal Birthing

A sense of safety is a baseline requirement for successful social behavior (Porges 2011), including childbirth (Buckley 2015). Feeling safe requires a two-step, two-pathway autonomic process. In Step 1, the "passive" pathway down-regulates sympathetic hypervigilance and up-regulates immobilization shutdown, increasing influence from the social engagement system. Through neuroception, visual and auditory cues of safety are detected from the environment. In Step 2, the "active" pathway involves conscious exercise of the vagus nerve through breathing, posture, and vocalization, such as chanting or singing (Porges 2017). Many homebirth midwives postulate a connection between the throat and the cervix, noting that deep guttural sounds help the cervix to dilate, while high-pitched tight sounds from a closed throat can inhibit labor progress (see Gaskin 2003), as was happening with Pam.

However, if Step 1—sensing safety—is not complete, and the sympathetic and/or dorsal vagal systems remain activated, Step 2—conscious exercise of the vagus nerve—may instead elicit a defensive response. The birthing body's attempt to engage the vagus nerve while in mobilization or immobilization (with fear) can create a sense of vulnerability, triggering a flight-or-fight reaction (Porges 2017). Without a sense of safety, sympathetic activation will rise and interfere with labor.

What makes a safe birthing environment? Such an environment is similar to a safe sexual environment—both are vulnerable states in which women open their bodies. Like all mammals, a birthing woman needs to feel private, safe, and undisturbed. Low lights and sounds, continuous support from trustworthy people, and consideration of her emotional well-being matter (Buckley 2010, 2015). Such an environment will activate the ventral vagal parasympathetic system and keep sympathetic activity in balance (Porges 2018).

Engaging the vagus from a place of safety may be beneficial in alleviating childbirth pain. Again, *the vagus nerve innervates both the uterus and the cervix.* Vaginocervical stimulation creates strong pleasurable *and* pain-relieving properties via the vagus nerve. The greater the pleasure, the stronger the analgesia (Komisurak and Sansone 2003); this may help to explain the pleasurable birth experiences described above.

Enderli (2017) explored the plausibility of vagus nerve stimulation (VNS) (an FDA-approved treatment for epilepsy and pharmacological-resistant depression) for labor pain. De Couck et al. (2014) suggest that vagal tone may protect against pain as the ventral branch of the vagus nerve reduces inflammation, oxidative stress, and sympathetic activity, and activates areas of the brain that modulate pain. Pregnant women receiving massage therapy, which stimulates the vagal nerve, experienced improved mood, reduced stress, lower labor pain, and labors averaging almost 3 hours shorter, speculated to be due to increased parasympathetic (ventral vagal) activity (Field et al. 1997).

Oxytocin and Immobilization without Fear

The hormone oxytocin plays a key role in social behavior. Oxytocin activates the parasympathetic social engagement system, increasing HRV (Reyes-Lagos et al. 2019). It is important in pair-bonding, attachment processes, and parental nurturing. The milk ejection reflex in breastfeeding is facilitated by oxytocin, as are labor, sexual arousal, and orgasm. Endogenous oxytocin increases throughout pregnancy, prepares the body for labor, causes uterine contractions, and helps to reduce stress during and after birth (Buckley 2015).

Ordinarily, the dorsal vagal immobilization pathway maintains homeostasis. Yet under perceived threat, immobilization can lead to behavioral shutdown. Oxytocin, often called "the hormone of love," modifies dorsal vagal function from a fear to a love system. Co-activation of the social engagement and immobilization systems (potentially with a small-to-moderate amount of sympathetic activation) appear central for reproductive behaviors, including sex, birth, and breastfeeding (Porges 2011).

Trust and safety are necessary for immobilization without fear. This state is where we can experience passionate, ecstatic pleasure during sex. When trust and safety are absent from a sexual encounter, pain and tissue damage may occur. Violations of trust switch the context and biology from safety to fear—stimulating sympathetic activation, or switching to immobilized shutdown if flight-or-fight is not an option. As explained above, should both the sympathetic (gas pedal) and immobilization (brake) systems be simultaneously activated, the "freeze" response can occur, as in rape. Oxytocin is thus the differentiating factor between affiliative immobilization without fear and defensive immobilization with fear; as potential threat is detected, the system switches. Porges (2018) describes this in the context of love and sexuality; however, given that these utilize the same autonomic systems as in labor, it seems logical that birth would follow a similar path. Notably, the synthetic oxytocin (Pitocin, or syntocinon) commonly administered in hospitals does not have the same effect as endogenous hormones; rather than supporting labor and breastfeeding, synthetic oxytocin may interfere (Olza-Fernandez et al. 2014; Buckley 2015).

Birth Trauma

While some women experience orgasm during birth, birth trauma is much more common. Acute postpartum PTSD affects 5%–8% of women, while clinically significant PTSD symptoms affect 9.6%-27.3% (Dekel et al. 2017). Traumatic births are associated with sense of loss, sexual dysfunction, difficulty bonding, family life challenges, suicidal ideation, and fear of having more children (Simpson and Catling 2016).

What makes a birth traumatic? Even when "the birth experience may appear uncomplicated to care providers…[the woman] may still find the event traumatic if she loses a sense of control or dignity" (Simpson and Catling 2016:2). The external environment, internal experience, and/or interpersonal interactions can each play a role. The physical and sociocultural environment of traumatic birth includes unsupportive hospital rules and routines and lack of privacy. The internal experience includes the emotions associated with severe pain, fears, delivery mode, complications, dissociation, trauma history, and mental health status. Interpersonal interactions include problems with healthcare providers, pressure for interventions, and lack of support/information (Simpson and Catling 2016; Dekel et al. 2017).

How does birth trauma develop? We can speculate by building on Polyvagal Theory. A laboring woman's neuroception may subconsciously detect threat from any of the above sources, activating the sympathetic nervous system. Her sympathetic arousal may stall labor, but in the hospital setting, this is an invitation for more intervention, and her ability to actually fight or flee is compromised. Perhaps this accounts for dissociative experiences in birth trauma—unable to act on her flight-or-fight mechanisms, immobilization with fear becomes her next option and dissociation ensues. In "inescapable shock," she can no longer use her voice, may feel hopeless, and may engage in "learned helplessness" (Seligman 1972), including submissive behaviors or passive compliance, such as agreeing to interventions she does not want. Further, the physiologic characteristics of the immobilization (with fear) state, including reduced heart rate, blood pressure, and oxygen (Porges 2011) may contribute to further complications, compounding the traumatic experience. Perinatal dissociation and delivery stress constitute a common pathway to PTSD (Thiel and Deckel 2020). One woman described dissociating during an emergency cesarean, "I felt like a head without a body, as if there was nobody in there" (quoted in Guittier et al. 2014:4).

The following sections describe sources and experiences of birth trauma in greater detail, emphasizing external environment, internal experience, and social interaction.

The External Environment: Fear and Safety in the Birth Setting

The cultural characterization of the hospital is one of safety and security. Yet numerous sources of data indicate that home and birth center births are just as safe, if not safer—with fewer complications and interventions, far less iatrogenic damage, and perinatal outcomes equal to those of low-risk hospital births (de Jonge et al. 2009, 2015; Stapleton et al. 2013; Cheyney et al. 2014). The juxtaposition between the hospital's image and its reality is maintained by an ideology that positions technology as safe and normalizes intervention, while truly normal physiology is deemed risky and unpredictable (Newnhan et al. 2016). Davis-Floyd (2003) terms this the "technocratic model of birth," wherein the female body is treated as a defective machine in need of technological surveillance and control.

Within the hospital setting, women may feel subjectively safe (ibid.). Yet simultaneously, many common hospital practices interfere with natural labor processes, which may be detected via neuroception both consciously and unconsciously. Lack of privacy, bright lights, loud sounds, hurried interactions with care providers, painful and unconsented vaginal exams, and time pressure can cause excess stress. Epidural analgesia, cesareans, and mother–infant separation have hormonal impacts that affect the normal progress of labor and attachment. Elevated sympathetic nervous system activation raises epinephrine-norepinephrine and inhibits oxytocin and beta-endorphins and their pain-relieving properties, increasing the risk of additional interventions (Buckley 2015).

The "cascade of interventions" often begins with inducing labor (Buckley 2015), which can have substantial effects long after birth for both mother and baby. Instrumental and unwanted cesarean births leave mothers at increased risk for depression, anxiety, somatization, obsessive-compulsive and PTSD symptoms (Dekel et al. 2017). Notably, infants born vaginally without epidural have significantly higher vagal tone than cesarean-born infants (Kozar et al. 2018). Infants with high vagal tone are more reactive to their environment at 5 months (positively and negatively), and more approachable and sociable at 14 months (Fox 1989).

In contrast to the technocratic model, the holistic model of birth centers the mental, emotional, physical, and spiritual needs of the birthing woman. The female body is honored as a source of intuition and wisdom, whether labor takes an hour or several days (Davis-Floyd and Davis 2018). The birth environment is sacred, as is the choice of who attends. The mother's sense of safety and of her own protagonism are paramount. These are significant reasons why the studies cited above show better outcomes for midwife-attended home and birth center births and the "midwifery model of care" (described in Davis-Floyd 2018).

Internal Experience: The Mental and Emotional Journey to and through Birth

A laboring woman carries her life experience into the birthing room. While birth will be difficult in an environment that feels unsafe, an otherwise safe environment may also feel compromised to a woman with a history of trauma and/or mental health concerns. Faulty neuroception involves difficulty discerning safe from unsafe environments and trustworthy from untrustworthy people, which may be at the root of many mental health ailments (Porges 2011).

Trauma and mental illness compromise autonomic functioning (ibid.), which can affect the birth experience. Pregnant women with anxiety have lower vagal tone compared to healthy pregnant women; such autonomic activity may play a role in pregnancy complications (Mizuno et al. 2017). Relatedly, women with a history of childhood sexual assault have longer labors, are 9.9 times more likely to have a cesarean, and 12.2 times more likely to have an instrumental (forceps or vacuum) delivery (Nerum et al. 2013).

A mother's experience of the moment of birth is also significant for her sense of self. Mothers' emotional experiences appear to differ by delivery mode. Guittier et al. (2014) observed many women with vaginal deliveries describe their births as magical or beautiful, while many with cesarean births described anxiety, fear, disappointment, or a sense of failure. Furthermore, fear of childbirth itself can have a significant impact on the experience. Fear of birth is associated with increased risk of epidural use, longer labor, and instrumental or cesarean delivery (emergency or elective), as well PTSD (Dencker et al. 2019; Chapter 9).

Social Interaction: Co-Regulation for Safety

Human birth is unique compared to most other species, as we typically birth in the presence of others for both physical and emotional support (see Chapter 1). From the perspective of the autonomic nervous system, social interaction can be supportive, activating the ventral vagal social engagement system and co-regulation, increasing oxytocin, and reducing excess stress. Alternatively, negative interactions can elicit defensive reactions activating the mobilization and/or immobilization with fear systems (Porges 2011).

Continuous support is associated with spontaneous vaginal birth and shorter labors, particularly with trained doulas. Support is linked to decreased risks for medication/epidural for pain, instrumental or cesarean births, low 5-minute APGAR scores, and negative birth experiences (National Partnership for Women & Families 2018). Midwife-attended women frequently develop personal relationships with the midwives who will be present at their births. In obstetrics, women often see a group of doctors and may not know who will be present at their labor, in addition to other "intimate strangers" working at the hospital (Chapter 1). The presence of unfamiliar care providers or hospital workers, particularly males, can create excess stress (Buckley 2015).

Disturbingly, women can be treated with disrespect or even abuse during labor (Sadler et al. 2016; Liese et al. 2021). Beck (2018) identified six main types of mistreatment, including failure to meet professional standards of care, poor rapport between women and providers, verbal abuse, physical abuse (including sexual abuse), health system conditions/constraints, and stigma/discrimination. Maltreatment is more common in low/middle-income countries, but happens everywhere (ibid.). Disrespect and abuse trigger a defensive reaction (Porges 2011), so for example, chastising a woman for not making fast enough progress will only traumatize her and stall her labor further.

A Polyvagal Perspective on Pam's Stalled Labor

Let's return to Pam's story—stuck at 5 centimeters in horrific pain for hours. Lucia enters, and within minutes Pam relaxes—and so does her cervix. What has happened?

Lucia enters quietly, honoring Pam's space. This is all about Pam; Lucia is there to support her mind, body, and spirit—all of which innately know how to birth her child. Physically, Lucia meets Pam where she is, positioned behind her, serving as a somatic support while respecting the instinctive movements of Pam's body. Never interrupting Pam, Lucia attunes to her. Synchronizing her breathing to Pam's, Lucia communicates to Pam's neuroception: I'm here *with* you. Sensing Lucia's calming presence, Pam begins to co-regulate to the state of Lucia's nervous system. Lucia speaks in rhythm with Pam's breathing, "Oh good." Pam's fast, high-pitched, "Oh God, oh God, oh God" reflects her body's memory of the trauma of her prior birth. With Lucia's intuitive support, Pam's "Oh God" cries gently give way to a slower, steadier, "Oh good." As her breathing slows, and her pitch drops, Pam's sympathetic nervous system down-regulates. The ventral branch of the vagus nerve has been activated, and her system senses safety. Immobilization with fear transforms into immobilization with love, and Pam's body releases oxytocin. "Oh gooooood," she chants gutturally, her cervix relaxing and opening as the pitch of her voice deepens. With Lucia's gentle attunement, Pam's neuroception detects safety, reduces defensiveness, and co-regulates with Lucia in trust and dignity. As described above, Pam later shared that during her last birth, her waters were artificially ruptured at 6 cm against her will, leading to excruciating pain, exacerbated by being forced to labor on her back (Roncalli 1997)—her body remembered. Despite being perfect strangers, Lucia was confident in Pam's birthing abilities, never attempting to rescue or control her. By supporting Pam's body through a point of prior trauma, Lucia helped Pam sense that this time was different—she was safe to let go and birth her baby, and she did.

Conclusion: Back to the Future

Porges calls Polyvagal Theory a "work in progress" (2011:iv), as is our understanding of the mysteries of birth. Technology is a tool; just as a hammer can help to build a loving family home, it can also serve as a cold-blooded weapon. So too can medicalized technology be used for good or harm (see Chapter 12); yet in an over-medicalized culture, it can be difficult to tell which is which (Liese et al. 2021). Yet to dispose of technology altogether would be shortsighted. After all, technology has not only saved lives, but has also brought us the ability to measure heart rate variability, which has shed light on the inner workings of the autonomic nervous system—a tool that can help uncover more deeply what it really means to be human.

In *Cyborg Babies: From Techno-Sex to Techno-Tots* (1998:11), Davis-Floyd and Dumit describe 8 theoretical constructs for cyborgs (see Introduction), one of which is "the cyborg as mutilator of natural processes." In the cyborgification of birth, technoscience fills a gap that was created by technoscience—the next intervention addresses a problem created by the previous intervention, the outcome of which will likely require an additional intervention—in what Reynolds (1991) has called the 1-2 Punch of technological mutilation and prosthesis (see Introduction and Chapter 1). The medicalized obsession with risk reduction creates its own risks, in the "obstetric paradox" described in Chapter 1. Gratitude is warranted for lives saved and suffering spared. Yet under the guise of safety, the laboring woman's body becomes an object of control. Ironically, the technocratic failure to center women's humanity in the birth process is precisely what compromises her safety, crippling her inherent birthing abilities and increasing the Punch 2 risk of "rescue" via intervention.

Yet safety is more than a discourse or ideology—it is physiologically, neuroceptively felt. Safety, privacy, and respect in birth are not—or should not—be privileges, but should be recognized as integral parts of being human and of humane care. How a society welcomes the next generation and honors women bringing humanity forth imprints on each new arrival, each mother, each family, and the culture at large. Whether newborns enter this world through women "immobilized" in love or in fear shapes those babies' foundational experience of life and the world they will help to create as they grow. To move toward our techno-sapiens future with happier, healthier women, babies, and families, we must—as Dr. Emmet Brown pleads with Marty McFly in the movie—go "back to the future," embracing the evolution-based neurobiology that generates our sense of being human: the core ways in which we are wired for safety, social connection, and healthy births.

References

Beck CT. 2018. "A Secondary Analysis of Mistreatment of Women During Childbirth in Health Care Facilities." *Journal of Obstetric, Gynecologic and Neonatal Nursing* 47(1):94–104.

Bolaza EB. 2020. "Birth Pleasure: Meanings, Politics, and Praxis." *Journal of the Motherhood Initiative for Research and Community Involvement* 11(1):123–135.

Buckley S. 2010. "Sexuality in Labour and Birth: An Intimate Perspective." In: *Essential Midwifery Practice: Intrapartum Care*, eds. D Walsh, S Downe. Oxford: Wiley-Blackwell, 213–234.

Buckley S. 2015. *Hormonal Physiology of Childbearing: Evidence and Implications for Women, Babies, and Maternity Care.* Washington, DC: Childbirth Connection Programs, National Partnership for Women & Families.

Cheyney M, M Bovbjerg, C Everson et al. 2014. "Outcomes of Care for 16,924 Planned Home Births in the United States: The Midwives Alliance of North America Statistics Project, 2004 to 2009." *Journal of Midwifery and Women's Health* 59(1):17–27.

Davis E, D Pascali Bonaro. 2010. *Orgasmic Birth: Your Guide to a Safe, Satisfying, and Pleasurable Birth Experience.* New York: Rodale.

Davis-Floyd R. 2003. *Birth as an American Rite of Passage*, 2nd edition. Berkeley, CA: University of California Press.

Davis-Floyd R. 2018. "The Midwifery Model of Care: Anthropological Perspectives." In: *Ways of Knowing about Birth: Mothers, Midwives, Medicine, and Birth Activism*, ed. R Davis-Floyd. Long Grove, IL: Waveland Press, 323–338.

Davis-Floyd R, E Davis. 2018. "Intuition as Authoritative Knowledge in Midwifery and Home Birth." In: *Ways of Knowing about Birth: Mothers, Midwives, Medicine, and Birth Activism* by Davis-Floyd R. Long Grove, IL: Waveland Press, 189–220.

Davis-Floyd R, J Dumit. 1998. *Cyborg Babies: From Techno-Sex to Techno-Tots.* New York: Routledge.

De Couck M, J Nijs, Y Gidron. 2014. "You May Need a Nerve to Treat Pain: The Neurobiological Rationale for Vagal Nerve Activation in Pain Management." *The Clinical Journal of Pain* 30(12):1099–1105.

de Jonge A, CC Geerts, BY van der Goes et al. 2015. "Perinatal Mortality and Morbidity up to 28 Days after Birth among 743,070 Low-Risk Planned Home and Hospital Births: A Cohort Study Based on Three Merged National Perinatal Databases." *BJOG: An International Journal of Obstetrics and Gynecology* 122(5):720–728.

de Jonge A, BY van der Goes, AC Ravelli et al. 2009. "Perinatal Mortality and Morbidity in a Nationwide Cohort of 529,688 Low-Risk Planned Home and Hospital Births *BJOG: An International Journal of Obstetrics and Gynecology* 116(9):1177–1184.

Dekel S, C Stuebe, G Dishy. 2017. "Childbirth Induced Posttraumatic Stress Syndrome: A Systematic Review of Prevalence and Risk Factors." *Frontiers in Psychology* 8:560.

Dencker A, C Nilsson, C Begley et al. 2019. "Causes and Outcomes in Studies of Fear of Childbirth: A Systematic Review." *Women and Birth: Journal of the Australian College of Midwives* 32(2):99–111.

Dick-Read G. 2006 [1942]. *Childbirth Without Fear: The Principles and Practice of Natural Childbirth.* London: Pollinger Limited.

Enderli T. 2017. *A Review of the Potential Therapeutic Application of Vagus Nerve Stimulation During Childbirth.* Master's Thesis. Melbourne, FL: Florida Institute of Technology.

Field T, M Hemandez-Reif, S Taylor, O Quintino, I Burman. 1997. "Labor Pain Is Reduced by Massage Therapy." *Journal of Psychosomatic Obstetrics and Gynecology* 18(4):286–291.

Fox NA. 1989. "Psychophysiological Correlates of Emotional Reactivity During the First Year of Life." *Developmental Psychology* 25(3):364–372.

Gaskin IM. 2003. *Ina May's Guide to Childbirth.* New York: Bantam.

Guittier MJ, C Cedraschi, N Jamei, M Boulvain, F Guillemin. 2014. "Impact of Mode of Delivery on the Birth Experience in First-Time Mothers: A Qualitative Study." *BMC Pregnancy and Childbirth* 14(1):254.

Komisaruk BR, G Sansone. 2003. "Neural Pathways Mediating Vaginal Function: The Vagus Nerves and Spinal Cord Oxytocin." *Scandinavian Journal of Psychology* 44(3):241–250.

Kozar M, I Tonhajzerova, M Mestanik et al. 2018. "Heart Rate Variability in Healthy Term Newborns Is Related to Delivery Mode: A Prospective Observational Study." *BMC Pregnancy and Childbirth* 18(1):264–273.

Laborde S, E Mosley, JF Thayer. 2017. "Heart Rate Variability and Cardiac Vagal Tone in Psychophysiological Research—Recommendations for Experiment Planning, Data Analysis, and Data Reporting." *Frontiers in Psychology* 8(13):1–18.

Liese K, R Davis-Floyd, K Stewart, M Cheyney. 2021. "Obstetric Iatrogenesis in the United States: The Spectrum of Disrespect, Violence, and Abuse." *Anthropology and Medicine*, in press.

Martin JA, BE Hamilton, MJK Osterman, AK Driscoll, TJ Mathews. 2017. "Births: Final Data for 2015." *National Vital Statistics Reports: From the Centers for Disease Control and Prevention, National Center for Health Statistics, National Vital Statistics System* 66(1):1.

Mizuno T, K Tamakoshi, K Tanabe. 2017. "Anxiety during Pregnancy and Autonomic Nervous System Activity: A Longitudinal Observational and Cross-Sectional Study." *Journal of Psychosomatic Research* 99:105–111.

National Partnership for Women & Families. 2018. "Continuous Support for Women During Childbirth: 2017 Cochrane Review Update Key Takeaways." *Journal of Perinatal Education* 27(4):193–197.

Nerum H, L Halvorsen, B Straume, T Sørlie, P Øian. 2013. "Different Labour Outcomes in Primiparous Women That Have Been Subjected to Childhood Sexual Abuse or Rape in Adulthood: A Case–Control Study in a Clinical Cohort." *British Journal of Obstetrics and Gynaecology* 120(4):487–495.

Newnham E, L McKellar, J Pincombe. 2016. "A Critical Literature Review of Epidural Analgesia." *Evidence Based Midwifery* 14:22–28.

Ogden P, K Minton, C Pain. 2006. *Trauma and the Body: A Sensorimotor Approach to Psychotherapy*. New York: W.W. Norton.

Olza-Fernández I, MAM Gabriel, A Gil-Sanchez, LM Garcia-Segura, MA Arevalo. 2014. "Neuroendocrinology of Childbirth and Mother–Child Attachment: The Basis of an Etiopathogenic Model of Perinatal Neurobiological Disorders." *Frontiers in Neuroendocrinology* 35(4):459–472.

Porges S. 2011. *The Polyvagal Theory: Neurophysiological Foundations of Emotion, Attachment, Communication, and Self-Regulation*. New York: W.W. Norton.

Porges S. 2017. "Vagal Pathways: Portals to Compassion." In: *The Oxford Handbook of Compassion Science*, eds. EM Seppälä, E Simon-Thomas, SL Brown, MC Worline, CD Cameron, JR Doty. Oxford: Oxford University Press, 189–202.

Porges S. 2018. "Polyvagal Theory: A Primer." In: *Clinical Applications of the Polyvagal Theory: The Emergence of Polyvagal-Informed Therapies*, by Porges S, Dana DA. New York: W.W. Norton, 50–69.

Reyes-Lagos JJ, CI Ledesma-Ramírez, AC Pliego-Carrillo et al. 2019 1437. "Neuroautonomic Activity Evidences Parturition as a Complex and Integrated Neuro–Immune–Endocrine Process." *Annals of the New York Academy of Sciences* 1(1):22–30.

Reynolds PC. 1991. *Stealing Fire: The Mythology of the Technocracy*. Palo Alto: California Iconic Anthropology Press.

Roncalli L. 1997. "Standing by Process: A Midwife's Notes on Story-Telling, Passage and Intuition." In: *Intuition: The Inside Story*, eds. R Davis-Floyd, PS Arvidson. New York: Routledge, 177–200.

Sadler M, MJDS Santos, D Ruiz-Berdún et al. 2016. "Moving Beyond Disrespect and Abuse: Addressing the Structural Dimensions of Obstetric Violence." *Reproductive Health Matters* 24(47):47–55.

Seligman MEP. 1972. "Learned Helplessness." *Annual Review of Medicine* 23(1):407–412.

Simpson M, C Catling. 2016. "Understanding Psychological Traumatic Birth Experiences: A Literature Review." *Women and Birth: Journal of the Australian College of Midwives* 29(3):203–207.

Stapleton SR, C Osborne, J Illuzzi. 2013. "Outcomes of Care in Birth Centers: Demonstration of a Durable Model." *Journal of Midwifery and Women's Health* 58(1):3–14.

Thiel F, S Dekel. 2020. "Peritraumatic Dissociation in Childbirth-Evoked Posttraumatic Stress and Postpartum Mental Health." *Archives of Women's Mental Health* 23(2):189–197.

14

FAMILY-CENTERED, EVIDENCE-BASED, PSYCHO-SOCIALLY SENSITIVE, AND CULTURALLY RESPECTFUL PERINATAL CARE:

Still a Futuristic Dream!

Beverley Chalmers

Introduction: Family-Centered Perinatal Care

Family-centered care during pregnancy, birth, and the postpartum period is defined in my book *Family-Centred Perinatal Care: Improving Pregnancy, Birth and Postpartum Care* (Chalmers 2017)—on which this chapter is based—as care that is evidence-based, psycho-socially sensitive, multi-culturally adapted, inter-and multi-disciplinary, and utilizing only essential and appropriate technology. Some might think that all our healthcare services fulfill this promise. We have, however, yet to implement our evidence-based guidelines, to truly integrate women and their families into care, and to understand that the woman giving birth is not only a uterus, vagina, and perineum carrying a fetus, but a person with hopes, wishes, expectations, feelings, and a family. Reinstating women, babies, and partners from the secondary, and primarily biological, role to which they have been assigned to a central, holistic role within perinatal care is still a future dream.

The mother, her partner, and her newborn are the sole reasons for the whole structure of perinatal healthcare services, and these should be totally directed towards best meeting their cognitive, emotional, social, cultural, and spiritual needs, in addition to their biological requirements. This is frequently forgotten, underplayed, or neglected. Our current emphasis on technological development benefits many, but lacks a humane perspective. As demonstrated in the preceding chapters in this section, providing humanistic techno-sapiens birth care remains a priority.

Care Should Be Based on the Best Available Evidence

Pregnancy and birth are healthy, normal life events during which caregivers must remain vigilant for deviations from normal. As discussed in detail in my book (Chalmers 2017), definitions of "normal birth" vary widely. For example, when comparing those of Canada (Society of Obstetricians and Gynaecologists of Canada 2008), the UK (Royal College of Obstetricians and Gynaecologists et al. 2007), and the World Health Organization (WHO 1994), most women's births do not meet the criteria specified in each of their own definitions for "normal birth." In addition, current trends towards referring to normal birth as "physiologic birth," downplaying psychological, social, and spiritual components, can reflect a clinical/medicalized/technologized approach that lacks recognition of these humanistic and holistic elements (Chalmers 2017).

Many technologies used in perinatal care confer no clinical benefit, and some are harmful. Two resources have reached similar conclusions regarding the effectiveness of perinatal technology: WHO (1985) debates, deliberations and published recommendations, and meta-analyses of randomized controlled trials resulting in evidence-based guidelines (Enkin et al. 1989; Cochrane Library 2015). Although over two decades have passed since this knowledge became available, and although evidence-based perinatal care has been accepted in principle, inappropriate technology is still used.

Childbirth practices and policies differ—sometimes widely—both among countries and across regions within countries. If evidence-based practices were implemented within a country, then rates of interventions should be similar across that country, yet this is often not the case. In Canada, rates of cesareans, epidurals, continuous electronic fetal monitoring, supine position for delivery, episiotomies, and perineal stitching, among others, differ considerably across its 13 provinces and territories (Chalmers et al. 2012). Similarly, in England, maternal characteristics and clinical risk factors accounted for little of the variability in cesarean rates across the country (Bragg et al. 2010). In both South Africa and Delhi, India, rates of interventions fall short of evidence-based guidelines, with overuse of interventions in private hospitals and deficiency of patient-centered practices, such as labor support, in public hospitals (Nagpal et al. 2014).

These wide variations suggest that the usage of interventions is not based only on evidence or medical need. Rather, other factors, including the types of healthcare providers in different regions, hospital size, availability of resources, maternal access to care, rural or urban residence, long-established ways of providing care, local cultural variations, medico-legal and economic concerns, availability of technology, and maternal demographic variables all influence practice. Practice is also affected by how maternity care is organized or reimbursed, how and where practitioners are trained, and prevailing attitudes toward pregnant women and their families (Chalmers et al. 2009).

Evidence-based practice should apply to all families regardless of socio-economic status or other discriminatory variables. Some procedures for which there are no medical indications, however, continue to be performed, sometimes in a discriminatory pattern (Public Health Agency of Canada 2009). In Canada, for example, where perinatal care is among the best in the world, and where equity in healthcare services is a matter of national pride, socially disadvantaged women are, nevertheless, more likely to have enemas, lie in a supine position for birth, and have their legs in stirrups—all unproven and potentially harmful practices (Chalmers et al. 2012). Among mothers having a vaginal birth, 19.1% have their perineal or pubic hair shaved and 15% report that someone pushed on their abdomen to push the baby down (Chalmers et al. 2012). Worse still, these procedures are performed more often on teenage mothers, poorly educated women, and low-income women than on those who are older, better off, and better educated. This is extremely concerning. We do not examine social determinants of health as mediators of abusive obstetric practices often enough, perhaps because it is unbelievable to think that such prejudices find outlet in practice, or because they are too embarrassing to expose.

Remuneration packages influence the use of technology. Where fee-for-service remuneration packages are in place for caregivers, the rates of technological interventions increase. Surveyed obstetricians in South Africa acknowledged that some cesareans were performed for financial incentives (Price and Broomberg 1990; Chalmers et al. 1991). In countries where both fee-for-service and salaried medical staff co-exist, the technological intervention rate can be almost twice as high in fee-for-service systems. This occurs frequently when there is private health insurance available to higher socio-economic groups, compared with salaried care services that care for families at lower socio-economic levels (Price and Broomberg 1990). It is obvious that where we financially reward caregivers for interventions, they, not surprisingly, intervene more.

Discrimination based on other variables also occurs. Many healthcare providers hold strong negative attitudes towards people with obesity that influence their judgment, interpersonal behavior, and decision-making and, consequently, the care they provide (Phelan et al. 2015). The management of labor for women with obesity differs from that of thinner women and leads to unnecessarily increased, non-evidence-based cesarean rates due to their negatively perceived BMI rather than to clinical need (Joy and Bittner 2015).

Interventions such as cesareans should be used only when clinically essential. Two global reports on optimal cesarean rates have found no reductions in maternal and neonatal mortality and morbidity when frequency of cesareans was more than 15% (Althabe et al. 2006, Villar et al. 2006). An increased rate of intervention was associated with higher mortality and morbidity in mothers and neonates (Villar et al. 2006). Many, if not most, technologically advanced societies have rates that far exceed this proportion, such as Canada (around 27%–28%), the US (around 32%) and China (around 45–50%) (Chalmers 2017). Some countries, however, have annual cesarean rates that are far too low, such as 1% of births or even less (Ethiopia, Burkina Faso, Niger, and Madagascar) (Gibbons et al. 2010). In a WHO survey, 54 countries reported rates below 10%, and 69 had rates above 15%. These figures indicate that 3.2 million additional cesareans are needed in countries where rates are below 10% and 6.2 million unnecessary sections are performed in countries where rates are above 15%.

Cesareans can also be performed with more psychological sensitivity. Having a companion of the mother's choice present, encouraging skin-to-skin contact from the moment of delivery, not separating mother and baby, breastfeeding when the baby shows signs of readiness for a feed, in as quiet and respectful an environment as possible, can make the experience of cesarean birth far more psychologically satisfying, and can facilitate parent-infant attachment and breast-feeding. I was asked by the World Health Organization Regional Office for Europe to develop a training program to introduce evidence-based, psychoso-cially sensitive, and culturally respectful perinatal care into the European region and particularly into the countries of the former Soviet Union. I and my co-trainers included this approach to cesareans in the multiple WHO-Euro training programs that we conducted in the 1990s and 2000s: it is now being termed "gentle cesareans" in Western countries but it is still by no means a routine prac-tice (Magee et al. 2014).

Families Need Support for Breastfeeding

We need to support breastfeeding of both normal term infants and babies requir-ing neonatal intensive care. Uninterrupted, skin-to-skin, mother- and/or par-ent-infant contact, for the first hour or more after birth, is the goal to strive for in both vaginal and cesarean birth to optimize breastfeeding. Most routine maternity and newborn care procedures, such as cord clamping, eye prophylaxis, and clothing of the infant can and should be delayed to allow for parent-infant time together, with both mother (or father/partner) and baby covered to ensure warmth. Thereafter, rooming-in 24/7, care by parents, and cue-based breast-feeding is the optimum approach. At present, this is not always practiced, even in the best of maternity services.

The *Baby Friendly Hospital Initiative* (BFHI) and the *Code of Marketing of Breastmilk Substitutes*—launched by WHO and UNICEF in 1991—are core components of family-centered care. The BFHI (Kramer and Kakuma 2012) promotes exclusive breastfeeding for the first six months of life and continued breastfeeding, together with complementary foods, for two years or longer (WHO/UNICEF 2003). Even though strong randomized control evidence sup-ports the BFHI (Kramer et al. 2001, 2008), very few hospitals in North America are accredited as Baby-Friendly and only some 20,000 to 30,000 worldwide. Many industrialized countries are aware of the BFHI and endorse its guidelines, although they are unable to implement it fully. One reason for this is a wide-spread lack of training for healthcare providers on the 10 Steps of the BFHI. All caregivers, including obstetricians, pediatricians, family doctors, nurses, and midwives need to be trained in the basic skills of breastfeeding that, judging from our less than ideal global outcomes, are lacking at present.

In addition, confusing advice is given to new mothers. Caregivers are will-ing to adamantly advise mothers not to smoke, drink, or use medications dur-ing pregnancy, yet hesitate to say that breastfeeding is best for fear of making mothers feel "guilty." We often imply that mothers are somehow to blame for not attempting to breastfeed, or not succeeding in breastfeeding, incurring feelings of guilt and, sometimes, anger towards the healthcare system that tends to equate breastfeeding with good mothering. We downplay the breastfeeding challenges faced by mothers who have cesarean births. These result in less mother-infant contact, less skin-to-skin contact, and less breastfeeding in the first two hours after birth, together with more pacifier use, more distribution of free formula samples, and more scheduled feeding than for mothers delivering vaginally, with subsequent poorer breastfeeding outcomes (Chalmers et al. 2010). There is still much to do to promote, support, and protect breastfeeding. It is not mothers who are failing to breastfeed their newborns, but caregivers who are failing mothers (Chalmers 2013).

Many benefits—both maternal and infant—accrue from breastfeeding (Lawrence and Lawrence 2011). The Canadian-led Promotion of Breastfeeding Intervention Trial (PROBIT), the largest randomized trial ever conducted in the field of breastfeeding, provides strong evidence that following the 10 Steps of the BFHI increases prolonged and exclusive breastfeeding, which in turn improves infant health in the first year of life and results in improved children's cognitive development at school-going age (Kramer et al. 2001, 2008). Other benefits include protection against child infections and malocclusion (misalignment of the upper and lower teeth), probable reductions in excessive weight gain and diabetes for children, and protection against breast cancer, ovarian cancer, and type 2 diabetes in mothers (Victora et al. 2016).

The 10 Steps of the BFHI apply to Neonatal Intensive Care Unit (NICU) care, although some modifications are needed. The NICU environment is clinically essential but frequently psychologically isolationist. It often involves separation of mother and baby, with minimal contact between them, and especially little skin-to-skin contact, as well as feeding with breastmilk substitutes either totally or in addition to breastmilk. In most of the industrialized world, these practices were accepted, for some decades, as essential care for the sick or preterm newborn. NICUs, however, do not have to be, and should not be, organized this way (Chalmers 2017; Chalmers and Levin 2001). The *Humane Neonatal Care Initiative* (HNCI) includes the mother, her baby, and her partner in a rooming-in NICU, with direct parent care of the sick or preterm newborn and close skin-to-skin mother- and/or father/partner-baby contact, with breastfeeding (or breastmilk feeding) 24/7, from birth until discharge (Chalmers and Levin 2001; Chalmers 2017). Except for technical medical and nursing care, under the HCNI, mothers who stay with their newborns in NICUs are encouraged and expected to provide all of the infant's care and to stay in the NICU until discharge. Mother/father-care of NICU babies has multiple physiological benefits. Extensive skin-to-skin care of NICU babies leads to fewer severe infections or sepsis, less hypothermia, earlier discharge, improved breastfeeding initiation and duration, and fewer severe illnesses at 6 months follow-up (Hall and Kirsten 2008, Moore et al. 2012, MJ Renfrew et al. 2009). Babies gain weight more rapidly, have enhanced immunological defenses against infection, have infection durations reduced by 3–5 days, have reduced needs for antibiotics, have 3–5 times fewer respiratory infections during the first year of life, have higher rates of physiological interferon that enhances the body's immune response, and have improved neurological development (Chalmers and Levin 2001). Reducing unnecessary technology and maximizing humane care leads to better outcomes for preterm and sick newborns. What is remarkable is not that these babies thrive with tender, loving care, but that caregivers, in the 21st century, still enforce separation of babies and mothers as well as institutionalization of the neediest of our infants, even in the best of units.

We Need Perinatal Psychologists

Perinatal psychologists play an important role in providing care. Psychologists with a thorough knowledge of perinatal practices, who are a part of the perinatal care team, and who focus on the emotional, intellectual, and interpersonal challenges faced by couples and caregivers are urgently needed. Every maternity care setting should have resident perinatal psychologists to provide support and care for women, their families, and their healthcare providers, as has been implemented by the government, on a national level, in the Republic of Moldova (Chalmers 2017) and in some units in Turkey (Çoker et al. 2015).

In addition to preparation for birth and parenthood through prenatal education classes, psychological support may be needed at many stages of the perinatal and parenting period (Chalmers and Levin 2001). Difficulties regarding adjustment to pregnancy, for example in a pregnancy following infertility treatments, after pregnancy loss, among teenagers and single women, after previous traumatic birth, or life, experiences, could be assisted with psychological support. In addition, women experiencing a pregnancy loss or the birth of a preterm or stillborn baby, or a baby with special needs, may benefit from counseling.

Healthcare providers too can benefit from the support of psychologists, who can help them deal with their own fears and emotions surrounding birth, during or after the birth (Chalmers and Levin 2001). In particular, those caring for babies or parents in difficulty, such as in NICUs, may value assistance. There is little formal training for perinatal psychologists available. We desperately need Departments of Psychology to educate students about psycho-social issues in health, and particularly perinatal health.

Families Need Prenatal Preparation

Ensuring that pregnant women and their families receive psychological and social preparation for pregnancy, birth, and the early months of parenthood is as important as providing good clinical care. The importance of preparation, not just for birth (e.g., pregnancy care, labor, birth, mother-infant contact and feeding, partners' needs, roles, and support), but also for parenthood (e.g., early child

development, infant nutrition, appropriate methods of discipline, marital adjustment, motherhood, conflict resolution, employment, and parenthood) cannot be
underestimated.

Preparation for parenthood is possibly even more important than preparation for birth and is a sadly neglected part of education globally. Although most
people become parents, there is no preparation for it other than the example set
by one's own family—which may or may not be helpful. We have also not yet
accepted that involving fathers or partners in this education is just as important
as including them at the birth. Encouraging a companion in labor and at birth is
strongly endorsed by randomized controlled trials (Hofmeyr et al. 1991; Hodnett
et al. 2012), although encouraging family support for women (and their babies)
in the post-birth period is as, if not more, important. If ever a mother needs assistance from others, it is in the hours, days, weeks, and months after giving birth.
Although nursing care is needed to care for the physical after-effects of birth,
practical and ongoing support with caring for the newborn is also needed. So too
is time to share the joys and wonders of new parenthood as a family. Postpartum
family support is desperately needed for all mothers, but is even more important
for women who have had cesareans.

We need innovative thinking to improve the transition to parenthood of all
new families, whether birth is vaginal or cesarean. Exciting models have been
developed in Scandinavian countries (Finland, Norway, Sweden, and Denmark),
called "patient hotels" where families stay together for a few days in postpartum
hotels adjacent to the maternity hospital, as part of their government-supported
postpartum care. Additionally, the growing availability in Canada and in the
United States of postpartum doulas who provide mother-baby and home care
for days or weeks after birth is welcome, although doulas are generally privately
paid, making access to them difficult for many. Internet-based support can have
mixed value: some sites are reputable while others may offer misinformation.
Mothers and families often cannot readily judge which are more reliable. An
evidence-based rating of pregnancy and birth websites (i.e., a "family-friendly"
website rating system) is sorely needed. Telemedicine networks or emergency
nursing pools that mothers could draw on for a day or night's assistance when
the going gets tough might well be valuable models to develop that may comple-
ment the network of community clinics and home visiting or telephone contact
services that currently exist, for example in Canada.

Care Must Not Be Abusive

All forms of abuse occur during perinatal care. Any form of abuse—psychological, social, sexual, physical, verbal, emotional, financial, or medical—is inappropriate and should never occur. A global review has established 7 categories of
abusive and disrespectful care of women during childbirth (also described in
Chapter 13). These include: physical abuse, sexual abuse, verbal abuse, stigma
and discrimination, failure to meet professional standards of care, poor rapport

between women and providers, and health system conditions and constraints (Bohren et al. 2015; see also Beck 2018).

Some procedures are regarded as abusive by women but are, or were at the time of their experience, considered necessary or beneficial by caregivers. These practices include: unconsented and painful vaginal exams; routine episiotomy; repair of minor perineal lacerations; manual exploration of the uterus; exteriorization (pulling it out) and examination of the cervix following vaginal delivery; swabbing of the vagina with antiseptic after birth; anal exploration after delivery; and lack of appropriate anesthesia or analgesia for such procedures. They also include less painful procedures such as routine perineal and pubic shaving, and enemas during labor. Even the embarrassing lithotomy position with its emotional and physical associations of helplessness and loss of control for the woman, its unconcerned exposure of psychologically and socially private bodily parts, and its compression of the pelvic outlet, may be considered abusive. Today, not being allowed a (desired) supportive companion during labor and birth is also abusive. In many countries these practices have, fortunately, been discontinued, although not completely and not everywhere.

Widespread lack of informed consent for common procedures occurring at the time of birth (non-consensual care), such as for episiotomies, hysterectomies, blood transfusions, sterilization, augmentation of labor, and even cesareans have been reported in many childbirth settings, with some women reporting lack of patient-doctor confidentiality (Chalmers 1998, Chalmers and Levin 2001). Worse still is the blatant physical abuse and non-dignified care of women during labor and birth in a number of countries through, for example, hitting or slapping with an open hand or instrument, pinching, particularly on the thighs, kicking, shouting at, or scolding the mother, exerting excessive pressure on her abdomen to expel the baby, repairing episiotomies without pain relief, or even tying the woman down during labor or using mouth gags (Bohren et al. 2015; Bowser and Hill 2010). Verbal abuse of women in childbirth is also commonly reported. This includes: the use of harsh or rude language, judgmental statements, threats of poor outcomes, or withholding treatment if women are noncompliant, most commonly from midwives and nurses and less often from doctors. Women from lower socio-economic groups, migrants, those from ethnic minorities, adolescents, and older mothers of high parity report discriminatory care (Bohren et al. 2015). Sexual abuse during labor has also emerged (Bowser and Hill 2010). For example, in Nigeria, sexual abuse of women by a healthcare worker is reported by 2% of women (Bohren et al. 2015).

A further abusive practice involves the payment of bribes to doctors, nurses, midwives, receptionists, and guards. These bribes take the form of money, food or drinks, jewelry, or other gifts and are expected in many countries around the world. Such payments may ensure better or more timely care, and/or the provision of medications.

Comments made and actions taken in the operating theater when a woman is anesthetized may be inappropriate and disrespectful of patients, harmful to students, and derogatory towards colleagues. Doctors sometimes "behave badly" in operating theaters (Singh and Posner 2015). In 2015, the *Annals of Internal Medicine* published an anonymous account of such behaviors, including the attending physician's comment, while swabbing a woman's labia and inner thighs prior to a vaginal hysterectomy, that he "bet she was enjoying this" (Anonymous 2015). Other inappropriate and derogatory, sometimes racist comments may be made and are often not countered by embarrassed—and often junior—colleagues, who in turn learn this behavior. Singh and Posner also report hearing openly homophobic, antisemitic, and sexually charged comments in operating theaters with little done to stop them (Singh and Posner 2015). These authors advise that "If you wouldn't say it with the patient awake and your mother in the room, don't say it." The patient should be cared for with the utmost respect whether awake or asleep.

Midwifery Care Is Beneficial

Why are we so surprised that studies confirm what we have known for decades: that women wish to be cared for with sensitivity, respect for their dignity, concern for their cultural, religious, or ethnic needs, and with gentleness as well as with evidence-based clinical care? Have we become so engrossed with technology that we have separated it from humanity? Are we just producing techno-caregivers?

The clinical birth environment is stressful (see Chapter 13), and midwifery care, despite its occasional abuses as noted above, is generally acknowledged as taking a more holistic, psycho-socially supportive approach that reduces this stress (Harvey et al. 1996). In addition, explorations of the value of supportive companions in labor have shown, with remarkable consistency and cross-cultural validity, the power of this psycho-social intervention to modify any negative impact of the clinical birth environment (Hofmeyr et al. 1991; Hodnett et al. 2012). Women want continuity of care, which midwives try to provide. This may also be one contributory factor to why women rate pregnancy and birth care by midwives more positively than for any other category of healthcare provider (Public Health Agency of Canada 2009). We also know that the more positive women's ratings are of their interactions with their caregivers, the higher their ratings of satisfaction with their labor and birth experiences (Chalmers and Dzakpasu 2015).

Research indicates that obstetricians (57%) and family doctors (36%) are most likely to regard birth as dangerous, although few midwives agree (4%) (Ratti et al. 2014). Randomized trials have clearly shown that intervention rates for mothers with similar levels of risk/complication are far higher among physicians than among their midwifery colleagues. Not surprisingly, outcomes of such midwife-managed births tend to be better than outcomes for physicians (see e.g. Harvey et al. 1996). Despite this, in some countries, including Canada and the United States, fewer than 10% of women are able to access midwifery care (Midwives Alliance of North America 2015; Canadian Association of Midwives 2015).

The Future of Perinatal Practice

Implementing change in perinatal practice is a slow process. The BFHI was launched in the early 1990s, yet almost 30 years later, we still have relatively few Baby-Friendly Hospitals globally and especially in North America. Application of the BFHI 10 Steps to NICU settings is in its infancy, although it has been in place in Estonia for approximately 40 years and endorsed by WHO for almost as many. Evidence-based care was first highlighted in 1989 and yet we still struggle to apply these recommendations widely today, with increasing use of such interventions as cesareans continuing to occur. How long will it take us to implement the ideas presented in this chapter? Perinatal Psychologists, proposed in the 1980s in South Africa, are few and far between, with little if any recognition of this professional branch in universities or in clinical practice. Midwifery care has yet, in some places, to achieve the appreciative recognition from co-workers that mothers have long attributed to it. Preparation of parents for birth has been a long-established, if undervalued, service while preparation for parenthood is almost non-existent. Providing care that respects women's privacy, dignity, and confidentiality was incorporated into WHO principles of care in the 1990s but has, instead, been replaced with increasing incidents of abusive care. Discriminatory and inappropriate care is provided to those with socially determined disadvantages, or based on prejudicial caregiver attitudes such as towards obesity, in place of care based on clinical need. Remuneration determines some aspects of clinical care linking corruption—one of today's global scourges—to perinatal care.

My book *Family Centred Perinatal Care* (Chalmers 2017) develops and examines principles of perinatal care that apply to both families (10) and caregivers (10). These 10:10 principles outline my futuristic recommendations for improved perinatal care, only some of which have been addressed in this chapter. I summarize them here:

Family-Centered Principles

1. Care addresses the needs of women, their newborn/s, and their family supports.
2. Care is sensitive to individual psychological and social needs of women and their families, including needs for knowledge, emotional support, and spiritual considerations.
3. Care is culturally sensitive and informed.
4. Care is individualized to meet each family's needs.
5. Families are cared for with respect and dignity.
6. Families are supported to be actively involved in the care of their newborn, whether a healthy term infant or a sick or preterm baby.
7. Families take an active role in decision-making, based on evidence-based information, provided without coercion, and with full knowledge about the potential adverse effects of any care procedure.

8. Families are offered knowledgeable care to support breastfeeding and, when needed, alternate feeding methods.
9. Feedback from families is encouraged and facilitated and is rigorously evaluated by caregivers and healthcare facilities.
10. Information about mothers, partners, and their infants is strictly confidential.

Caregiver-Centered Principles

1. Care is based on the best available evidence.
2. Pregnancy and birth are regarded as healthy, normal events with caregivers remaining vigilant for deviations from normal.
3. Interventions are used only when essential.
4. Care is interdisciplinary.
5. A holistic approach is expected of all care providers.
6. Education of caregivers should include the principles of family-centered care.
7. Families are entitled to full, open, and honest communication about their care and are entitled to apology in the event of avoidable negative outcomes.
8. Care respects the reproductive and sexual rights of women and their families.
9. Care is always non-abusive.
10. Aggregated information about family-centered care outcomes is made publicly available and accessible, regardless of socio-economic or educational background.

Other initiatives that focus on the rights of the mother during pregnancy and childbirth, discussed in more detail in *Family-Centred Perinatal Care* (Chalmers 2017), include: The White Ribbon Alliance's *Respectful Maternity Care Charter*; Childbirth Connection's *Rights of Childbearing Women*; New York State's *Breastfeeding Mother's Bill of Rights*; the Unites States *Center for Reproductive Rights* declarations; and the Canadian *Charter of sexual and reproductive rights and health*. A further development is the *International Childbirth Initiative (ICI): 12 Steps to Safe and Respectful MotherBaby-Family Maternity Care*. These rights-based reproductive health initiatives and programs have been predominantly directed towards women in keeping with the "woman-centered" approach to care that has superseded previous "physician-centered" or "baby-centered" attitudes. With the exception of the ICI, there is still a dearth of attention being paid to a rights-based approach that is truly "family-centered."

Our perinatal healthcare future—techno-sapiens birth—is on the threshold of change: will it continue to flounder in the face of narrow-minded, technocratic perspectives, or will we benefit from our knowledge of best practices that support a humanistic approach combined with only essential technological intervention? This latter is the futuristic dream toward which we must strive.

References

Althabe F, C Sosa, JM Belizán, L Gibbons, F Jacquerioz, E Bergel. 2006. "Cesarean section rates and maternal and neonatal mortality in low-middle- and high-income countries: An ecological study." *Birth* 33(4):270–277.

Anonymous. 2015. "Our family secrets." *Annuls of Internal Medicine* 163(4):321. doi:10.7326/M14-2168.

Beck CT. 2018. "A secondary analysis of mistreatment of women during childbirth in health care facilities." *Journal of Obstetric, Gynecologic and Neonatal Nursing* 47(1):94–104.

Bohren M, JP Vogel, EC Hunter, O Lutsiv, SK Makh, JP Souza, C Agular, FS Coneglian, AL Araujo Diniz, O Tuncalp, D Javadi, OT Oladapo, R Khosia, MJ Hindin, AM Gulmezoglu. 2015. "The mistreatment of women during childbirth in health facilities globally: A mixed-methods systematic review." *PLOS Medicine* 12(6). doi:10.1371/journal.pmed.1001847.

Bowser D, K Hill. 2010. *Exploring Evidence for Disrespect and Abuse in Facility-Based Childbirth: Report of a Landscape Analysis*. Washington, DC: USAID-TRAction Project. Harvard School of Public Health and University Research Co.

Bragg F, DA Cromwell, LC Edozien, I Gurol-Urganci, TA Mahmood, A Templeton, JH van der Meulen. 2010. "Variation in rates of caesarean section among English NHS trusts after accounting for maternal and clinical risk: Cross sectional study." *British Medical Journal* 341:c5065.

Canadian Association Midwives. 2015. "Midwifery in Canada is growing." *The Pinard: Newsletter of the Canadian Association of Midwives* 5(1):5–6.

Chalmers B. 1998. "Psychosomatic obstetrics and gynaecology in the new millenium: Some thoughts and observations." *Journal of Psychosomatic Obstetrics and Gynaecology* 19(2):62–69.

Chalmers B. 2013. "Breastfeeding unfriendly in Canada?" *Canadian Medical Association Journal* 185(5):375–376. doi:10.1503/cmaj.121309.

Chalmers B. 2017. *Family-Centred Perinatal Care: Improving Pregnancy, Birth and Postpartum Care*. Cambridge: Cambridge University Press.

Chalmers B, S Dzakpasu. 2015. "Interventions in labour and birth and satisfaction with care: The Canadian maternity experiences survey findings." *Journal of Reproductive and Infant Psychology* 33(4):374–387.

Chalmers B, J Kaczorowski, E Darling, M Heaman, D Fell, B O'Brien, L Lee, Maternity Experiences Study Group of the Canadian Perinatal Surveillance System. 2010. "Cesarean and vaginal birth in Canadian women: A comparison of experiences." *Birth* 37(1):44–49.

Chalmers B, J Kaczorowski, C Levitt, S Dzakpasu, B O'Brien, L Lee, M Boscoe, D Young, Maternity Experiences Study Group of the Canadian Perinatal Surveillance System, Public Health Agency of Canada. 2009. "Use of routine interventions in vaginal labor and birth: Findings from the maternity expereinces survey." *Birth* 36(1):13–25.

Chalmers B, J Kaczorowski, B O'Brien, C Royle. 2012. "Rates of interventions in labor and birth across Canada: Findings of the Canadian maternity experiences survey." *Birth* 39(3):203–210.

Chalmers B, A Levin. 2001. *Humane Perinatal Care*. Tallinn: TEA Publishers.

Chalmers B, J McIntyre, D Meyer. 1991. "South African obstetricians' views on caesarean section." *South African Medical Journal = Suid-Afrikaanse Tydskrif vir Geneeskunde* 82(3):161–164.

Cochrane Library. 2015. *The Cochrane Database of Systematic Reviews.* John Wiley and Sons. www.cochranelibrary.com/cochrane-database-of-systematic-reviews/index.html, accessed April 17, 2020.

Çoker H, N Karabekir, S Varlik. 2015. "Birth with no regret birth model and team." *Journal of Obstetric and Womens Health and Disease* 1(3):27–34.

Enkin M, M Keirse, I Chalmers. 1989. *A Guide to Effective Care in Pregnancy and Childbirth.* Oxford: Oxford University Press.

Gibbons L, JM Belizán, JA Lauer, AP Betrán, M Merialdi, F Althabe. 2010. *The Global Numbers and Costs of Additionally Needed and Unnecessary Caesarean Sections Performed per Year: Overuse as a Barrier to Universal Coverage.* World Health Report (2010) Background Paper, No 30. Geneva: World Health Organization.

Hall D, G Kirsten. 2008. "Kangaroo mother care—A review." *Transfusion Medicine* 18(2):77–82.

Harvey S, J Jarell, R Brant, C Stainton, D Rach. 1996. "A randomized control trial of nurse-midwifery care." *Birth* 23(3):128–135.

Hodnett ED, S Gates, GJ Hofmeyr, C Sakala. 2012. "Continuous support for women during childbirth." *Cochrane Database of Systematic Reviews* 10:CD003766.

Hofmeyr J, C Nikodem, W-L Wolman, B Chalmers, T Kramer. 1991. "Companionship to modify the clinical birth environment: Effects on progress and perceptions of labour and breastfeeding." *British Journal of Obstetrics and Gynaecology* 98(8):756–764.

Joy SB, K De, Bittner. 2015. "Obesity stigma as a determinant of poor birth outcomes in women with high BMI: A conceptual framework." *Maternal and Child Health Journal* 19(4):(693–699). doi:10.1007/s10995-014-1577-x.

Kramer M, F Aboud, E Mironova, I Vanilovich, PW Platt, L Matush, S Igunov, E Fombonne, N Bogdanovich, T Ducruet, J-P Collet, B Chalmers, E Hodnett, S Davidovsky, O Skugarevsky, O Trofimovic, L Shapiro, S Shapiro, Promotion of Breastfeeding Intervention Trial (PROBIT) Study Group. 2008. "Breastfeeding and child cognitive development: New evidence from a large randomized trial." *Archives of General Psychiatry* 65(5):578–584.

Kramer M, B Chalmers, E Hodnett, Z Sevkovskaya, I Dzikovitch, S Shapiro, J-P Collett, I Vanilovich, I Mezen, T Ducruet, G Shishko, V Zubovish, D Miknuik, E Gluchanina, V Dombrowsky, A Ustinovich, T Kot, N Bogdanovich, L Ovchinikova, E Helsing. 2001. "Promotion of Breastfeeding Intervention Trial (PROBIT): A cluster-randomized trial in the Republic of Belarus." *Journal of the American Medical Academy* 285:413–420.

Kramer M, R Kakuma. 2012. "Optimal duration of exclusive breastfeeding." *Cochrane Database of Systematic Reviews* 8.

Lawrence RA, RM Lawrence. 2011. *Breastfeeding: A Guide for the Medical Profession.* 7th ed. USA: Elsevier, Mosby.

Magee SR, C Battle, J Morton, M Nothnagle. 2014. "Promotion of family-centered birth with gentle cesarean delivery." *Journal of the American Board of Family Medicine: JABFM* 27(5):690–693.

Midwives Alliance of North America. 2015. *What Is a Midwife?* http://mana.org/about-midwives/what-is-a-midwife, accessed 24 June.

Moore ER, GC Anderson, N Bergman, T Dowswell. 2012. "Early skin-to-skin contact for mothers and their healthy newborn infants." *Cochrane Database of Systematic Reviews* 5.

Nagpal J, A Sachdeva, R Sengupta Dhar, VL Bhargava, A Bhartia. 2014. "Widespread non-adherence to evidence-based maternity care guidelines: A population-based cluster randomised household survey." *British Journal of Obstetrics and Gynaecology* 122(2):238–247. doi:10.1111/1471-0528.13054.

Phelan SM, DJ Burgess, MW Yeazel, WL Hellerstedt, JM Griffen, M van Ryn. 2015. "Impact of weight bias and stigma on quality of care and outcomes for patients with obesity." *Obesity Reviews: An Official Journal of the International Association for the Study of Obesity* 16(4):319–326.

Price M, J Broomberg. 1990. "The impact of fee-for-service reimbursement system on the utlization of health services: Part III. A comparison of caesarean section rates in white nulliparous women in private and public sectors." *South African Medical Journal = Suid-Afrikaanse Tydskrif vir Geneeskunde* 78(3):136–138.

Public Health Agency of Canada (PHAC). 2009. *What Women Say: The Maternity Experiences Survey.* Ottawa, ON: Public Health Agency of Canada.

Ratti J, S Ross, K Stephanson, T Williamson. 2014. "Playing nice: Improving the professional climate between physicians and midwives in the Calgary area." *Journal of Obstetrics and Gynaecology Canada: JOGC = Journal d'Obstetrique et Gynecologie du Canada: JOGC* 36(7):590–597.

Renfrew MJ, D Craig, L Dyson, F McCormick, S Rice, SE King, K Misso, E Stenhouse, AF Williams. 2009. "Breastfeeding promotion for infants in neonatal units: A systematic review and economic analysis." *Health Technology Assessment* 1(40):1–146.

Royal College of Obstetricians and Gynaecologists, Royal College of Midiwves and National Childbirth Trust. 2007. *Making Normal Birth a Reality: Consensis Statement from the Maternity Care Working Party.* London: Matenrity Care Working Party.

Singh S, G Posner. 2015. "Doctors behaving badly and the tyranny of peer pressure." *Journal of Obstetrics and Gynaecology of Canada* 37(12):1113–1115.

Society of Obstetricians and Gynaecologists of Canada. 2008. "Joint policy statement on normal birth." *Journal of Obstetrics and Gynaecology of Canada* 30(12):1163–1165.

Victora C, R Bahl, A Barros, G Franca, S Horton, J Krasevic, S Murch, M Sankar, N Walker, N Rollins, Lancet Breastfeeding Series Group. 2016. "Breastfeeding in the 21st century: Epidemiology, mechanisms and lifelong effect." *The Lancet* 387(10017):475–490.

Villar J, E Valladares, D Wojdyla, N Zavaleta, A Shah, L Campodónico, A Shah, L Campodónico, V Bataglia, A Faundes, A Langer, A Narváez, A Donner, M Romero, S Reynoso, KS de Pádua, D Giordano, M Kublickas, A Acosta, WHO 2005 Global Survey on Maternal and Perinatal Health Research Group. 2006. "Caesarean delivery rates and pregnancy outcomes: The 2005 WHO global survey on maternal and perinatal health in Latin America." *Lancet* 367(9525):1819–1829.

WHO. 1994. *Safe Motherhood Package—Implementing Safe Motherhood in Countries.* WHO, Maternal Health and Safe Motherhood Programme.

WHO/UNICEF. 2003. *Global Strategy for Infant and Young Child Feeding.* Geneva: World Health Organization; United Nations Children's Fund.

World Health Organization Human Reproduction Programme. 2015. "WHO Statement on Caesarean Section Rates." *Reproductive Health Matters* 23(45):149.

15

FLEXIBLE HELPERS:

Re-Scribing Obstetric Technologies to Generate More Viable Futures for "Good" Pregnancies and Births

Annekatrin Skeide

Introduction

Obstetric technologies have often been conceived in deterministic terms by both their supporters and their critics. The shared assumption is that these technologies are direct applications of obstetric science, tools that straightforwardly realize what they are intended to do. Enthusiasts have emphasized that obstetric technologies are "good" and helpful because they save lives and preserve health. Critics have warned against the overpowering obstetric ideology and discourse these technologies form part of, colonizing "natural," understood as inherently "good" pregnant and birthing experiences.

Instead of assuming to know what obstetric technologies are—"good" for saving lives or "bad" for their inescapably alienating and disruptive effects on "natural" processes—I suggest studying what these technologies (help to) do. Building on Donna Haraway's material semiotics and its uptakes in feminist science and technology studies of care practices, I plead for carefully attending to obstetric technologies' specificities in practice. Instead of prescribing or describing obstetric technologies as stable and bounded applications of science, added to "social" situations and inflicted upon human bodies, I *re-scribe* obstetric technologies' becomings in relation to other participants—for example, fetuses, bodies, practitioners, and care environments such as hospitals and people's homes (for "rescription" see Harbers 2005:265; Pols 2014, 2015; Yates-Doerr 2017). Re-scribing emphasizes that specific technologies, situations, or practices cannot be neutrally described but are written anew in and through research. Scholars studying midwifery care (or any other) practices together with the bodies and technologies enacted therein are necessarily involved in their becomings. I analyze how technologies-in-practice can actually contribute to shaping "goodness" in pregnant, fetal, and birthing lives and to improving midwifery care.

Midwifery has often figured as the "natural," "social," "warm," and "female" counterpart to "male" obstetrics and its "cold" technologies, especially in anthropological and midwifery research. My ethnographic study of midwifery care practices in Germany shows that no matter in which surrounding midwives work, from a clinical labor ward to a home, midwives also "do obstetrics." They use obstetric techniques and technologies such as, among many others, abdominal palpations, called Leopold's maneuvers, named after the German obstetrician Christian Gerhard Leopold, and fetal stethoscopes, called Pinard horns, named after the French obstetrician Adolphe Pinard, to surveil pregnancies and births. Midwives stick to obstetric standards, norms, and goals as realized through these technologies, while also expanding and redefining obstetric repertoires and the norms established therein. The Leopold's maneuvers, for example, serve to diagnose the fetus' growth and position in the womb and to build up trust in midwifery care situations; both aims mutually inform each other.

In this chapter, I show the diversity and creativity of midwifery care relationships that give rise to "medical," "technical," and "social" repertoires that run through classic binaries: nature-culture, medical-social, and bodies-technologies. I develop three interdependent analytical steps: (1) to understand "obstetric," "technological," and "social" genres as parts of one another; (2) to "unnaturalize" pregnant, fetal, and birthing bodies; (3) to study the various, changing, and contradictory sets of values that obstetric technologies help to craft, thereby shaping different kinds of "good" pregnant, fetal, and birthing lives.

Material Semiotic Tools: Practices and Their Values

My analysis is inspired by a set of analytical sensitivities and tools coined "material semiotics" by feminist philosopher of science Donna Haraway (1991a, b, c). Material semiotics takes the idea that words obtain meaning in relation to other words from the linguistic study of signs (semiotics) and extends it to material entities, such as bodies or (other) technologies. Haraway (1991a:163) argues that what is, or rather what becomes, is an effect of the relations in which it is located. Matter and meaning are not separate but co-produce each other.

Empirical philosopher Annemarie Mol (2002:31–33) called for studying ethnographically, or more specifically "praxiographically," what "entities" such as technologies or bodies become, how this happens, and the kinds of material semiotic relations in which they are "enacted" in practice. Praxiography is a methodology created by intersecting (medical) anthropological concerns and analytical tools for science and technology studies (STS). Pivotal to the praxiographic approach is to understand entities such as humans, technical devices, or medical standards as effects of their relationships *done in practice*. Realities are *enacted* in midwifery care practices as much as in the research practices relating thereto. Like Haraway (1991b:201), Mol urges considering how realities—"the conditions of possibility we live with" (1999:75)—are shaped in medical and scientific practices, understood as *reality-generating* practices (2002:153).

"Material semiotics" has been utilized to study practices in health care and other environments together with their political and ethical normativities (Pols 2003, 2005; Mol 2008; Moser 2008, 2011; Mol et al. 2010). These studies demonstrate how, in care practices, lives (and deaths) are shaped through attentively experimenting with what might work best in a specific situation. This involves needing to compromise among different, possibly conflicting "goods" within care practices, as Jeannette Pols (2015:82) shows. Healthcare technologies—often staged as "cold," as instrumental and alienating "others," in opposition to social and thus "warm" care relations—play an important role in shaping meaningful affective and aesthetic care relations (Pols 2012:25–44). Technologies, Pols (2017:2) argues following Haraway, together with other care participants, people, things, and words, "get their meaning, and ultimate function in the way they are put to use."

A Material Semiotic Analysis of Obstetric Technologies

Inspired by these material semiotic insights, I address the question: How can obstetric technologies be studied in ways that can help to achieve more viable futures for "good" pregnancies and births?

To answer this question, I draw on praxiographic fieldwork that I carried out between February 2015 and March 2016 in various sites where midwives work in Germany, in which pregnancy, birth, and postpartum care are fragmented, taking place in different surroundings such as hospitals and homes, midwife-led birthing places, and ob-gyn practices, and often involving several midwives, obstetricians, and nurses. The common path starts with monthly, later biweekly, prenatal care provided by obstetrician-gynecologists (ob-gyns), sometimes assisted by midwives. It continues with childbirth and prenatal classes taught by midwives. Birth in Germany normatively takes place in a clinical labor ward, accompanied by both midwives and obstetricians. After the 3 days that new mothers and babies spend on the maternity ward, looked after by a team of nurses, midwives, and doctors, a midwife makes home visits to check on the mother's health and the child's development until 12 weeks after birth. Six weeks after birth, an obstetrician conducts a follow-up office examination. Only in so-called "out-of-hospital" or "community" modes of care do midwives provide assistance during pregnancy, birth, postpartum, and breastfeeding, continuously and independently from obstetricians. These are rare exceptions: in 2017 it was estimated that in Germany no more than 1.3% of all births took place outside the hospital (QUAG 2019).

During my fieldwork, I attended approximately 50 prenatal care visits, 30 births, and 50 postpartum care visits in homes and midwife-led birthing places, in ob-gyn practices, and on labor wards. After having "observingly participated" in specific prenatal, birth, and postpartum care situations and having had many informal conversations with my interlocutors, I conducted 20 semi-structured interviews with midwives and pregnant and postpartum people. Comparing and contrasting different midwifery care arrangements created by technologies, environments, midwives, fetuses, pregnant and birthing people, and their partners, I developed 3 interconnected analytical steps for understanding how obstetric technologies may contribute to creating more viable futures for "good" pregnancies and births: (1) studying the sociotechnical relations of midwifery care; (2) unnaturalizing pregnant, fetal, and birthing bodies in midwifery care practices; (3) comparing midwifery care values and their effects.

Step 1: Studying the Sociotechnical Relations of Midwifery Care

In order to show how in obstetric technologies "the obstetric," "the technological," and "the social" come in different shapes and are mixed with each other, and to study which kind of sociotechnical relations and identities are shaped, I employ the case of fetal heartbeat monitoring technologies. Midwives use three different devices to listen to fetal heart sounds during pregnancy and birth. Two are electronic devices that audibly amplify the fetal heartbeat—the portable Doppler fetal monitor called the Doptone and the cardiotocograph (CTG) (often called the electronic fetal monitor [EFM] in the US and elsewhere). The third, non-electronic, instrument is the Pinard horn. In the following, I will compare uses of the CTG, the Pinard horn, and the Doptone in midwifery prenatal and natal care.

A CTG as used in Germany is a machine of the size of small home printers, usually placed on a trolley standing next to a cot or bed on which a pregnant or birthing person lies during the monitoring. Nearly all pregnant people in Germany get CTGs during pregnancy to check on the fetal heartbeat, and also during hospital labors. Two wired transducers, attached to the belly with two large rubber straps, register the fetal heartbeat via ultrasound and measure the frequency of uterine contractions as tensions of the abdominal wall. Along with highly audible sounds, CTGs transcribe the fetal heart rate as a jagged curve on scaled paper, which is printed out simultaneously with the recording.

In Germany, obstetricians, as well as midwifery and public health researchers, emphasize that without indications, CTGs in pregnancy are unnecessary and potentially harmful interventions that facilitate further unnecessary and potentially harmful interventions (DGGG 2012:7; Schäfers and Kolip 2015:6), creating what Cheyney and Davis-Floyd (2019; Chapter 1) call "the obstetric paradox"—intervening in birth to keep it safe, thereby causing harm.

The midwives I accompanied were quick to point out that CTG recordings were no more than "snapshots" whose predictive value is quite limited. According to the midwives, the (re)assurance that CTGs may provide to pregnant people is based on a "false faith," as the heartbeat registered in the moment cannot guarantee fetal health in the future. However, CTG scripts also serve as juridical and medical evidence for fetal health at the time of the CTG (Grivell et al. 2015:1). The CTG scripts' visible and durable materiality bestows them with strong probative force. That might explain why midwives apply a panoply of inventive strategies in order to craft "beautiful CTGs" depicting a "good" fetal heart rate in the form of a continuous curve running within the ideal range and showing the variations defined as normal. If "the child moved away from the transducer," as midwives suggested, the transducer is moved to other spots on the belly to "catch the child," and thereby get a continuous curve. Another trick is having the pregnant person turn around and positioning the transducer on the other side of the belly. If the heart rate curve is either wide or flat—read as signs of an "overly active" fetus or a fetus that "takes a rest" or "sleeps"—the midwife tries "to wake it up" by clapping her hands or wiggling the pregnant belly.

Producing a CTG script depicting a "good" fetal heart rate, "beautiful" evidence of the fetus' "well-being" thus creates specific relationships between a fetus enacted as an unruly child, a pregnant person enacted as a parent, and a midwife, jointly taming and disciplining this child for the sake of its own—and the other participants'—good. Whereas many pregnant people think of the CTG as a "necessary evil" that needs to be used in order to "assure that the child is doing well," others look forward to "the best part of the prenatal care visit." The heartbeat listening is their occasion to relax during the otherwise rather hasty prenatal care appointments, while being lulled by the steady and soft beating of "the child's heart"—"the loveliest music" to her ears, as Anna called it. Bathing in the heartbeat music the CTG produced, Anna appreciated not only the intimate one-to-one-encounter with "the child" that the heart sounds provided but also that the cardiotocography promoted her sense of wellbeing.

These examples show that devices usually designated as obstetric and used predominantly in ob-gyn practices and hospitals, such as the CTG, are never merely "obstetric" or "medical." They co-create "social" relationships between the CTG and its products, script and sounds, between the fetus listened to as a child and a pregnant person already becoming a considerate parent.

Whereas the CTG is often considered a classic obstetric instrument of surveillance (Cartwright 1998), the Pinard horn is considered, especially by midwives providing out-of-hospital care, to be the social midwifery tool *par excellence*, a supposedly non-obstetric but "social" and "natural" instrument. The Pinard horn is a cylindrical device that resembles a champagne flute. One end is placed on the belly, as close as possible to the fetus's back, at heart level, and on the other end a midwife's ear listens. Small, simple, and seemingly ordinary, the device is made of wood and hence feels "warm" to the touch. It is claimed to be modest and flexible, as instead of electricity and abstract curves to interpret, the Pinard horn "only" needs a skillful midwifery ear to listen. Preceded by abdominal palpations, this fetal heartbeat listening tool helps to bring the midwife's hands onto and the midwife's head close to the pregnant belly, thereby creating an intimate physical proximity between midwife, fetus, and pregnant person. Robbie Davis-Floyd (2001, 2018) describes this intimate proximity as part of the "holistic model of birth," in which the "energy fields" of mother and midwife are merged, allowing for "intuitive diagnosis" to arise. The intimate listening with the Pinard horn that I re-scribe also brings about a "reasoned" and "authoritative" way of diagnosing.

The Pinard horn is a good example of the intricacies of the intertwined "obstetric" and "social" relations that a specific fetal heartbeat monitoring device co-produces. Compared to other, more sophisticated technologies such as the CTG, which keeps on monitoring even in the absence of medical staff, the physical closeness that the use of the Pinard horn creates may entail a social closeness as well. There is, however, a "cold" and asocial side to this charmingly "warm" midwifery technology, as the one listening is the midwife, not the childbearer. It can be interpreted as a classic medical device, with the professional as the authorized expert listener, and the pregnant person making their body available to the listener by lying still and silent on their back. The necessary physical proximity is thus a sociotechnical orchestration that is at once intimate and openly surveillance-oriented. It creates a social and epistemological disparity between a midwife acting as an authoritative and skilled expert who knows, a pregnant person as a patient who just passively undergoes an examination as a body that is helping to make knowing possible—as well as a fetus as an object of surveillance that is known as such by the midwife alone. Thus in practice, technologies such as the Pinard horn, mostly employed in midwife-led environments and commonly understood as social, may indeed show "medicalizing" effects.

The Doppler fetal monitors, called "Doptones," that I encountered at my field sites were composed of a wired transducer and the device itself. The transducer is held to the woman's belly with one hand while the device, equipped with a small electronic display and a loudspeaker, is held in the other. The Doptone, used in both midwife-led and obstetric settings, is a practical and user-friendly device, which can also be purchased for home use by laypeople: hand-sized, it is easy to transport and handle; battery-run, it does not depend on infrastructural electricity. The Doptone detects the fetal heartbeat via ultrasound and makes the sounds it produces audible to everyone in hearing distance through the integrated loudspeaker, allowing pregnant people and their companions, including their children, to participate in the listening process. Before listening, midwives usually carry out Leopold's maneuvers in order to know where to place the transducer. The object of listening is directly addressed, verbally and haptically (via touch), as "the child" and the sounds are announced as fetal "heartbeats." The listeners are thus equipped with particular genres of knowing that guide their attentive listening.

While how to listen and what to listen to are framed and directed beforehand, they take concrete shape in shared sensorial practice. Fetal heart sounds produced with the help of a Doptone become artifacts of obstetric surveillance *and* of socio-emotional expressions and symbolic communication (see Howes-Mischel 2016). Those present listen to the heartbeats of a fetus they jointly get to know and learn to relate to. The diagnostic and social meanings that are collectively generated are inseparable and inform each other.

In Germany, fetal heartbeat listening via the Doptone is also a way to anticipate and train for parenting through learning to become attentive to children's aural expressions: "Listening to the fetal heart sounds, I can point out to parents that their ears also need to prepare themselves for becoming parents," as Stadelmann (2005:29–30), a midwife, suggests in her alternative birthing manual. The sonic enactments of "the child" stage the fetus as a biosocial entity-in-action-and-in-relation that should be loved and cared for. In Doptone orchestrations, the focus often lies on educating pregnant people addressed as future parents in how to listen and what to (learn to) hear.

Studying these devices in practice shows how CTGs, Pinard horns, and Doptones co-shape social relations while also serving as instruments of medical surveillance. In order to understand how obstetric technologies work and for whom or for what they help to bring about improvements, I argue that an analysis that avoids opposing "obstetric" and "technical" against "social" repertoires, but rather shows how these repertoires inform each other, is indispensable.

Step 2: Unnaturalizing Pregnant, Fetal, and Birthing Bodies in Midwifery Care Practices

The second analytical step I suggest is to articulate the kinds of pregnant, fetal, and birthing bodies that are enacted by and through obstetric technologies. As part of a cyborgian analysis of obstetric technologies, I unnaturalize bodies in midwifery practices through studying bodies-in-labor as collective, distributed, and heterogeneously composed actors and effects.

In all surroundings, an overarching goal of midwifery birth attendance is to help the mother handle labor pains in ways that allow birth to progress and that help to avoid obstetric complications such as slow or obstructed labor. In obstetric terms, "good" labor pains are uterine contractions that are effective in provoking an opening of the cervix and in pushing the fetus down through the pelvis and vagina within a certain timespan, measured by vaginal examinations. Birth progresses regularly if the cervix opens up continually and the child descends progressively, and if these happen within a defined space of time. However, midwifery birth attendance is also guided by how and to what extent these pains are livable (bearable) for the person giving birth, for the fetus, for the partner, for the midwife, and for whomever else may be present during birth and concerned with it. Supporting the regular proceeding of birth while also rendering labor pains livable are intertwined goals in tension with each other when effective pains are not livable and livable pains are not effective.

In Germany, the repertoire of midwifery techniques and technologies for dealing with—and thereby co-enacting—bodies-in-labor reaches from vaginal examinations through walking, bathing, massaging, breathing, and relaxation techniques to various pain medications such as spasmolytic suppositories, intramuscular injections with opiates, or epidural anesthesia. Each of these midwifery techniques involves specific surroundings, devices, knowledges, bodies, and worlds. Crafting particular socio-material relations between these various participants, each labor pain intervention brings about particular versions of bodies-in-labor.

When Tina gave birth to her second child in the hospital, the vaginal examinations performed at her arrival and then regularly throughout her lengthy birthing trajectory, which ended in a cesarean, enacted labor pains as objectively measurable effects of biological processes. Labor pains were located within a body as a biological system, and more specifically in its reproductive organs—the uterus and its cervix. How the pains felt and how they acted upon Tina's body-in-labor other than dilating the cervix was not at stake when this technique was used. Here the pains' effectiveness in terms of "obstetric" standards was foregrounded.

After the initial vaginal examination, Tina took a bath in the "pre-labor" room. Bathing was introduced for diagnosing and guiding labor while also soothing Tina's pains: immersion in warm water can help to alleviate or even stop contractions if they are not signs of labor or to intensify them if they are, while also easing the pain (see Chapter 11). Immersing herself in water represented a compromise that met Tina's request for pain relief, thereby acknowledging her sensations while also aiming to make her body produce effective uterine contractions. In water, livable labor pains were aligned with effective labor pains, staging them as co-dependent: livable pains have the potential to become effective. In the bathing arrangement, in which Tina and her partner Karl "were laboring and bathing and laboring and bathing," as Tina explained, the body-in-labor was inhabited as an activity, which was laboring in a relaxing situation in which Tina and Karl "felt comfortable." While bathing, the body-in-labor was not bounded by its skin but incorporated pleasurable environmental qualities such as warmth, calm, and intimacy.

As the bathing proved ineffective in terms of a measurable progress of birth, the midwife who took over the morning shift "proposed something homeopathic, something to relax," because Tina "was very tense," as she herself emphasized. This time, the labor pains were staged as products of bodily tensions that were both ineffective and unbearable. Thus labor pains were situated in an individual biological body and an operating psyche or mind was added to the tableau. Labor pains viewed as pathological were interpreted as symptoms of a fearful mind provoking an overall muscular tension that prevented the cervix from opening. These pains hurt excessively and were not effective because they were not adequately "coped with" by the embodied psyche-in-labor. This resonates with Grantly Dick-Read's "fear-tension-pain" cycle (1961:18), which conceives of individual women's psyches as unruly, yet educable, actors in directing birthing bodies and which has formed part of the teaching of generations of German midwives and inspires both their birth preparation courses and their birth attendance.

After several further interventions, Tina finally had regular contractions that provoked an ongoing opening of the cervix and the descent of the child—"so that one could finally do something." Tina was administered an epidural, combined with an infusion of oxytocin. Here, the aim was to render labor pains livable through backgrounding the hurting as much as possible while also increasing their effectiveness as much as possible. As labor pains felt less like pains but more as uterine contractions in this arrangement, Tina described them as a "working" of her uterus that did not hurt. Because now diagnostic examinations and the "objective" data they provided were needed for managing labor, Tina's body-in-labor was shaped into an obstetric object, distributed over complex medical and technical infrastructures, and directed quasi-independently from the subject-in-labor.

Depending on the surroundings in which bodies-in-labor are situated, on which techniques are used to handle labor pains and on the goals they foreground—such as rendering labor pains more effective, more livable, or both—bodies take various shapes in labor pain arrangements. As "material-semiotic…nodes" (Haraway 1991b:200), bodies may, for example, become biological systems, helpful activities, or obstetric objects. This second analytical step—unnaturalizing pregnant, fetal, and birthing bodies—shows that bodies-in-labor are not naturally given but actively engage in and are acted on by midwifery techniques constituted of mixed "obstetric" and "social" repertoires.

Step 3: Comparing Midwifery Care Values and Their Effects

My third analytical step for understanding how obstetric technologies can contribute to "good" pregnancies and births is to compare values-in-practice in order to learn about "good" midwifery care practice. Midwifery practices are normative. They are directed at "doing good"—at stabilizing or improving life situations. What exactly is "good" for whom or what and in which terms is not decided beforehand but enacted in practice. Midwifery care practices are also structured by overarching values—ideals, standards, and goals. These may belong to specific surroundings such as hospitals or homes that afford certain options but not others, or may come from other places and practices, such as scientific ones. These institutionalized values are dealt with—integrated, adapted, or counteracted—in concrete midwifery care situations. To study how midwives do this offers lessons about the effects of such values.

To demonstrate the analytic strategy of comparing values-in-practice in order to evaluate their effects, I take up an influential ideal that shapes midwifery care in Germany: woman-centered care. Woman-centered care foregrounds a pregnant and birthing person's (a "woman's") right and duty to make choices and to be in control of the care situation. Firstly, I ask what this ideal does. What are its effects and limitations? Secondly, I contrast it with a more marginal goal-in-practice, which is creating long-term care relationships.

Woman-centered care resonates with the famous medical ethical principle of autonomy. This principle assumes competent individuals who, after having been informed about their possibilities, make the most reasonable choice according to what is available to them and in line with their preferences. But midwives do not only attend to pregnant and birthing people but also to fetuses. And these are physically and vitally interdependent—thus far at least. Interventions such as continuous CTG during birth have been shown to bring risks and benefits for both the birthing person and the child-to-be (Grivell et al. 2015; Alfirevic et al. 2017). What would a reasonable choice look like when a birthing person has to decide if they want to be monitored or not? The ideal of woman-centeredness hides these complex and challenging physical, obstetric, and moral relationalities between pregnant and birthing people and fetuses. While overburdening childbearers with the need to be competent and responsible and while eclipsing fetuses and the affec-tivities with which they and their (future) lives are equipped, woman-centeredness also makes of midwives service providers whose appreciations and doubts do not matter and are not allowed to form part of their working relationships. Another problem is thus that "woman-centeredness," widely advocated by birth activists everywhere, does not capture the relational, collective, and contingent endeavors that attending to pregnancies and birth in midwifery care practices become.

An alternative to woman-centeredness is enacted in homebirth environments and their long-term care relationships, despite the frequent invoking of the ideal of woman-centeredness in these surroundings: A childbearer ("woman") has made the brave choice to opt for the homebirth alternative, so the credo goes. However, in homebirth midwifery practices, notions of choice and autonomy are not enacted as individual competencies but as situational and relational events. Pregnant and birthing people and midwives are in this together. What matters in these homebirth care relationships is ongoing communication and contact through words, touches, devices, and physical proximities in homey and inti-mate surroundings in which obstetric surveillance examinations are routinized and multiplied. As does the ideal of woman-centeredness, the relationship-based goals in homebirth surroundings also come at a cost, as they require quite some physical, emotional, and social investments on the part of both mother and midwife, along with long-term training and discipline on the part of everyone involved. In other words, the midwife and woman have to "train" together—to become co-responsive to each other, to the techniques, and to the homebirth environment that offers certain possibilities and limits others (Skeide 2019).

I seek for my analysis to provide tools and insights that help to evaluate mid-wifery practices in terms of their sociomaterial effects and to allow the participants to adapt technologies, techniques, ideals, and goals in ways that best fit specific pregnancy and birth situations. The ways of shaping and addressing care prob-lems and values are informed by how obstetric technologies are put into practice as well as by the surroundings in which midwifery care takes place. In ob-gyn practices and hospitals, ideals, standards, and goals partly overlap and partly dif-fer from those in midwife-led birthing places or peoples' homes. The various relationships between obstetric technologies, childbearing bodies, and midwives entail different rationales and values of what constitutes "good" midwifery care.

Conclusion: Flexible Helpers for Viable Birthing Futures

In order to avoid a deterministic approach to obstetric technologies, I have devel-oped three analytical steps that focus: (1) on the particularity of midwifery care situations; (2) on the heterogeneous, embodied, technological, and discursive participants they configure; and (3) on the values they incorporate. Instead of generalizing obstetric technologies, I insist on attending to the specificities of technologies-in-practice.

The analytical shifts I have introduced suggest that the question of which kinds of pregnancies and births to strive for and to promote in the future cannot be answered once and for all, although other chapters in this volume attempt to do so. The various technologies used for surveilling pregnancies and births that I have analyzed here give differing shapes to pregnant, fetal, and birthing lives. Studying obstetric technologies-in-practice makes it possible to show the diversity of values—goals, ideals, standards—these technologies help to realize, to articulate dominant and marginal values, and to demonstrate the effects of different values that shape "good" midwifery care relations with technologies. The values obstetric technologies may help to enact differ from one midwifery care arrangement to another; yet one specific arrangement of which one specific technology forms a part may also attend to various, sometimes contradictory, "goods."

Each technology brings along particular promises and limitations that need to be thought about, compared, and weighed. Which technologies to cultivate (and how exactly), and which to keep at bay, is a matter of carefully attending to the hopes and possibilities, the fears and difficulties that may be encountered in the course of being (which is rather a doing) pregnant and giving birth.

In order to generate more viable futures for good pregnancies and births, the challenge is to stick to the messy, "not transcendent and clean" (Haraway 2004:236) realities of obstetric technologies-in-practice as well as to the different goods and bads that need to be lived and dealt with. Putting obstetric technologies in practice in ways that improve fetal, pregnant, and birthing lives is an ongoing *co-responding* between various heterogeneous participants within situated events. Not only obstetric technologies and midwifery techniques, but also research technologies and techniques, emerge in my analysis as *flexible helpers* that give rise to fetal, pregnant, and birthing realities-in-becoming. "Sapient" human-technological relations are able to co-shape "good" pregnancies and "good" births, whatever that may encompass in specific pregnant and birthing situations.

References

Alfirevic Z, D Devane, GML Gyte, A Cuthbert. 2017. "Continuous Cardiotocography (CTG) as a Form of Electronic Fetal Monitoring (EFM) for Fetal Assessment during Labour." *Cochrane Database of Systematic Reviews* 2. https://doi.org/10.1002/14651858 .CD006066.pub3.

Cartwright E. 1998. "The Logic of Heartbeats: Electronic Fetal Monitoring and Biomedically Constructed Birth." In: *Cyborg Babies: From Techno-Sex to Techno-Tots*, eds. R Davis-Floyd, J Dumit. New York: Routledge, 240–54.

Cheyney M, R Davis-Floyd. 2019. "Birth as Culturally Marked and Shaped." In: *Birth in Eight Cultures*, eds. R Davis-Floyd, M Cheyney. Long Grove, IL: Waveland Press, 1–16.

Davis-Floyd R. 2001. "The Technocratic, Humanistic, and Holistic Paradigms of Birth." *International Journal of Gynecology & Obstetrics* 75(1):S5–S23. doi: 10.1016/S0020-7292(01)00510-0.

Davis-Floyd R. 2018. "The Technocratic, Humanistic, and Holistic Paradigms of Birth and Health Care." In: *Ways of Knowing about Birth: Mothers, Midwives, Medicine, and Birth Activism*. Long Grove, IL: Waveland Press, 3–44.

Deutsche Gesellschaft für Gynäkologie und Geburtshilfe (DGGG). 2012. *Anwendung Des CTG während Schwangerschaft und Geburt*. www.dggg.de/leitlinien-stellungnahmen/leitlinien/leitlinie/anwendung-von-ctg-waehrend-schwangerschaft-und-geburt-321/.

Dick-Read G. 1961. *Childbirth without Fear. The Principles and Practice of Natural Childbirth*. 4th edition. London: William Heinemann.

Gesellschaft für Qualität in der außerklinischen Geburtshilfe (QUAG). 2019. *Geburtenzahlen in Deutschland*. www.quag.de/quag/geburtenzahlen.htm.

Grivell RM, Z Alfirevic, GML Gyte, D Devane. 2015. "Antenatal Cardiotocography for Fetal Assessment." *Cochrane Database of Systematic Reviews* 9. https://doi.org/10.1002/14651858.CD007863.pub4.

Haraway D. 1991a. "A Cyborg Manifesto: Science, Technology, and Socialist-Feminism in the Late Twentieth Century." In: *Simians, Cyborgs, and Women: The Reinvention of Nature*, ed. Haraway D. London: Free Association Books, 149–81.

Haraway D. 1991b. "Situated Knowledges: The Science Question in Feminism and the Privilege of Partial Perspective." In: *Simians, Cyborgs, and Women: The Reinvention of Nature*, ed. Haraway D. London: Free Association Books, 183–201.

Haraway D. 1991c. "The Biopolitics of Postmodern Bodies: Constitutions of Self in Immune System Discourse." In: *Simians, Cyborgs, and Women: The Reinvention of Nature*, ed. Haraway D. London: Free Association Books, 203–30.

Haraway D. 2004. "Modest_Witness@Second_millenium." In: *The Haraway Reader*, ed. Haraway D. New York: Routledge, 223–50.

Harbers Hans. 2005. "Epilogue: Political Materials—Material Politics." In: *Inside the Politics of Technology: Agency and Normativity in the Co-Production of Technology and Society*, ed. Hans Harbers. Amsterdam: Amsterdam University Press, 257–72.

Howes-Mischel Rebecca. 2016. "'With This You Can Meet Your Baby': Fetal Personhood and Audible Heartbeats in Oaxacan Public Health." *Medical Anthropology Quarterly* 30(2):186–202.

Mol A. 1999. "Ontological Politics. A Word and Some Questions." *Sociological Review*. Oxford. https://doi.org/10.1111/j.1467-954X.1999.tb03483.x.

Mol A. 2002. *The Body Multiple: Ontology in Medical Practice*. Durham, NC: Duke University Press.

Mol A. 2008. *The Logic of Care: Health and the Problem of Patient Choice*. London: Routledge.

Mol A, I Moser, J Pols eds. 2010. *Care in Practice: On Tinkering in Clinics, Homes and Farms*. VerKörperungen 8. Bielefeld: transcript Verlag.

Moser I. 2008. "Making Alzheimer's Disease Matter. Enacting, Interfering and Doing Politics of Nature." *Geoforum* 39(1):98–110. https://doi.org/10.1016/j.geoforum.2006.12.007.

Moser I. 2011. "Dementia and the Limits to Life: Anthropological Sensibilities, STS Interferences, and Possibilities for Action in Care." *Science, Technology, & Human Values* 36(5):704–22. https://doi.org/10.1177/0162243910396349.

Pols J. 2003. "Enforcing Patient Rights or Improving Care? The Interference of Two Modes of Doing Good in Mental Health Care." *Sociology of Health & Illness* 25(4):320–47. https://doi.org/10.1111/1467-9566.00349.

Pols J. 2005. "Enacting Appreciations: Beyond the Patient Perspective." *International Journal of Health Care Philosophy & Policy* 13(3):203–21. https://doi.org/10.1007/s 10728-005-6448-6.

Pols J. 2012. *Care at a Distance*. Amsterdam: Amsterdam University Press.

Pols J. 2014. "Radical Relationality. Epistemology in Care and Care Ethics for Research." In: *Moral Boundaries Redrawn: The Significance of Joan Tronto's Argument for Political Theory, Ethics of Care*, eds. G Olthuis, H Kohlen, J Heier. Leuven: Peeters, 175–94.

Pols J. 2015. "Towards an Empirical Ethics in Care: Relations with Technologies in Health Care." *Medicine, Health Care & Philosophy* 18(1):81–90. https://doi.org/10.1007 /s11019-014-9582-9.

Pols J. 2017. "Good Relations with Technology: Empirical Ethics and Aesthetics in Care." *Nursing Philosophy: An International Journal for Healthcare Professionals* 18(1):1–7. https://doi.org/10.1111/nup.12154.

Schäfers R, P Kolip. 2015. *Zusatzangebote in der Schwangerschaft: Sichere Rundumversorgung Oder Geschäft mit der Unsicherheit?* Gütersloh: Bertelsmann Stiftung. www.bertel smann-stiftung.de/fileadmin/files/Projekte/17_Gesundheitsmonitor/Newsletter _Ueberversorgung_in_der_Schwangerschaft_20150727.pdf.

Skeide A. 2019. "Enacting Homebirth Bodies: Midwifery Techniques in Germany." *Culture, Medicine, & Psychiatry* 43(2):236–55. https://doi.org/10.1007/s11013 -018-9613-8.

Stadelmann I. 2005. *Die Hebammen-Sprechstunde*. Ermengerst: Stadelmann Verlag.

Yates-Doerr E. 2017. "Counting Bodies? On Future Engagements with Science Studies in Medical Anthropology." *Anthropology & Medicine* 24(2):142–58. https://doi.org/10 .1080/13648470.2017.1317194.

16

COMING HOME:

Re-Visioning Place of Birth in the 21st Century

George Parker and Suzanne Miller

Prelude: Birth in the Time of COVID-19

When we first conceived the idea for this chapter about a world in which home birth is the norm, we could not have imagined the world in which we found ourselves when we actually came to write it. Surely, when we pitched an essay centered around an imagined near future where there had been a reversal in discourses of risk and safety about place of birth, resulting in the normalization of home birth, there were many portents from the future that made this idea at least conceivable. Mounting evidence of Climate Catastrophe was adding pressure to the fault lines running through global security and economic stability. There were also ongoing warnings about pandemics and superbugs and the ever-present threat of natural disasters. All of these threatened to wreak significant havoc on hospital-centric Western healthcare systems and infrastructures.

Yet, despite these portents of future calamity, and pleas for the political, social, and economic transformations needed to tackle them, the procedures of modern life were continuing more or less as normal, including near-wholesale hospitalization of birth under a technocratic ideology. Despite at least four generations of challenge by birth activists, practitioners (especially midwives), and scholars (e.g., Jordan 1978; Davis-Floyd 1992; Cheyney 2011; Chalmers 2017), this paradigm has persisted and the choice to birth outside of hospitals has remained severely marginalized. We thus embraced the task of imagining a near future when the technocratic paradigm's hold on birthplace had begun to unravel.

As it transpired, this process would be underway before we even put fingers to keys. In the months between conceiving of and actually sitting down to write this chapter, COVID-19 swept the globe, massively disrupting our lives and the logics that underpin them. One of these logics was that hospitals are the commonsense place to give birth. Yet as the pandemic took hold, hospitals were transformed overnight from places of safety and companionship for birth to places of fear and separation. In tandem, home birth with midwives was elevated as a safe and desirable choice where families could stay intact and where exposure to contagion could be limited (Davis-Floyd, Gutschow, and Schwartz 2020). At this time of writing (September 2020), it is unclear whether COVID-19 represents a permanent or temporary disruption to the cultural consensus about hospitalized birth. Whatever the future of birth, one of the lessons of COVID-19 and the central theme of this chapter is that the current paradigm of hospital-based, medically managed birth is flawed, mutable, and unsuitable for maternity disaster care and will inevitably be transformed by the challenges we face in our 21st-century world.

The Chapter Ahead: Back to the Past and Forward to the Future

In the chapter ahead, we combine speculative fiction with critical analysis to transport the reader both back into the past and forward into an imagined near future to examine the changing cultural meanings assigned to place of birth. We first look back to examine the social and political forces implicated in the whole-sale shift in Aotearoa New Zealand (now so called to acknowledge the Indigenous name for New Zealand) of birth from home to hospital during the 20th century. We show the current cultural consensus about hospital birth as safer to be a historical-social construct created under the influence of power and politics.

Then, in Kae's story, we imagine a near future in which home birth, instead of being marginalized, is normative and hospital birth is considered risky, dangerous, and irresponsible. We critically examine the limitations of the technocratic model of birth (Davis-Floyd 2001, 2018a) for meeting future challenges. We conclude by affirming the potential for transformation in both cultural understandings about birth, and birth practices, in order to meet the coming challenges of the 21st century.

Leaving Home: Power, Politics, and Place of Birth in the 20th Century

The story of midwifery across the 20th century in Aotearoa New Zealand, where we live and work, reflects the narratives of other Western nations, particularly those of the UK and US (Carter and Duriez 1986). As the century dawned, moves towards state regulation of midwifery practice were gaining momentum. Ostensibly, regulation would improve midwifery education by establishing state-run maternity hospitals to oversee it (NZ Govt. 1904). To an extent this vision was achieved, but ultimately it proved costly to midwifery autonomy.

The progressive industrialization of birth moved it from being a family and community event that took place at home or on the *marae* (an Indigenous communal sacred space) and set it down in institutions where birthing women became "clinical fodder" for student doctors and midwives (Tracy and Grigg 2019). High maternal and infant mortality rates were drivers for change, and the professionalization of midwifery was one strategy to address this issue. Professionally educating midwives meant that they could not only improve the safety of birth, but could also act as agents of the state in the lives of mothers (de Souza 2013). The practice of lay midwifery, and for *Māori* (New Zealand's Indigenous people) the common practices of having *whānau* (family) and *tohunga* (expert practitioners of the healing arts) supporting birth were effectively criminalized, reducing women's choices and undermining the *mana* (respect and prestige) of established cultural birthing practices. For rural Indigenous communities, birthing in urban hospitals represented a cultural dislocation and disrupted Indigenous babies' birthright to the connection to ancestral lands so integral to their cultural and spiritual wellbeing. While poverty, racism, and classism diminished the wellbeing of Indigenous children, bringing Indigenous mothers' reproductive capacities under State control provided a means to absolve the State of its responsibility for the high mortality problem (de Souza 2013). As in other colonized countries, *pākehā* (non-Māori) women were exhorted to breed "for King and country," especially in the aftermath of World War I.

To support women's task to replenish the population postwar, the burgeoning medical specialty of obstetrics brought with it a promise of pain-free childbirth from the use of anesthetics (Guilliland and Pairman 2010). Midwives were increasingly used to restrain women experiencing the effects of scopolamine ("twilight sleep"), reducing both women's and midwives' autonomy. The increased use of forceps on women laboring "in the twilight zone" further resulted in widespread sepsis, which required even more medical intervention.

Until the late 1930s, the state-run maternity hospitals were led by midwives, who educated student midwives and supported laboring women, providing low-cost care to women across the socio-demographic spectrum. But legislative change as a result of medical lobbying saw the entry of medical students into these midwife-led hospitals. Women could receive free care if it was provided by a doctor, introducing professional competition for midwives. As hospitals grew bigger during the 1950s and 1960s, maternity care became fragmented; antenatal, labor, and postnatal care was provided in separate spaces (Guilliland and Pairman 2010). Midwives often specialized in one aspect of care provision, reducing the scope of practice for some, and eroding midwives' vision of pregnancy to parenthood as a continuum. Midwifery was increasingly subsumed into nursing management structures, rendering midwives even more invisible to obstetric powerbrokers. Further legislative change in 1971 brought midwives firmly under the control of doctors by prohibiting them from practicing without medical supervision.

The safety of home birth continued to be contested between midwives and doctors throughout this time period. Advances in medical technology and pharmacology undoubtedly improved some aspects of safety, and birth in hospitals provided access to timely intervention, especially useful for higher risk pregnancies. However, the closing 20 years of the century in ANZ witnessed a remarkable renaissance of political allegiance between women (who demanded increased choice and more humanized birth) and midwives (who fought successfully to wrest themselves from obstetric control), which expanded possibilities for birth at home. As the sun set on the 20th century, ANZ midwives were again the primary care providers for the vast majority of women, as they remain today, and home birth was once again fully funded and endorsed by the government for eligible women with low risk pregnancies.

Despite this enabling environment, which includes seamless obstetric referral and transfer systems, home birth has remained a counter-cultural choice, with just 3% of families currently exercising this option. While 10% choose freestanding birthing centers, midwife-attended hospital birth with access to analgesic and surgical services remains the choice of the majority (87%) of birthing families (Ministry of Health [MoH] 2019). Although based on an illusion of increased safety, the technocratic birth environment can lead to increased rates of harmful and unnecessary interventions due to risk-aversion and the need for rapid throughput (Miller 2020). Cesarean rates continue to climb in Aotearoa New Zealand—the last 10 years have seen a significant rise, from 23.6% in 2008 to 27.9% in 2017, a rate which is even higher (31%) for first births (MoH 2019).

Ultimately, leaving home to birth has proved detrimental in multiple ways. Reflecting on the ANZ politics of birthplace over the 20th century makes it clear that colonialist interests, the forces of modernization, and the obstetric ambition to control the birthing sphere all were implicated in the wholesale shift of birth into hospitals. If place of birth reflects the interplay of the power and politics of the time, what then for the next century?

Kae

Kae parked the electric bug at the charging yard on Customs St, past the crumbling Quay and the old ferry terminal, disused since the harbor had swelled around and under, leaving it a relic of the 20th century. It was almost 9 o'clock and already the morning felt too hot to be outside. Kae glanced around nervously. The last thing she needed was someone noticing her entering the hospital. She knew what people fear, but this used to be normal, and she missed the *old* normal.

Kae stepped around a fresh ruffle of split concrete. The city was scarred from flash floods, although much of the time the ground looked so baked, it was hard to believe it ever rained. She couldn't help glancing around again before stepping up to the shiny entrance of the building. Almost immediately, the hum of the day was hushed by the heavy door of the clinic closing behind her.

The aesthetic of the reception space was sterile. Every surface was either wipeable or disposable, including the limited seating. Kae had never been in a place so uniformly frictionless yet so disturbingly un-tranquil. As she passed through the doors of the infection control airlock, she steadied herself and stared into the eye-D® camera, the doors opening into a changing room where she placed her own clothes and belongings in a compartment and donned the pale blue scrubs left for her by unseen staff. A voice from the ceiling ushered her through the next set of doors and into the clinic, where she was immediately disoriented by the shock of warm, human color.

Risk factors. Two words that had formed a second caul around this baby. The whole point of this final scan was not, as touted, to make her comfortable with "the team" and go through the birth plan. No, this was a health screen to check if she was fit to be allowed entrance to the birthing suite on Level 9, eligible to use the hospital's resources, and to rule her out as a contaminant.

A smiling person in similar scrubs, although pale pink, approached Kae chattering a welcome while leading her along a hallway to a smaller room where the obstetrician and anesthetic technician were waiting for her. The consult took about an hour, but Kae couldn't have described it well to anyone later if she'd been asked. For a while she was sitting answering questions, then lying on a firm bed, then her legs were in stirrups, then she was lying on her side while they inspected her lower back and felt along her spine. At one point, an unspeaking person in red scrubs performed an ultrasound while the doctor and technician talked to the screen. They all seemed proficient and skilled, and Kae somehow felt reassured, even as she as a person disappeared. Would she meet the threshold for hospital access? It wouldn't matter how convincing her application letter had been if she failed these final tests...

Kae came back to herself at home, which she recognized as clean but lived in, familiar, mammalian. She dropped her clothes into the sterilizer and began preparing for the afternoon's tea party, the gathering that Clare insisted on calling a "baby shower." Kae hadn't talked to her mother about her decision yet, even when Clare would start excitedly again with stories of her own birth, of friends arriving in the night, lighting candles, and filling up the birthing pool.

Kae well knew the changes in her lifetime, and not just around the places of birth. It wasn't the viruses, so much. People had quickly relearned the old arts of managing a fever, of sweating and retching on astringent brews, of being held through the night. What choice did they have? But the bacteria were shapeshifters, and people sometimes got sicker in hospitals, even died from secondary infections. For those who could afford it, home visits by medics or nurses grew to be commonplace again. Professions returned that had once almost disappeared—herbalists, bonesetters, independent midwives. But the pandemics started overlapping, the remaining antibiotics were rationed, and cesareans were a last resort; it was then that people began staying home to have their babies if they could. During the early days, it was hard to find a homebirth midwife, but then the midwives and nurses started leaving the hospitals, too, when the tide fully turned.

Soon the doorbell rang and Kae buzzed up the first of her friends. Before she knew it, she had been hugged and touched and fed and sung to by a dozen joyful nieces, cousins, friends. She understood, then, why it was called a "shower"; Kae felt bathed in love and kindness.

"What's this?" A sharp question from her friend Misha pierced the warm hum of the room. Misha was looking at a photo on the tablet Kae had been sharing around. She held up an image of Kae's 30-week scan.

"What do you mean?" replied Kae nervously.

"Have you never seen a scan before?" someone laughed. Since medical imaging had become readily available at home, the thrill of the first scan had largely given way to commonplace scans of everything.

"Not that, *this*," said Misha firmly, pointing to the words along the top left of the image: Kae's name, her date of birth, the date of the scan. And the name of the OB/GYN clinic.

Kae shuddered and it spilled out. "I've been seeing an obstetrician. I'm planning to have the baby in hospital."

The small gathering fell silent, a sea of shocked faces, and then a tumble of questions.

"Really?!" "But why would you do that? It's so UNSAFE."

"What if there's a power cut?" "Or a new spike in infections?" "The hospital shut down for days after that last big storm, remember?"

"Did you even qualify to birth there?"

"I was born in hospital," Aunt Jade announced matter-of-factly.

"Really?"

"Well, of course. By the start of the 21st century, only 5% of births happened at home. Maybe less."

"I knew it was kind of normal," said cousin Nita, "but that's...well, that's almost everyone."

"Sure, it was seen as unsafe to give birth at home," continued Jade, all eyes turning to her. "It wasn't until later that we realized that it wasn't, well not usually. In some ways I feel like we were cheated out of having our babies at home, with our families around, our own things, our music, grandma's pie." The women laughed, as Jade's eyes drifted to the photo of her grandmother on the altar the gathering had created earlier. "Some, like your brave mum, did it at home when that was still considered weird."

"Well, I wouldn't take a baby into a hospital unless I had to, let alone give birth there," blurted out Kae's teenage niece.

Kae stared down at the floor, her baby shower now feeling less like a blessing and more like a courtroom. She felt herself disappearing for the second time that day.

"Honey, don't cry," said Clare gently. "I know you will have given this a lot of thought and then some."

Kae sobbed a thank you into her mother's shoulder, as the others cleared up quietly around them. She heard someone say, softly—"Sorry, Kae we're just worried."

Someone else—"We'll be there for you. We'll visit you as soon as you're home and out of quarantine."

"She's just like you, Clare," said Aunt Jade to her sister, shaking her head as she placed coffee mugs in the sink. "No one could tell you what to do, either. Kae will do what she's decided to do and that's that. But they all come home in the end."

Coming Home: The Future Place of Birth

Kae's story offers us a portal into an imagined near future when the technocratic dominance of hospital-based birth has unraveled. This is, of course, a playful twist on the current status quo, in which those choosing to birth at home have to defend themselves against the norm of hospitalized birth and the technocratic model of risk and surveillance that underpins it (Davis-Floyd 2001, 2018b). Yet the risks inherent in the practice of this technocratic paradigm of birth itself are largely ignored. These include the iatrogenic harms arising from the routinized use of medical procedures (Davis-Floyd 2018b; Liese et al. 2021), exposing birthing people and their babies to environments provided for the sick, and subjugating them to a model of medically interventionist birth that is neither environmentally nor economically sustainable (Chadwick and Foster 2014). As a result, birth at home is currently constructed as the outsider choice for the "selfish" and "irresponsible" few who are willing to "risk" both their own and their baby's safety to have an empowering birth experience.

However, as our recent experience of COVID-19 has illuminated, dominant cultural understandings about safety and risk in relation to place of birth are mutable and subject to changing logics and forces. What then for the politics of birthplace as we head towards a future in which we will likely experience pressures such as those wrought by the coronavirus pandemic in greater frequency and severity? Evidence pointing to future impacts of the Climate Crisis is now considered indisputable (United Nations 2020). The effects of rising global sea and land temperatures leading to accelerating sea level rise and melting ice are already being felt and are set to intensify in coming decades, fueling environmental degradation, (un)natural disasters, weather extremes, food and water insecurity, economic disruption, and conflict (World Meteorological Organization 2020).

The resulting effects on human health and healthcare systems will likely be dramatic (Royal Society 2017). Direct health effects will result from extreme temperatures and an increase in "natural" disasters, including severe storms, floods, wildfires, droughts, and their resulting infrastructure damage and displacement of peoples (Royal Society 2017). Indirect health effects will result from an increase in vector-borne and other diseases, meaning greater likelihood of future pandemics. We will face food insecurity, poor air quality, migration of tropical species, human conflict resulting from migration and from social, political, and economic instability, as well as declining mental health and well-being (Royal Society 2017; see also the Conclusions to this volume).

Thus it is not hard to imagine that healthcare systems and infrastructure in all countries will come under severe pressure in the coming decades. Indeed, the model of medically dominated and technology-intensive hospital-based health care has been described as unsustainable and ill-suited to meeting the long-term health needs of humanity (Schroeder et al. 2012; Gutchow, Davis-Floyd, and Daviss 2021). For example, even for high-resource countries, the ever-expanding panoply of technologies, including pharmaceuticals, is making health care unsustainably expensive (WHO 2020). Carbon-intensive Western-style healthcare systems (Schroeder et al. 2012; Tomson 2015) consume large amounts of energy to power buildings and machines, for transport to and from hospitals, and for the procurement of goods and services to use within them. They also produce large amounts of waste (Sustainable Development Unit 2016). As fossil fuel and water scarcity increase under climate change, energy-intensive health care will become both unsustainable and unjustifiable (Schroeder et al. 2012). We can also anticipate greater access challenges through disruptions to transportation infrastructure, and that healthcare services will periodically become overwhelmed by those injured during disasters and/or suffering infectious diseases, as they were during COVID-19.

To return to our earlier question, will dominant cultural views on place of birth shift as we begin to experience growing effects of the Climate Crisis? Recent evidence drawn from disaster zones including the 2004 Aceh Tsunami, the superstorm Hurricane Haiyan that hit the Philippines in 2013, and the 2011 Great Japanese Earthquake and tsunami, suggest that a midwifery model of care is best suited to meet the challenges generated by disaster and upheaval (Ivry et al. 2019; Davis-Floyd et al. 2021; Lim and Davis-Floyd 2021). Despite extremely challenging environments and circumstances, implementing "low-tech, skilled-touch" midwifery practices in disaster zones has been found to offer flexible, low resource-intensive, safe, and high-quality care and to produce excellent outcomes that rival those under normal conditions (see Davis-Floyd et al. 2021). For example, in the wake of the 2004 Aceh Tsunami, the not-for-profit, midwife-led Bumi Sehat team partnered professionally trained and traditional midwives to provide non-interventionist localized midwifery-led care in devastated communities. Bumi Sehat found that despite the high risk/low resource environment, almost all women could safely manage to birth without clinics, hospitals, obstetricians, or extensive medical technology and with skilled, supportive home-based midwifery care (Lim and Davis-Floyd 2021). In "Sustainable Birth Care in Disaster Zones: Low-Tech, Skilled Touch," Davis-Floyd et al. (2021) argue that overall disaster preparedness must include the *decentralization of maternity care*, which should include greatly increased governmental support and full integration for autonomous, community-based midwives and large increases in their numbers.

Our recent global experience of the COVID-19 pandemic has provided further insight into the viability of home-based midwifery care when Western-style healthcare systems come under crisis. As discussed in our chapter Prelude, the pandemic resulted in rapid and fairly dramatic changes in cultural attitudes toward place of birth. In particular, birthing at home was transformed into a much more mainstream choice for families afraid of exposure to contagion in hospitals and reluctant to acquiesce to hospital policies intended to curb virus transmission—through, for example, allowing only one support person or excluding them altogether (Nicol-Williams 2020; Davis-Floyd, Gutschow, and Schwartz 2020). In a survey conducted by the Women's Health Action Trust (WHA) in ANZ during the country's month-long lockdown, over 40% of the pregnant people surveyed said they had changed their plans from hospital birth to birth at home or in a freestanding birth center (WHA 2020).

Yet a major challenge during the COVID-19 pandemic was the ability to access a homebirth midwife or to find a birth center with availability. In Aotearoa New Zealand, the midwifery workforce is integrated into mainstream maternity care, and all birthplace options are publicly funded. Thus, the workforce was at least partially equipped to respond to this influx of interest in home birth, despite being strained to meet the demand (Burrows 2020). In countries such as the US, where the independent midwifery workforce and the option of home birth are further marginalized by legal and funding barriers, there were much greater constraints to meeting the popular demand for community/out-of-hospital (OOH) birth care (Davis-Floyd, Gutschow, and Schwartz 2020). There were simply not enough OOH providers. As a consequence, well women who wished for OOH birth and their babies were placed at risk of viral exposure and the psychological trauma of lack of birthing companions by having to birth in hospitals (ibid.). Others chose unassisted births at home.

Intelligent Life: Reflecting on the Techno-Sapiens Birthplaces of the Future

Increasing technologization is synonymous with the Western cultural tradition of imagining the future. The entire genre of science fiction imagines a future defined by advancements in science and technology and the brave new frontiers of human existence and exploration opened up as a result (see Chapter 17). Indeed, the inevitability of human-technology co-evolution is assumed as the starting point for this volume, along with the questions it begs about what shapes and forms human-technology co-evolution will take in regards to reproduction and whether or not those forms can be as holistic and organic as they are technological. Our answer to the latter question is affirmative. The birthing future we imagine is one in which the technocratic paradigm of hospital-based birth has been disrupted. As we have imagined in Kae's story, the administrative barriers once faced by those seeking birth outside of hospitals are now faced by those wishing to birth within them. In Kae's world, birth in hospitals is no longer the social-cultural norm. In our imagined world that is navigating the challenges wrought by climate change and pandemics, the cultural consensus that birth in hospital is lower risk, safer, and therefore logical has been upended. Birth has returned home under the care of midwives, and those still intent on pursuing a planned hospital birth must defend this choice against a new cultural norm that finds this decision irresponsible and reckless, at best.

Returning to the question of what shapes and forms human-technology co-evolution will take in regards to reproduction in the future, we assert that *a break from technocratic birthing does not equate to a rejection of science or technology.* In fact, quite the contrary, we contend that our imagined near future of normative home birth will help bring birth care into alignment with scientific evidence about optimum childbirth care. The contemporary construction of the hospital as the only safe space for birth misrepresents the reality. Most high quality studies that have compared outcomes for planned home birth in healthy populations with low-risk hospital births have concluded that there is no difference in perinatal mortality, that common birth interventions are less frequently applied at home (therefore reducing maternal morbidity), and that parents are more satisfied with their care (see Fleming et al. 2016; Scarf et al. 2018). Further, as shown above, where Western-style healthcare infrastructure and systems break down in disaster and conflict zones and birth simply can't take place in hospitals, the midwifery model of care delivers sound outcomes. Midwifery care for home birth is also sustainable, as it offers a lower resource, lower cost, lower carbon model of care that minimizes intervention (Daellenbach et al. 2010).

In this way, we might think of the return home not as a break from technology but rather as *a technology in its own right*. We agree with the authors of Chapter 11 (on water as a valuable birthing technology) that framing a midwifery model of care as a technology is consistent with the WHO definition of health technology as "the application of organized knowledge and skills in the form of devices, medicines, vaccines, procedures and systems developed to solve a health problem and improve quality of lives" (WHO n.d.). Conceptualized in this way, midwifery care for home birth constitutes the application of knowledge and skills that solve a health problem (the iatrogenic harms of technocratic birth) and improve quality of lives (increased agency and satisfaction with the birthgiving experience). Further, physiologic birth care that causes minimal ecological disruption is consistent with the definition of "eco-technologies." Smart and sustainable low-carbon birth care at home that minimizes unnecessary intervention and waste, and limits the spread of infections, is surely the blueprint for techno-sapiens reproduction in a near future fully in the grip of the Climate Crisis and facing future pandemics.

Given that the weight of evidence supports the safety, acceptability, and sustainability of midwifery care for home birth, and that we are being called on *now* to both try to mitigate and prepare for the Climate Crisis ahead, it is primarily technocratic ideology and logic that is standing in the way of coming home to birth. Certainly, the COVID-19 pandemic has offered a rupture in the logics of hospital-based birth that we might utilize to wrestle back from the technocratic paradigm some power to re-define risk and safety in birth. We can nurture the insights gained about the safety, pleasure, and family empowerment of birth at home from those who may otherwise have attended hospitals into counter-stories of sustainable and safe birthing futures at home for the majority.

However, we should also not be naïve in assuming that the technocratic paradigm of birth will cede its power willingly. The idea that birth at home outside of medical control is dangerous remains deeply embedded in the hearts and minds of the medical community, who continue to hold great sway over birth practices. For example, half of the doctors in a study exploring health practitioner support for publicly funded home birth in Australia felt home birth was unsafe for babies (McLachlan et al. 2016). Obstetric professional bodies such as ACOG (2017) and RANZCOG (Australia and Aotearoa New Zealand) continue to assert opposition to home birth in their position statements. We should be alert to and challenge the ways in which the technocratic model of birth becomes entrenched and intensifies in times of crisis. For example, even as the COVID-19 pandemic exponentially elevated the risks of birthing in hospital, ACOG (2020) reasserted its position that hospitals remain "the safest setting for birth." Meanwhile within hospitals, efforts were being made to expedite birth and thus shorten the length of hospital stays by intensifying medical interventions such as inductions and cesareans, rather than supporting women to birth out of the hospital altogether (Davis-Floyd, Gutschow, and Schwartz 2020).

There is much to fear in a near future in which the effects of the Climate Crisis will be mounting. However, we offer this chapter to suggest that when it comes to the future of birth, there may also be *less* to fear if we embrace birth at home under the care of midwives as an obvious eco-technology for a techno-sapiens future.

Acknowledgments

Thanks are due to Garrick Martin for generously sharing your creative writing talents to help us craft Kae's story.

References

American College of Obstetricians and Gynecologists. 2020, April. *Planned Homebirth (Committee Opinion Number 697)*. www.acog.org/-/media/project/acog/acogorg/clinical/files/committee-opinion/articles/2017/04/planned-home-birth.pdf.

American College of Obstetricians and Gynecologists. 2020, April 20. *ACOG Statement on Birth Settings*. www.acog.org/news/news-releases/2020/04/acog-statement-on-birth-settings.

Burrows M. 2020, May 13. *Coronavirus: Midwives Leaving Their Jobs in Droves as COVID-19 Exposes Culture of Overwork, Stress, Poor Pay*. www.newshub.co.nz/home/new-zealand/2020/05/coronavirus-midwives-leaving-their-jobs-in-droves-as-covid-19-exposes-culture-of-overwork-stress-poor-pay.html.

Carter J, Duriez T. 1986. *With Child: Birth Through the Ages*. Edinburgh: Mainstream Publishing.

Chadwick RJ, Foster D. 2014. Negotiating risky bodies: Childbirth and constructions of risk. *Health, Risk & Society* 16(1):68–83.

Chalmers B. 2017. *Family-Centred Perinatal Care: Improving Pregnancy, Birth and Postpartum Care*. Cambridge: Cambridge University Press.

Cheyney M. 2011. Re-inscribing the birthing body: Homebirth as ritual performance. *Medical Anthropology Quarterly* 25(4):519–542.

Daellenbach R, Davies L, Kensington M. 2010. Introduction. In: *Sustainability, Midwifery and Birth*, eds. Davies L, R Daellenbach, M Kensington. London: Routledge, 1–8.

Davis-Floyd R. 1992. *Birth as an American Rite of Passage*, 1st edition. Berkeley, CA: University of California Press.

Davis-Floyd R. 2001. The technocratic, humanistic, and holistic models of birth. *International Journal of Gynecology & Obstetrics* 75(Supplement 1):S5–S23.

Davis-Floyd R. 2018a. The technocratic, humanistic, and holistic paradigms of birth and health care. In: *Ways of Knowing about Birth: Mothers, Midwives, Medicine, and Birth Activism*, ed. R Davis-Floyd. Long Grove, IL: Waveland Press, 1–44.

Davis-Floyd R. 2018b. The rituals of hospital birth: Enacting and transmitting the technocratic model. In: *Ways of Knowing about Birth: Mothers, Midwives, Medicine, and Birth Activism*, ed. R Davis-Floyd. Long Grove, IL: Waveland Press, 45–70.

Davis-Floyd R, Gutshow K, Schwartz D. 2020. Pregnancy, birth and the COVID-19 pandemic in the United States. *Medical Anthropology* 39(5):413–427.

Davis-Floyd R, Lim R, Penwell V, Ivry T. 2021. Sustainable birth care in disaster zones: Low-tech, skilled touch. In: *Sustainable Birth in Disruptive Times*, eds. Gutschow K, R Davis-Floyd, BA Daviss. Springer Nature, in press.

De Souza R. 2013. Who is a "good" mother?: Moving beyond individual mothering to examine how mothers are produced historically and socially. *Australian Journal of Child & Family Health Nursing* 10(2):15–18.

Fleming S, Donovan-Batson C, Burduli E, Barbose-Leiker C, Hollins Martin C, Martin CR. 2016. Birth satisfaction scale/birth satisfaction scale-revised (BSS/BSS-R): A large scale United States planned home birth and birth centre survey. *Midwifery* 41:9–15.

Guilliland K, Pairman S. 2010. *Women's Business: The Story of the New Zealand College of Midwives 1986–2010*. Christchurch: New Zealand College of Midwives.

Gutchow K, Davis-Floyd R, Daviss BA, eds. 2021. *Sustainable Birth in Disruptive Times*. Switzerland: Springer Nature.

Ivry T, Takaki-Einy R, Murotsuki J. 2019. What disasters can reveal about techno-medical birth: Japanese women's stories of childbirth during the 11 March, 2011 earthquake. *Health, Risk & Society* 21(3–4):164–184.

Jordan B. 1978. *Birth in Four Cultures: A Crosscultural Investigation of Childbirth in Yucatan, Holland, Sweden, and the United States*, 1st edition. Montreal: Eden Press.

Liese K, Davis-Floyd R, Stewart K, Cheyney M. 2021. Obstetric iatrogenesis in the United States: The spectrum of disrespect, violence, and abuse. *Medicine's Shadowside*, a special issue, eds. Varley E, S Varma. *Anthropology & Medicine*, in press.

Lim R, Davis-Floyd R. 2021. Implementing the International Childbirth Initiative (ICI) in disaster zones: Bumi Sehat's experience in Indonesia, Haiti, the Philippines, and Nepal. In: *Birthing Models on the Human Rights Frontier: Speaking Truth to Power*, eds. Daviss B. and Davis-Floyd, R. London: Routledge.

McLachlan H, McKay H, Powell R, Small R, Davey M, Cullinane F, Newton M, Forster D. 2016. Publicly-funded homebirth in Victoria, Australia: Exploring the views and experiences of midwives and doctors. *Midwifery* 35:24–30.

Miller S. 2020. *Moving Things Forward: Birthing Suite Culture and Labour Augmentation for Healthy First-Time Mothers* (Unpublished PhD thesis). Wellington: Victoria University of Wellington.

Ministry of Health. 2019. *Report on Maternity 2017*. Wellington: Ministry of Health.

New Zealand Government. 1904. *Midwives Act* (4 EDW VII 1904 No 31) 1904. www.n zlii.org/nz/legis/hist_act/ma19044ev1904n31210/.

Nicol-Williams K. 2020, March 29. *More Kiwi Women Considering Home Births as COVID-19 Rules Put Them under Pressure*. www.tvnz.co.nz/one-news/new-zealand /more-kiwi-women-considering-home-births-covid-19-rules-put-them-under-pres sure-v1.

Royal Australian and New Zealand College of Obstetricians and Gynaecologists. 2017. *Home Births*. https://ranzcog.edu.au/RANZCOG_SITE/media/RANZCOG-MEDIA/Women%27s%20Health/Statement%20and%20guidelines/Clinical-Ob stetrics/Home-Births-(C-Obs-2)-Review-July-17.pdf?ext=.pdf.

Royal Society. 2017. *Human Health Impacts of Climate Change for New Zealand*. www.r oyalsociety.org.nz/assets/documents/Report-Human-Health-Impacts-of-Climate-Change-for-New-Zealand-Oct-2017.pdf.

Scarf V, Rossiter C, Vedam S, Dahlen H, Ellwood D, Forster D, Foureur MJ, McLachlan H, Oats J, Sibbritt D, Thornton C, Homer C. 2018. Maternal and perinatal outcomes by planned place of birth among women with low-risk pregnancies in high-income countries: A systematic review and meta-analysis. *Midwifery* 62:240–255.

Schroeder K, Thompson T, Frith K, Pencheon D. 2012. *Sustainable Healthcare*. Hoboken, NJ: John Wiley & Sons.

Sustainable Development Unit. 2016. *Carbon Footprint Update for NHS in England 2015*. London, UK: Sustainable Development Unit.

Tomson C. 2015. Reducing the carbon footprint of hospital-based care. *Future Hospital Journal* 2(1):57.

Tracy S, Grigg C. 2019. Birthplace and birth space. In: *Midwifery: Preparation for Practice 4E*, eds. Pairman S, S Tracy, H Dahlen, L Dixon. Amsterdam: Elsevier, 131–145.

United Nations. 2020. *The Climate Crisis: A Race We Can Win*. www.un.org/en/un75/c limate-crisis-race-we-can-win.

Women's Health Action. 2020, April. *Summary Report: Information and Support Needs of Pregnant People and Caregivers of Infants and Young Children during Covid-19*. Auckland: Women's Health Action. https://womens-health.org.nz/health-topics/maternity/.

World Health Organization. 2020. *Countries—New Zealand*. www.who.int/countries/ nzl/en/.

World Health Organization. n.d. *What is a Health Technology?* www.who.int/health-t echnology-assessment/about/healthtechnology/en/.

World Meteorological Association. 2020. *WMO Statement on the State of the Global Climate in 2019*. World Meteorological Association. https://library.wmo.int/doc_nu m.php?explnum_id=10211.

17

CREATING LIFE IN *STAR TREK*:

Future Imagineering

Dana Solomon and Beverley Chalmers

Introduction: *Star Trek*, Technology, and Humanism

Star Trek (*ST*) is arguably the most successful television franchise of all time. Gene Roddenberry created *The Original Series* (*TOS*) in the 1960s; since then the *ST* universe has expanded to include an additional 7 existing spin-off series: *The Animated Series*, *The Next Generation* (*TNG*), *Deep Space Nine* (*DS9*), *Voyager* (*VOY*), *Enterprise* (*ENT*), *Discovery*, and *Picard*. In addition, *ST* has an ongoing series of shorts called *Short Treks* with several new series in development, including *Strange New Worlds* and the animated *Lower Decks*. There are also 13 feature films, hundreds of novels, graphic novels, audiobooks, and computer games. *ST* is a popular culture icon, with even those who have never seen an episode recognizing quotes like "Beam me up, Scotty" (incidentally, a line that was never used in any of the original episodes or movies).

The influence of *ST* on scientific innovation can be seen in everything from the design of the first flip phones (based on the *TOS* "communicator") to the look and function of an iPad. As one character in a different science fiction franchise so aptly phrased it "I don't know how you can call yourself a scientist and not worship at the altar of Roddenberry" (Wood 2002). *ST* has inspired technological innovations from cellphones to tablets, touchscreens to voice interfaces (like Siri and Alexa), real time translators to directed energy weapons. It continues to inspire technological innovation, with international teams racing to develop the first tricorder. Only a few years ago, the Qualcomm Tricorder XPRIZE competition offered a multi-million dollar reward to challenge research teams to develop a tricorder; a process resulting in significant advancements in the development of this device (Weekly 2017). While warp drive, replicators, and transporters may be out of our grasp (for now), much of the technological world that *ST* imagined has become reality far sooner than even Roddenberry might have dreamed.

The medical advances envisaged by *ST* have been no less influential. NASA developed technology for a low vision enhancement system, which they named the JORDY (Joint Optical Reflective Display), an homage to Geordie LaForge, *TNG*'s blind chief engineer who wore a VISOR to enable him to see (Heiney 2005). The Borg—a species that combines organic life with technology, named for "cyborgs"—inadvertently inspired advances in cybernetic technology, such as mind-controlled robotic limbs. MRIs were in their earliest conceptual stages in the 1960s, with *ST* elaborating on the concept, creating a realm of non-invasive medical technologies such as bio-beds, scanners, and tricorders, many of which we strive to develop today.

The technology of *ST*, however, plays a relatively minor role in the series. One of *ST*'s primary goals has always been to oppose prejudice and discrimination. While the 1960s *TOS* is, from today's perspective, rife with outdated gender and cultural stereotypes that are almost painful to watch, for its time, it was revolutionary—pushing far beyond the boundaries that were acceptable. At the same time as Samantha Stephens in *Bewitched* was suppressing her witching abilities in order to be the model demure housewife her husband desired, Lieutenant Uhura was one of the first Black female characters to hold a position of authority on a television show—in Uhura's case, the chief communications officer on the bridge of the Federation's flagship. She served as a role model for many other Black women, including Whoopi Goldberg and former NASA astronaut Mae Jemison. When segregation was still common practice in the US, and less than a year after interracial marriage became legal, *ST* aired the first[1] interracial kiss between a Black woman and a white man on television (Alexander 1968). It has tackled controversial issues such as genocide, environmentalism, religious and sexual freedom, racism, and intolerance, and continues to do so today. *ST*'s vision is of the future of humanity, and its vision of the future of reproduction exemplifies this focus. *ST*'s focus on the personal, interactional, and ethical aspects of care should be central components of advancements in reproduction as we move into the future. The technological innovations, as fun and remarkable as they may be, are merely the backdrop to the bigger issues—ethics, relationships, and the concept of life itself.

Imagined Technology in Familiar Contexts

Most of *ST*'s image of the future of medical technology appears to be based on the premise that medical care should be evidence-based, non- or minimally invasive, and respectful. Healing a broken bone, cut, or abrasion is simply a matter of passing a device over the affected area (Auberjonois 1996). A heart transplant (with an artificial heart) is depicted as a routine procedure requiring only

---

1 There is some debate over whether this was, in fact, the first interracial kiss on television, but it is usually identified as such.

4 hours of recovery time (Landau 1989). *ST*'s imagined future of birth (at least human birth) involves similar approaches.

In some cases, this means presenting birth in a way that evidence already shows is beneficial, but that clinical practice has yet to adopt. For example, many births in *ST* are depicted with women giving birth in an upright position (Bowman 1988a) (except when a character, Keiko, gives birth on a bar table with the support of a panicked Klingon, Worf, in the middle of a ship-wide emergency [Beaumont 1991]). While this is hardly a great technological innovation, this kind of birth it is something for which we have yet to gain acceptance in most countries in which birth has been medicalized, despite widespread evidence of its value (Gupta et al. 2017).

ST also briefly introduces a device that simultaneously cuts and heals the umbilical cord (Beaumont 1991). Even a cesarean can be done non-invasively, with a doctor beaming the distressed baby out of the uterus (Livingston 1996). In *VOY*, one episode proposes an advancement on ultrasound imaging in which a 3-dimensional holographic image of a fetus is created and even aged to predict what the child might look like later in life (Lauritson 2001). *ST* creates a future in which technologies far beyond our current abilities are commonplace. *DS9* imagines a fetal transplant to save both mother and baby; Dr. Julian Bashir must transplant a fetus from an injured human mother (Keiko O'Brien) into a Bajoran surrogate (Kira Nerys) (Brooks 1996).

In *VOY*, The Doctor is confronted with a fetus containing a common genetic abnormality, which he corrects *in utero* (Lauritson 2001). While we are beginning to explore medical treatments at the genetic level, in *ST*, not only is this a common procedure, but it can be done during early pregnancy. Scientists today continue to strive to achieve such remarkable advancements, from a hand-held diagnostic scanner through to genetic manipulation and non-invasive cesareans.

Ethical Dilemmas

There are multiple directions in which the technological enhancement of reproduction can develop. One such avenue is to address issues related to infertility—to create ordinary people through extraordinary means. A second is to enhance humanity (or other species)—to create extraordinary people.

One of the first references to infertility in *TNG* is an episode that emphasizes its social and emotional implications. The Aldeans, a highly technologically advanced society, are faced with extinction when their fertility rates drop to zero (Manners 1988). They kidnap children from the *Enterprise*, hoping that new genetic material will solve their problem. The Aldeans' infertility was due to radiation from the destruction of their ozone layer caused by the planetary shield and cloak the civilization had employed for centuries. This episode aired in 1988, a time when the destruction of Earth's ozone layer was one of the primary environmental danger narratives. Once the *Enterprise* crew reveals the cause of the Aldean's fertility problems, they re-seed the planet's ozone layer, cure their infertility, and return the kidnapped children to their families on the *Enterprise*. These technological marvels are almost an afterthought of the episode itself. The main focus of the story is on the societal level fears of extinction and the intensely personal desperation and despair that comes with the combination of a desire for children and the inability to have them.

One cannot imagine future reproductive technologies without mentioning cloning. When looking at the technology of cloning, *ST* seems to envision a process similar to the ones already in development—that of using a sample of genetic material to create an embryo that is then allowed to develop into a clone. In *ST*, this process does not require a surrogate womb, but can be completed entirely through technology and even accelerated to speed up the development process. Cloning in *ST* seems to have the same pitfalls as cloning in most other science fiction—that of diminishing returns. In this case, a single clone creates a fairly effective copy; however multiple clones, and clones of clones, create genetic abnormalities resulting from making copies of copies: the accuracy eventually deteriorates. This problem is most effectively introduced in *Up The Long Ladder* (Kolbe 1989b), an episode of *TNG* in which we learn that a group of human colonists calling themselves the Mariposans crashed on a planet with only five survivors—too few people to build a population with sufficient genetic diversity. They used cloning to build their civilization. Unfortunately, with time, the clones faced the problem of diminishing returns and the civilization needed an influx of new genetic material. At first, they asked the *Enterprise* crew for donations, but when none were forthcoming, they stole the samples. When the crew discovered this theft, they destroyed their own clones before they were completed, stating that they were unique and would not allow themselves to be replicated. The *Enterprise* crew proposed a solution: another small human colony needed a new planetary home and were relocated with the Mariposans. Dr. Crusher of the *Enterprise* calculated that each woman from this group would have to have three husbands to ensure sufficient genetic diversity; they agreed.

ST also proposes another, less familiar, cloning approach: using "Lyssarian Desert Larvae" which, when injected with DNA from another organism, will evolve into a clone of that organism. The clones develop, mature, and die within 15 days and, unexpectedly in the case of humans, also share the memories of the individual from whom they had been cloned. In the episode of *ENT* in which this creature is introduced, it was used to create a clone of the ship's chief engineer, Commander Tucker, specifically for the purpose of growing the clone to maturity and then harvesting its neural tissue to treat Tucker after what would otherwise have been a fatal accident (Burton 2003). This episode occurs after Earth has been attacked, with millions murdered. The attack was a test of a larger weapon intended to be used to eliminate humanity. The *Enterprise* is on a mission, months away from any support, to find the attackers and stop the creation of this genocidal weapon. It is in this context that Tucker—a crew member with expertise essential to the success of the mission—is injured and left in a coma. Dr. Phlox and Captain Archer are forced into this ethical dilemma: do they let him die and risk the failure of their mission and the consequent destruction of humanity? Or do they commit the abhorrent ethical violation of creating a life with the express intention of destroying it?

These examples share a common ethical concern: the commodification of life and of genetic material. The Aldeans attempted to trade technology for children, the Mariposans stole genetic material, and Dr. Phlox and Captain Archer were willing to create a life to harvest its neural tissue. This concept recurs in many other episodes, including in *DS9* when someone creates a clone of himself in order to murder it and frame the station's security chief for that murder (Lynch 1993). Further, in *DS9* the Dominion includes a species of clones called the Vorta. While the leaders of the Dominion, who are Changelings (shapeshifters), hold little regard for the lives of "Solids," the Vorta seem to be particularly disposable, with one Vorta being killed and replaced by its clone with remarkable frequency.

ST goes beyond asking whether a technology will work, or even how it will work; *ST* assumes that it will work, but then questions what we do with that technology. Should we be able to clone a living entity for the purpose of treating illnesses in a different being? Who owns our genetic material? Today, with massive DNA databases, we have yet to clarify ownership of our genetic data and, in turn, the genetic data of our relatives who can be connected through our own DNA. In short, who owns a life? In the case of the Mariposans, it was clear that each member of the *Enterprise* crew had the right to control their own genetic material. In *DS9*, the man who murdered his own clone was still charged with murder—it was his genetic material, yet nevertheless a life separate from his own (Lynch 1993). In *Similitude*, Dr. Phlox and Captain Archer regret their choice to create the clone, yet under the circumstances, they could not find another alternative. This episode is actually one of several that explore the ethical sacrifices made when one's species is under the threat of genocide. It explores morality *in extremis* and the choiceless choices that emerge in such situations (Langer 1982).

Genetic Manipulation

Another ethical concern common to much of science fiction is that of genetic engineering or manipulation; the attempt to "improve" humanity. Science fiction has explored this concept repeatedly, often by using genetic engineering to create enhanced humans. In some cases, this is portrayed as a positive contribution to the world. In many examples, however, the attempt to enhance humanity is depicted as highly dangerous, with strong historical precedent to support this hypothesis.

The scientific precursor to genetics was eugenics. In *TNG*'s *The Masterpiece Society*, the *Enterprise* encounters a planet of human colonists who developed their society based on eugenic principles. They believed that through controlled procreation they could breed out the flaws that are so common in humanity. When the colony finds itself at risk of destruction from an outside force, they are unable to find a solution to the problem. Eventually, the solution emerges out of the technology from Geordie LaForge's VISOR (which allows him to see, despite being born blind) (Kolbe 1992). The technology needed to save this genetically engineered society would never have been developed in a world without disability and "flaws."

Perhaps the most memorable series of episodes around genetic engineering is a complex storyline that was initiated in *TOS* in 1967, in which the *Enterprise* discovers a group of cryogenically frozen people (Daniels 1967). One man, Khan Noonien Singh, is revived and, over the course of the episode, we learn that he is a remnant from the late 20th century (based on predictions from the 1960s), when humans conducted a series of experiments to create "augments" or augmented humans. Their efforts resulted in a group of genetic "supermen," among whom Khan was a leader. This group of augments assumed control of the majority of Earth, with Khan as a tyrannical ruler. This resulted in the Eugenics Wars, during which the augments were defeated. Many disappeared from Earth, and it was these individuals whom the *Enterprise* encountered. Khan attempted to take over the *Enterprise*, freeing his comrades in the process, but was ultimately banished, along with his followers, to a planet where they could build their own civilization. He returns in the second *ST* movie, *The Wrath of Khan* (and again in the rebooted movie series depicting an alternate timeline, *Into Darkness*) where he was ultimately defeated, but not before murdering Captain Kirk's son (in *The Wrath of Khan*) (Meyer 1982).

Khan and the 20th-century augments were engineered to have superior strength, intellect, immune systems, and overall functioning. *ST* predicted that enhancing strength and intellect would also affect other characteristics, like ambition and aggression. Any group of people believing themselves to be superior will predictably oppress, dominate, and disregard the value of individuals they deem to be inferior. This perspective is indicative of a recurring theme in *Star Trek*'s depiction of genetic augmentation, which, when taken as a whole, reflects an uncharacteristically (for *ST*) conservative approach to the technology. There are very few positive examples of genetic enhancement, and even those are presented as exceptions. For instance, Dr. Julian Bashir of *DS9* was illegally genetically enhanced when he was a child because he was "slow" and his parents wanted a child who excelled. Eventually their secret was discovered and Julian's father went to prison for this crime (Livingston 1997).

ST also recognizes that humanity does not always learn from its errors. Almost 150 years after the Eugenics Wars, a geneticist named Arik Soong believed that he could create augments without the aggressive, psychopathic, megalomaniacal tendencies of Khan's generation. He took advantage of an ethical dilemma that faced Earth after the Eugenics Wars—the question of what to do with the remaining frozen embryos used to create the augments. In 20th century Earth, the questions surrounding these embryos remained too complex to parse, so humanity decided to store the embryos indefinitely. Arik Soong stole a number of them, attempted to "correct" the faults in their genetic engineering that he assumed resulted in the instability of the original augments, and raised the newly engineered augments as his children. Predictably, most of his augments exhibited the same instability, cruelty, aggression, and psychopathy as their ancestors (Livingston 2004; Vejar 2004; Burton 2004).

The unintended side effects of genetic engineering are discussed in several other episodes. In *DS9*, we encounter a group of people who were genetically augmented as children with disastrous results, ranging from catatonia through to severe emotional instability, coupled with an unshakable belief in their own superiority (Williams 1997). In *TNG*, a group of scientists created genetically enhanced children, whose "improved" immune systems created an airborne virus that was deadly to all other humans. As a result, the children were forced to spend their lives in isolation (Lynch 1989). In *VOY*, The Doctor attempts to dissuade a pregnant crewmember from genetically altering her daughter by citing the potential for unintended consequences that would affect personality and behavior (Lauritson 2001).

The inadvertent consequences of genetic manipulation are a problem that could, potentially, be resolved by technology; however, *ST* recognizes that the social implications of technological advancements are not that simple to solve. Many of the genetic engineering examples explored in *ST* are based on 3 fundamental premises: that it is possible to create a "superior" race; that humanity is flawed; and that those flaws, disabilities, and genetic variations should be eliminated. These concepts represent two sides of prejudice—the belief in one's own superiority, and the belief in the inferiority of others.

Belief in the superiority of one group over another frequently, if not always, leads to violence and oppression, including the dominance of men over women; white supremacy and colonialism that resulted in slavery and centuries of oppression and genocide; Christian supremacy that fueled the Crusades and the Inquisition; Islamic fundamentalism that inspires some extreme terrorist groups; or Aryan superiority that resulted in genocides against Jews, the Roma and Sinti, people with disabilities, homosexuals, and anybody else deemed "life unworthy of life," by specifically manipulating birth in addition to murder (Chalmers 2015), to name only a few examples. It is hardly surprising that with such a wealth of historical precedent, *ST* would recognize the risk of any group believing itself to be inherently better than another.

The desire to eliminate "flaws" is a more insidious aspect of the philosophy behind genetic engineering. It is easy to believe that, in finding ways to eliminate disabilities and genetic abnormalities, we are helping people—and in many instances that may well be true. *ST,* however, identifies the complexity behind this premise and challenges it in multiple ways. For example, one of the tenets of Vulcan philosophy (the species to which Spock belongs), is that of the value of IDIC: Infinite Diversity in Infinite Combinations. *ST* does not simply tolerate diversity; it embraces it as one of the greatest strengths of the Federation. In addition to *TNG*'s blind engineer, Geordie La Forge (Roddenberry 1987–1994), *ST* includes a renowned negotiator, Riva, who is deaf and can only speak through sign language or telepathy (Shaw 1989); and a brilliant scientist, Melora, who requires the use of a wheelchair anywhere other than on her home world, which has lighter gravity (Kolbe 1993). In *ST*, these "flaws" or disabilities become sources of strength and advancement. Geordie's VISOR and subsequent ocular implants allow him to see far better than any human being. When, as previously mentioned, he is confronted by members of a society that has bred out disability, they say, with arrogance and disparagement, that nobody in their society would ever be born blind. Geordie responds "I can see you just fine" (Kolbe 1992). When the ambassador who is both deaf and silent finds himself without his interpreters, he chooses to turn his disadvantage into an advantage, by teaching warring communities to speak his sign language—to create a new common language between them as part of the first essential steps of any peace process (Shaw 1989). When Melora is offered a treatment that would allow her to walk but would make it impossible for her to return to her home world (with its lighter gravity), she declines the treatment. For her, the unique experiences she could have when in a lighter gravity, and the ability to return to her home, outweighed the immense obstacles she faced in the heavier gravity in which she worked (Kolbe 1993).

In a society that genuinely values diversity, some characteristics that are commonly regarded as disadvantages can become advantages and opportunities for tremendous development. This is the warning that *ST* provides: that we should use our technological advancement with critical self-awareness, being sure not to allow good intentions to mask discrimination. As we move forward into a world that increasingly embraces the idea of techno-sapiens, this is an ideal to which we can aspire.

Relationships

Birth is an inherently social aspect of life. Conception (at present) requires interaction (including via IVF); there are physiological and psychological benefits to having support during labor (Hodnett et al. 2011); and raising a child requires the interaction of multiple individuals. Imagining the future of birth should also require imagining the future of the relational aspects of the experience.

Increasingly we are focusing our attention on person- and family-centered, psychosocially and culturally sensitive, and respectful care practices (Chalmers 2017). The relationship between a caregiver and care recipients is a central component of developments in the research and practice of perinatal care, with growing recognition that this relationship influences outcomes as much as any treatment they offer or fail to offer (Chalmers and Dzakpasu 2015a; Vedam et al. 2019). *ST* explores the nature of such relationships. In a *TOS* episode, a woman in labor declines medical care from Dr. McCoy, yet he continues to offer care despite her resistance. She becomes violent and slaps him; to her surprise, he slaps her back. This interaction, combined with McCoy's expertise, results in the establishment of mutual trust and this woman's willingness to accept Dr.

McCoy's care. In today's world, this series of events—even ignoring the exchange of slaps—raises some highly topical questions on ethical medical practice. To what extent can people refuse medical care? Can a woman refuse a cesarean or an induction? Can someone refuse to labor on their back, or refuse fetal monitoring? To what extent is it acceptable for a caregiver to pressure families into accepting medical interventions? These questions are raised by this *TOS* episode, but are not adequately answered. In later *ST* series, similar issues emerge, with a far clearer set of answers: doctors are not allowed to perform interventions without informed consent—a principle that theoretically exists today, but is actually practiced in *ST*. Even within *ST*, however, there are debates around medical ethics, with different caregivers taking different approaches, sometimes with ethically ambiguous results. The principle of client-centered informed, not coerced, care, however, remains a consistent focus.

Generally, the caregiver-client relationship depicted in *ST* is a model to emulate. Doctors in *ST* are typically highly respectful, empathetic, culturally sensitive, and acutely aware of the needs of each individual to direct their own care. Even when doctors disagree with a patient's choice, they are respectful of their needs and abide by their wishes (Chalmers 1992). For example, when Dr. Pulaski initially questions Data's (an android) ability to act as a companion to Deanna Troi during labor, Troi disagrees and Dr. Pulaski immediately responds by saying it is Troi's choice (Bowman 1988a).

That said, not all doctors in *ST* are perfect. The Doctor on *Voyager* is an Emergency Medical Hologram who was never designed to act as the ship's physician for the long term. The result is that he was initially programmed with only a minimal bedside manner. This creates numerous opportunities for *VOY* to explore the importance of empathy, compassion, and kindness in addition to competent or even exceptional clinical care. In one early episode, The Doctor is dismissive of a pregnant crew member when she comes in with sciatic nerve pain resulting from her pregnancy. The Doctor tells her that "pregnancy causes its fair share of discomforts, and you'll have to learn to live with them" (Singer 1995). When he is challenged on his lack of compassion, he says he will not "coddle" the crew. In time, The Doctor learns that his programming is deficient and begins to update it. By the 7th season, The Doctor is a highly compassionate entity and is trusted, liked, and respected enough by the crew that when a different crew member goes into labor and her husband cannot accompany her, she says "Don't worry, The Doctor will be here with me" (Kroeker 2001).

Medical care today is often more like The Doctor in Season 2 of *VOY* than the humanistic practice he develops by Season 7. A wealth of research, including that focused on clients' experiences of care, makes it evident that we—as caregivers and as the medical system as a whole—are failing many families. Only 54% of women in Canada consider their experiences of labor and birth to be "very positive" (Public Health Agency of Canada 2009). Likewise, in the US, only 35% rate the quality of their care as "excellent" (Declercq and Chalmers 2008). Some families are so distrustful of the care they expect to receive in hospitals or even with homebirth midwives that they choose to give birth without any skilled birth attendants present (Chalmers 2017).

Our current technocratic model of care often prioritizes technology over sensitivity; "good intervention is seen as good medicine" (Chalmers 2017:76). It is an approach that is comfortable for caregivers who are trained to accept a medicalized approach. Mothers, however, make it clear that higher intervention rates decrease satisfaction with their experience of birth (Chalmers and Dzakpasu 2015b). Moreover, some over-medicalized perinatal care is abusive (Liese et al. 2021; Chalmers 2017:119–127). Like *VOY*'s Doctor, some caregivers see no advantage to sensitive care; they see no need to "coddle" their patients.

Beyond the doctor-client relationship, *ST* also explores other relationships surrounding pregnancy and birth. In *DS9*, when Major Kira Nerys acts as a surrogate for the human Keiko O'Brien, Kira, a Bajoran, chooses to give birth in a traditional Bajoran way, including with rhythmic chimes and a traditional birth attendant. While Dr. Bashir checks on her labor progress periodically (a necessity given that the child is a different species than the surrogate mother), he abides by the cultural conventions Kira has requested. This includes adding elements of traditional attire over his uniform, adopting the appropriate demeanor, and aside from the occasional discreet, non-invasive exam, he leaves the delivery to Kira and the traditional birth attendant (Treviño 1997). In fact, this birth scenario is a superb model of the integration of two different approaches to perinatal care. Both caregivers treat each other respectfully, focusing entirely on the needs of the family, which consists of Kira, her partner Shakaar, and Keiko and Miles, the baby's parents. There is no push for greater intervention or medicalization, despite the complications and potential for risk presumably inherent in an inter-species birth. Cultural traditions are treated with as much dignity and reverence as the medical care—as should be the case. While there is conflict between Miles, the baby's father, and Shakaar, Kira's boyfriend, the other caregivers, Keiko, and Kira work together well and respectfully, and evict Miles and Shakaar when their jealous bickering disrupts the peaceful harmony of the birth. Unfortunately, today, even the integration of midwifery and obstetrics—based on two different but overlapping knowledge systems (Davis-Floyd 2018)—appears to be almost beyond our abilities (Chalmers 2017:87).

Major Kira's pregnancy also provides the opportunity to examine the complex relationships surrounding parenthood and surrogacy. As mentioned, Kira becomes the surrogate for Keiko's baby when Keiko is injured during an accident. Through this scenario, *ST* explores the relationship between a surrogate and the birth parents. In this case, the O'Briens invite Kira to live with them, out of a desire not to miss the development of their baby (Brooks 1996). While Keiko is happy that Kira was willing to be a surrogate, she also experiences an intense sense of loss, knowing that she will not give birth to her own child. Kira and Miles find their relationship becoming far closer, resulting in both volatile arguments and some romantic feelings that both manage to resist. The complications of this kind of relationship emerge over several episodes and continue after the baby's birth, when Kira feels tremendous loss for the child she carried but will not be able to raise. During the pregnancy, there is also discussion over how much control Miles should have over the actions of the woman carrying his child. Should he be able to dictate how much caffeine she drinks or whether she can play her favorite sport? While this leads to some heated arguments between Miles and Kira, it also contributes to a humorous discussion in which Quark—a Ferengi—states that in his culture, pregnancy is viewed as a "rental," thus providing the father with the rights of a lessee (Friedman 1996). It is also notable that when it comes to the birth, Kira's and the parents' needs are treated with respect, and the birth takes place in the manner that Kira—the surrogate—desires, with the full support of Keiko and Miles. As is the case with so much of *ST*, the technological marvels of a fetal transplant and inter-species surrogacy are barely mentioned, while the interpersonal implications of those technological feats become the focus of multiple episodes.

Artificial Life—Beyond AI

ST explores reproduction from pregnancies and labors with some enviable technology, to artificial reproduction such as cloning, through to eugenics and genetic engineering. In all these examples, the foundation for the creation of life is the same: genetic material from one or more individuals is used to create another, related life. *ST* goes beyond this concept to the creation of life without the contribution of living genetic material—artificial life.

Perhaps the most complete, even ideal, example of artificial life in *ST* is Lieutenant Commander Data. Data is a sentient, humanoid android with a deep sense of curiosity, an unwavering moral compass, and a combination of confidence and vulnerability that makes him both a competent commander and an eternal student of life and of human behavior. A notably bad poet (his *Ode to Spot*, his cat, being particularly painful), Data represents an idealized image of what artificial intelligence could become. He has flaws and imperfections that are endearing representations of his inherent humanity (for want of a more inclusive term), alongside the superior strength and intelligence that we imagine will be part of any artificially created lifeform in the future. He learns, grows, and aspires to be more than the sum of his programming. In fact, becoming human is one of his greatest desires.

Artificial life on *ST* is not limited to Data. In one episode, a science experiment gone wrong results in the creation of a civilization of intelligent, living nanites, who evolve within the ship's computers until eventually negotiating with the crew, who then facilitate the establishment of a home for the nanite civilization (Kolbe 1989a). In another, a series of robotic devices called "exocomps," created to help with construction and repair, evolve to become alive and sentient (Frakes 1992), with one exocomp even sacrificing itself so the others can survive. In *DS9*, an artificial lifeform moves into the station computer, demanding attention (in a manner similar to a puppy) and disrupting the ship's systems until Chief O'Brien designs a virtual "dog house" for it, where it could get the attention it wanted without causing further problems (Landau 1993). *ST* also includes holographic life, with *VOY*'s holographic doctor as the most memorable example. A hologram of Professor Moriarty also gains sentience in an episode of *TNG*, and takes over the ship, demanding to be made real along with his paramour. Since that is impossible, the crew designs a holographic universe for them to explore, believing they are in the real world (Singer 1993). One also cannot forget Data's family: Lore—Data's evil, genocidal older brother (Bowman 1988b); B-4—a prototype android that was one of three failed prototypes before the construction of Lore (Baird 2002); and Lal—Data's daughter (Frakes 1990).[2] In *Picard*, we learn that, after Data dies while saving Picard, an entire community of androids (synths, or synthetic lifeforms)—in this case, organic androids—was created using a single positronic neuron from a parent android—Data. In a sense, these synths are Data's descendants (Goldsman et al. 2020).

While not an exhaustive list of every artificial lifeform depicted in *ST*, these examples indicate a range of possibilities for the creation of artificial "technosapiens." More importantly, however, *ST*'s inclusion of artificial life made it possible to explore some of the most complicated questions surrounding the advancement of reproduction and the technological creation of life. How does one determine when something is alive? How do we define sentience? Does artificial life have the same rights as other life forms? Who is responsible for the actions of an artificially created intelligence?

When Data asks Dr. Crusher to define life, her response is: "Life is what enables plants and animals to consume food, derive energy from it, grow, adapt themselves to their surroundings, and reproduce." Data responds by asking "What about fire? [...] It consumes fuel to produce energy, it grows, it creates offspring" (Frakes 1992). He then points out that he himself neither grows nor reproduces (though he did later create his daughter Lal), yet he is alive. *ST*'s inclusion of artificial life in its universe forces us to question fundamental concepts of life that we, perhaps, believed to be self-evident. We accept that humans, animals, bacteria, and viruses, for example, are alive. Likewise, despite chapter author Solomon's father treating his Roomba like a badly behaved, untrainable pet, we accept that the Roomba, computerized toys, and smartphones are not alive—no matter how many jokes Siri tells.

In a trial to determine whether Data has rights or is the property of Star Fleet, *ST* also tackles the challenge of defining sentience—possessing "intelligence, self-awareness, and consciousness" (Scheerer 1989), according to the episode.

---

2 Doctor Juliana Tainer—the wife and assistant of Data's creator, Dr. Noonian Soong—was referred to as Data's mother. Dr. Soong transferred his wife's memories into an android body without her knowledge after she was severely injured in an attack on their planet. Since Dr. Tainer was originally human, she is not included in this list of artificial beings.

The same trial raises the question of whether artificial life is property, and if so, would a race of artificial beings become slaves? While the judge of this trial determines that Data is not, in fact, property, and does have the same rights as other sentient beings, the same question is re-visited when Data identifies another artificial lifeform—the exocomps (Frakes 1992)—and when The Doctor's holonovel[3] is stolen by the publisher on the grounds that The Doctor is not a person and therefore has no rights to the novel he created (Livingston 2001). Even Data has to face the same challenge later in his life; when he attempts to reproduce, he is challenged by Captain Picard and Starfleet as to why he did not seek permission before creating another android, his daughter Lal. He responds by saying, "I have not observed anyone else on board consulting you about their procreation, Captain" (Frakes 1990).

In *Picard*, the concept of artificial life is explored at length. By that point in Federation history, synthetic lifeforms had been banned after a group of "synths" committed a mass atrocity on Mars. All research into cybernetic life was halted, other than theoretical explorations. Even the use of a positronic net (the foundation for Data's brain) for medical research had been halted, resulting in the death of Troi's and Riker's son of a disease that would otherwise have been curable. Just as some blame all Muslims for the atrocities committed by a few, the responsibility for the actions of the synths on Mars was laid upon all synths, and not on the individuals themselves or the programmers who caused their actions (Goldsman et al. 2020).

Artificial intelligence (AI) research continues its rapid progression, and while the invention of artificial life is beyond our current abilities, the creation of cars driven by AI, for example, is raising questions that go far beyond the car's ability to navigate the roads. If a self-driving car causes an accident, who is responsible? Is it the owner of the car? Perhaps the programmers who designed the car's software? Can the car itself be held responsible? If that is the case, is the car alive and is it ethical to enslave it by forcing it to drive us around? As far as we know, self-driving cars are not alive, but the creation of a machine with that much responsibility raises numerous ethical and practical questions that beg answers.

The Future: *Star Trek's* Vision

ST's vision of the future of creating life is a wealth of extraordinary potential coupled with difficult questions and cautious warnings. Imagine a future of medicine that is non-invasive, respectful, culturally and psychologically sensitive, and evidence-based. It is a future with remarkable technologies that can cure infertility, perform a cesarean without an incision, transfer a fetus in danger from a mother to a surrogate, and treat genetic abnormalities *in utero*. Imagine a

---

3 A story played out on a holodeck—an artificial environment that looks and feels real while inside, but is comprised entirely of holograms.

future that embraces caring medical professionals, a variety of birth companions when they are desired, and multiple approaches to caregiving. In this future, the creation of life is both biological and artificial.

ST's vision of the future contains extraordinary technological potential, including creating techno-sapiens through genetic engineering and artificial life, yet the true focus is not on the gadgets, but on the people themselves—the multi-species "humanity" that should, but does not always, underlie perinatal care. As much as we can learn from the imagined technological future *ST* presents, so should we learn from the extraordinary socially, culturally, and psychologically sensitive care that *ST* demonstrates. We should seek to emulate not only the tricorder, but also the inclusive and respectful care offered by the person wielding it.

References

Alexander, David. 1968. "Plato's Stepchildren." In: *Star Trek*. USA: Paramount Pictures.

Auberjonois, Rene. 1996. "The Quickening." In: *Star Trek: Deep Space Nine*. USA: Paramount Pictures.

Baird, Stuart. 2002. *Star Trek: Nemesis*. USA: Paramount Pictures.

Beaumont, Gabrielle. 1991. "Disaster." In: *Star Trek: The Next Generation*. USA: Paramount Pictures.

Bowman, Rob. 1988a. "The Child." In: *Star Trek: The Next Generation*. USA: Paramount Pictures.

Bowman, Rob. 1988b. "Datalore." In: *Star Trek: The Next Generation*. USA: Paramount Pictures.

Brooks, Avery. 1996. "Body Parts." In: *Star Trek: Deep Space Nine*. USA: Paramount Pictures.

Burton, LeVar. 2003. "Similitude." In: *Star Trek: Enterprise*. USA: Paramount Home Entertainment.

Burton, LeVar. 2004. "The Augments." In: *Star Trek: Enterprise*. USA: Paramount Home Entertainment.

Chalmers, Beverley. 2015. *Birth, Sex, and Abuse: Women's Voices Under Nazi Rule*. Guildford: Grosvenor House Publishing Limited.

Chalmers, Beverley. 2017. *Family-Centred Perinatal Care: Improving Pregnancy, Birth and Postpartum Care*. Cambridge: Cambridge University Press.

Chalmers, Beverley, and Susie Dzakpasu. 2015a. "Interventions in Labour and Birth and Satisfaction with Care: The Canadian Maternity Experiences Survey Findings." *Journal of Reproductive and Infant Psychology* 33(4):374–387. doi:10.1080/02646838.201 5.1042964.

Chalmers, Beverley, and Susie Dzakpasu. 2015b. "Interventions in Labour and Birth and Satisfaction with Care: The Canadian Maternity Experiences Survey Findings." *Journal of Reproductive and Infant Psychology*, in press.

Chalmers, Chip. 1992. "Ethics." In: *Star Trek: The Next Generation*. USA: Paramount Pictures.

Daniels, Marc. 1967. "Space Seed." In: *Star Trek*. USA: Desilu Productions. National Broadcasting Company.

Davis-Floyd, Robbie. 2018. *Ways of Knowing about Birth: Mothers, Midwives, Medicine, & Birth Activism*. Long Grove, IL: Waveland Press.

Declercq, Eugene, and Beverley Chalmers. 2008. "Mothers' Reports of Their Maternity Experiences in the USA and Canada." *Journal of Reproductive and Infant Psychology* 26(4):295–308.

Frakes, Jonathan. 1990. "The Offspring." In: *Star Trek: The Next Generation*. USA: Paramount Pictures.

Frakes, Jonathan. 1992. "The Quality of Life." In: *Star Trek: The Next Generation*. USA: Paramount Pictures.

Friedman, Kim. 1996. "…Nor the Battle to the Strong." In: *Star Trek: Deep Space Nine*. USA: Paramount Pictures.

Goldsman, Akiva, Michael Chabon, Kirsten Beyer, and Alex Kurtzman. 2020. In: *Star Trek: Picard*. USA: CBS All Access, Amazon Prime Video, Bell Media.

Gupta, Janesh K., Akanksha Sood, G. Justus Hofmeyr, and Joshua P. Vogel. 2017. "Position in the Second Stage of Labour for Women Without Epidural Anaesthesia." *Cochrane Database of Systematic Reviews* 5: CD002006.

Heiney, Anna. 2005. *A Second Set of Eyes*. Accessed 15 June 2020.

Hodnett, Ellen D., Simon Gates, G. Justus Hofmeyr, Carol Sakala, and Julie Weston. 2011. "Continuous Support for Women During Childbirth." *Cochrane Database of Systematic Reviews* 2:CD003766.

Kolbe, Winrich. 1989a. "Evolution." In: *Star Trek: The Next Generation*. USA: Paramount Pictures.

Kolbe, Winrich. 1989b. "Up the Long Ladder." In: *Star Trek: The Next Generation*. USA: Paramount Pictures.

Kolbe, Winrich. 1992. "The Masterpiece Society." In: *Star Trek: The Next Generation*. USA: Paramount Pictures.

Kolbe, Winrich. 1993. "Melora." In: *Star Trek: Deep Space Nine*. USA: Paramount Pictures.

Kroeker, Allan. 2001. "Endgame." In: *Star Trek: Voyager*. USA: Paramount Pictures.

Landau, Les. 1989. "Samaritan Snare." In: *Star Trek: The Next Generation*. USA: Paramount Pictures.

Landau, Les. 1993. "The Forsaken." In: *Star Trek: Deep Space Nine*. USA: Paramount Pictures.

Langer, Lawrence L. 1982. *Versions of Survival: The Holocaust and the Human Spirit*. Albany: State University of New York Press.

Lauritson, Peter. 2001. "Lineage." In: *Star Trek: Voyager*. USA: United Paramount Network.

Liese, Kylea, Robbie Davis-Floyd, Karie Stewart, and Melissa Cheyney. 2021. "Obstetric Iatrogenesis in the United States: The Spectrum of Disrespect, Violence, and Abuse." *Anthropology & Medicine Special Issue on "Medicine's Shadowside."* eds. Emma Varley and Saiba Varma, in press.

Livingston, David. 1996. "Deadlock." In: *Star Trek: Voyager*. USA: Paramount Pictures.

Livingston, David. 1997. "Doctor Bashir, I Presume." In: *Star Trek: Deep Space Nine*. USA: Paramount Pictures.

Livingston, David. 2001. "Author, Author." In: *Star Trek: Voyager*. USA: Paramount Pictures.

Livingston, David. 2004. "Borderland." In: *Star Trek: Enterprise*. USA: Paramount Home Entertainment.

Lynch, Paul. 1989. "Unnatural Selection." In: *Star Trek: The Next Generation*. USA: Paramount Pictures.

Lynch, Paul. 1993. "A Man Alone." In: *Star Trek: Deep Space Nine*. USA: Paramount Pictures.

Manners, Kim. 1988. "When the Bough Breaks." In: *Star Trek: The Next Generation*. USA: Paramount Pictures.

Meyer, Nicholas. 1982. "Star Trek II: The Wrath of Khan." In: *Star Trek*. USA: Paramount Pictures.

Public Health Agency of Canada, and PHAC. 2009. *What Women Say: The Maternity Experiences Survey*. Ottawa, ON: Public Health Agency of Canada.

Roddenberry, Gene. 1987–1994. In: *Star Trek: The Next Generation*. USA: Paramount Pictures.

Scheerer, Robert. 1989. "The Measure of a Man." In: *Star Trek: The Next Generation*. USA: Paramount Pictures.

Shaw, Larry. 1989. "Loud as a Whisper." In: *Star Trek: The Next Generation*. USA: Paramount Pictures.

Singer, Alexander. 1993. "Ship in a Bottle." In: *Star Trek: The Next Generation*. USA: Paramount Pictures.

Singer, Alexander. 1995. "Tattoo." In: *Star Trek: Voyager*. USA: Paramount Pictures.

Treviño, Jesús Salvador. 1997. "The Begotten." In: *Star Trek: Deep Space Nine*. USA: Paramount Pictures.

Vedam, Saraswathi, Kathrin Stoll, Tanya Khemet Taiwo, Nicholas Rubashkin, Melissa Cheyney, Nan Strauss, Monica McLemore, Micaela Cadena, Elizabeth Nethery, Eleanor Rushton, Laura Schummers, G. Eugene Declercq, and VtM-US Steering Council, and GVtM- U. S. Steering Council The. 2019. "The Giving Voice to Mothers Study: Inequity and Mistreatment during Pregnancy and Childbirth in the United States." *Reproductive Health* 16(1):77–18. doi:10.1186/s12978-019-0729-2.

Vejar, Michael. 2004. "Cold Station 12." In: *Star Trek: Enterprise*. USA: Paramount Home Entertainment.

Weekly, Telecommunications. 2017. *Family-Led Team Takes Top Prize in Qualcomm Tricorder XPRIZE Competition for Consumer Medical Device Inspired by Star Trek[R]*. NewsRX LLC.

Williams, Anson. 1997. "Statistical Probabilities." In: *Star Trek: Deep Space Nine*. USA: Paramount Pictures.

Wood, Martin. 2002. "The Other Guys." In: *Stargate SG-1*. MGM Worldwide Television Productions.

CONCLUSIONS:

Birthing Techno-Sapiens in Disruptive Times

Beverley Chalmers and Robbie Davis-Floyd

The Overall Contributions of This Book

The forerunner to this book—*Cyborg Babies*—was seen as "an enormously influential, highly regarded, and widely cited volume discussing cutting edge research on reproductive technologies in the late 1990s" (Lisa Mitchell, reviewer, 2020). Our volume continues some of the powerful ideas initiated in the earlier volume and adds complexity and originality to how we might think about reproduction, reproductive technology, the relationships between culture and biology, and what it means to be human as we move into the second quarter of the 21st century. Our chapters offer approaches to reproductive lives that are empirically grounded in ethnographic material and richly theorized from diverse disciplines. We intend to have presented visions and possibilities that will engage researchers and scholars looking for empirical work and big ideas. Our material is provocative; we trust that it will generate debate, ideas, and future research and, most importantly, have potential to shape ethical policy and practice in reproductive health care.

In this Anthropocene Era, characterized as the time in which the collective activities of *homo sapiens* began to substantially alter Earth's surface, atmosphere, and oceans, there is clearly considerable interest in the topic of "human-technology co-evolution"; in this volume, we have employed the term *techno-sapiens* to capture the essence of this evolutionary direction. Having seen a part of the vast range of possibilities for becoming techno-sapiens, we can now ask, have we always been so? Did we become techno-sapiens the first time a woman thought to use a stick to dig up tubers and roots, or the first time she thought to sharpen it and stick it through a hole in a rock to give it more force? Or carve that hole herself? Or the first time a man sharpened a similar stick of wood to make it into a spear? Can human bodies themselves be coded as "technologies," given that they are things that make things happen in the world?

Reviewer Lisa M. Mitchell summed up what we have sought to achieve with this volume better than we could ourselves:

> The editors are offering a bold and forward-looking perspective on the ways in which humans and their reproductive lives are transformed through our engagement with diverse forms of technology. The authors... offer an evolutionary, "big picture" perspectives...at the same time as they pay close attention to the empirical, on the ground, lived experiences of people using and refusing reproductive technologies. This ability to tack back and forth between the local and the global, the specific and the broad, the present and the past/future, is a hallmark of anthropology and is critical to developing new ways of framing our thinking, policies, and caring practices around reproduction.
>
> Further, the book adopts an updated, enlivened and nuanced view of cyborgs, of human-technology co-dependencies. In their conceptualization, cyborgs are not reducible to human-machine interactions but are complex, multifaceted intercalations and interdependencies of biology, technology, sensation, emotion, meaning, and spirituality. This conceptualization avoids both a narrow object-oriented approach to technology and a deterministic view of human-technology relationships. Instead, the chapters in this volume stretch our thinking to consider not only how human reproductive lives are constrained and enabled by technology but also how our cyborg lives are also about sensation, feelings, and spirit.

This diversity in our chapters reflects the multitude of issues, ideas, approaches, wishes, knowledges, and fantasies that—like all human behavior—are closer to the truth than any single discipline or approach could achieve. To state the obvious, human beings are complex. We function on multiple levels simultaneously, from the micro-biological to the individual, the social, the political, the societal, the spiritual, and the generational. We ignore any one of these at our peril.

Findings from Our Chapters and Further Developments: Human-Technology Co-Evolution in the Anthropocene Era

Here we both present some of the findings of our chapters and consider further developments, some of which are not mentioned in those chapters, presenting opportunities for future thinking and action.

Part I: From Biocultural Evolution to Human-Technology Co-Evolution

Our chapters begin at the beginning of human evolution. In Chapter 1, Melissa Cheyney and Robbie Davis-Floyd describe the relevance of human biocultural evolution for childbirth, showing that premodern norms across cultures shared many physiologically sound practices that were undone during the Industrial

Revolution and the later development of technocratic societies, and, as there is now strong scientific evidence for their efficacy, should be recaptured in these postmodern times, for which the authors set out a racial- and gender-egalitarian future. And their futuristic story about Kiri the Cyborg points to possible techno-evolutionary innovations such as the computer chip embedded in Kiri's baby's brain.

Marcia Inhorn's Chapter 2 on what she terms "egg-freezing activists" argues that the advent of egg freezing has made possible reproductive futures for three groups of people: (1) young women with fertility-threatening medical conditions or therapies (e.g., cancer patients); (2) older women with age-related fertility decline but (usually) no reproductive partners; and (3) transgender men who can preserve eggs before transitioning. Inhorn's analysis of reasons for freezing one's eggs is an important pushback against stereotypes about women, reproduction, and technology and a strong and inspiring indication of what individual activists can accomplish.

While Inhorn's chapter deals with people who really need to freeze their eggs in order to biologically reproduce, Lucy Van der Wiel shows in Chapter 3 that the financialization of and easier access to egg freezing are driving even young, fertile, and cancer-free women to freeze their eggs for a future in which they may wish to have children. The increasing demand for egg-freezing, driven by the marketing efforts of various companies, makes the industry hugely profitable, not only because the numbers of such women are growing but also because they often incur debt that they may pay interest on for years. Yet they are aided in these endeavors by the work of the activists Inhorn describes, who played instrumental roles in getting employer insurance to cover oocyte cryopreservation.

In Chapter 4, Noémie Merleau-Ponty describes researchers' work on exploring in vitro gametogenesis (IVG)—the use of embryonic or adult cells to make spermatozoa and eggs, also known as "stem cell derived gametes," and "artificial or synthetic gametes." IVG has the potential to become a cure for infertility and for enabling any human, regardless of fertility, sexuality, or disability status, to conceive children. Theoretically, same-sex partners could have (presently impossible) children who are genetically related to both. All this, as Merleau-Ponty shows, could lead to "the democratization of reproduction." But thus far IVG is not for human use, as that would involve the morally and ethically fraught artificial production of human embryos for research. Merleau-Ponty shows that most researchers in the field do not perceive IVG—which *could* eventually entail the actual making of artificial human gametes—as a *reproductive* technology but rather as a potentially *regenerative* system for studying gametes' biological development and for advancing understanding of epigenetic reprogramming. Regenerative potentials include eliminating the inheritance of genetic diseases (described by Kaur in Chapter 7 as supported by many with such diseases while contested by others). Yet the possibility for using artificial gametes for the more futuristic, "democratizing" ventures mentioned above remains, and might someday be realized, resulting in the creation of genetically modified babies. As a way of dealing with such dilemmas, Merleau-Ponty offers the concept of "sociology as technology." She insists that sociology can, and should, "be practiced as a technology for the democratization of biotechnology," meaning that tools should be created in interdisciplinary collaboration to include alternative perspectives in biotech conception, instead of bioscience researchers translating their research into publications and applications without such perspectives.

The Racialization of Reproduction

Tessa Moll (Chapter 5) shows that in South Africa, while the embryos of (usually white) middle- and upper-class people are carefully protected from outside contamination, many Black people on the other side of the country are subject to reproductive damage to ovaries and semen from chemical spraying to eliminate malaria. Moll argues that *logics of attrition,* whether intentional or unintentional, are built into reproductive neoliberal futures, even in the new South Africa, and points to these as underlying logics that create "superfluous" lives—of both embryos thrown out as waste, and of the Black children not born—as "sacrificial." This damaging racialization of reproduction is also addressed in other chapters, and today remains a reality that must be eliminated in the future.

Lurking in the background of such discussions is the ominous specter of both old ideas of eugenics and newer variations on this theme, raised by Margaret Eby and Meghna Mukherjee in Chapter 6. They posit that selection for desirable characteristics in reproductive processes is fraught with ethical and moral uncertainty and reminiscent of the days of the Better Babies and Fitter Families State Fairs of the early 20th century, in which only white children were admitted as contestants. And they imagine a futuristic World Fair in which people who can and can't afford it pay for enhanced embryos with selected-for characteristics and abilities, expecting that the initial high cost will be recovered via their enhanced child's contributions later on. Tragically, so high is the general cultural valuation of whiteness that, as clearly documented in Eby's and Mukherjee's interviews and fieldnotes, some people of darker skin would choose lighter skin for their children, if they could. *Such devaluation of darker skin must be culturally undone.*

Yet here we note that the supervaluation of whiteness extends far beyond skin color. It has long been reflected, for just two examples, in the artificial creation of white rice and white bread, which have no nutritional value while brown rice and bread have plenty. Yet many prefer the seeming "purity" of the whiteness, with highly detrimental effects. For example, world-renowned midwife Robin Lim (2021) has written about the effects of the advent on the island of Bali of the white techno-rice that supplanted the nutritious red rice native to the island, because the genetically modified white rice can be grown in three crops per year instead of the previous two. It makes bellies feel full while generating severe malnutrition that leads to cases of postpartum hemorrhage, which previously were scarce but are now common there. And the highly nutritious red rice has now become a limited, boutique commodity available only to the wealthier, as many reproductive options are. Just as the Climate Crisis may soon turn our world upside down (see below), so we must turn our cultural color valuations sideways, equally valuing all.

At a large Women Deliver conference, Robbie once heard a keynote speaker from India state, "What white people fear most are hordes of Black and Brown people descending on their shores," and sadly, there is truth in that statement. Protests against immigrant refugees have already swept some European countries and added fuel to the fire of the "alt-right" movement in the US. Yet, again, humanitarianism demands the accommodation of *everyone*. As the current social movement reminds us all, "Black Lives Matter." Thus white people will just have to get over their racism and their fears and accept that all of us will live in multi-cultural, multi-ethnic, and multi-racial societies if we are to survive and thrive as a species. *Techno-sapiens should be color-blind, or rather multi-colored in a rainbow of human and technological possibilities.* Achieving a non-racialized world presents a massive challenge: as Moll described in Chapter 5, even South Africa's "rainbow nation" is still struggling with racial discrimination, almost 30 years after the end of Apartheid and despite a globally admired, non-racialized constitution. Whiteness must cease to be a criterion for "better."

Projecting Techno-Scientific Possibilities

Our chapters on genome editing and in-vitro gametogenesis both consider the ground-breaking concepts underlying gene modification and its societal implications. Chapter 7, by Amarpreet Kaur, notes that the genome editing technology CRISPR-Cas9 has brought mass attention to the possibilities such editing opens for furthering the development of techno-sapiens. These include preventing the inheritance of genetic diseases, "redesigning" humans, and, scarily, military applications. Despite the unilateral condemnation of the work of Chinese scientist Dr. He (who broke the assumed scientific consensus on not using embryonic genome editing to produce human children), there are countries in which legislation and regulation of human germline genome editing do not exist or are not clear nor robust; thus such work could conceivably proceed in such countries. Kaur questions the "tech-sumptions" that underlie such work, concluding that presently there is "weak impetus to redesign or enhance humans in the foreseeable future." And we are grateful for that, for, as mentioned in the Introduction and in our *Star Trek* chapter, technologically "enhanced" humans could and would be quite likely to challenge the democratic principle that all humans are created equal.

As Kaur notes in her chapter, efforts to enhance humans can be viewed as a form of "biohacking," which generally refers to the efforts of laypeople to alter their own biology or that of others to generate, for examples, better health, enhanced intelligence, and longer lives. Many such attempts are made via nutritional supplements and pharma- or nutra-ceuticals and careful attention to diet—all relatively harmless. Yet we can predict that, as envisioned in the World Fair of the future imagined in Chapter 6, many biohackers would jump at the chance to alter their genes and their DNA to ensure such results for themselves and/or their children, selecting for precisely those technological enhancements that seem so eugenically dangerous and morally questionable to others.

Famed entrepreneur Elon Musk apparently disagrees about such dangers. The most recent example of biohacking, created by Musk and his colleagues, is a "brain-hacking" device—a working brain-to-machine interface that forms part of Musk's very real plans to give people superhuman powers. This interface "could allow people with debilitating neurological conditions to control phones or computers with their minds," but the long-term ambition is to usher in what Musk calls "superhuman cognition," in which people merge with artificial intelligence (AI)—"in part to avoid a scenario in which AI becomes so powerful that it destroys the human [species]" (BBC News 2020). The device, in development by Musk's company Neuralink, consists of a tiny probe containing more than 3,000 electrodes attached to flexible threads thinner than a human hair, which can monitor the activity of 1,000 brain neurons" (ibid.). Neuralink said it had "carried out tests on a monkey that had been able to control a computer with its brain" (ibid.). Certainly Elon Musk and his colleagues seem hell-bent on technologically enhancing humans—the consequences to democracy and the moral principle that "all humans are created equal" be damned!

Moving on in this summary section on "Projecting Techno-Scientific Possibilities," in Chapter 8, Suki Finn and Sasha Isaac address (an equally frightening) one of these possibilities—growing babies in artificial wombs. They speculate that removing fertility from humans altogether via "ecotegensis" may become an option for some people desiring to have children without anyone having to bear them. These authors describe the Fetal Containment Model, which insists that gestators are simply containers for fetuses, and therefore ectogenesis should become a viable technology. They also describe the Parthood Model, which in contrast insists that fetuses form parts of their gestators and are therefore intimately connected to them. While the Fetal Containment Model does make sense of surrogacy, we, and the chapter authors, argue that it is not a ticket to women's liberation, but rather represents a further devaluation of women's (still) essential roles in reproduction. And we ask, as we also did in the Introduction, would a fetus gestated externally in a machine, with no connection to its mother's emotions, know how to love? What kind of person would that baby become? Honestly, we do not wish to find out! Yet at least partial research into this possibility continues, bolstered somewhat by the Fetal Containment Model.

Just as Chapter 1 shows the importance of the development of "obligate midwifery"—Wenda Trevathan's term for women's needs for physical and emotional support during labor from a trusted companion—Emaline Reyes' findings in Chapter 9 that fear drives prospective mothers' preferences for cesarean birth, and Sarah Melancon's in a later chapter that fear can immobilize women during labor, illuminate the importance of support people who can help women cope with their fears prior to and during labor, and of disseminating informed perspectives about the frightening birth scenarios that potential parents often see depicted in the media.

Cross-cultural differences impinge on all discussions of reproductive manipulation. For example, the meanings of such bodily functions as menstruation, childbearing, and menopause differ considerably across cultures. As Rebecca Irons details in Chapter 10, changes in the normal function of any of these processes can raise alarm, such as occurs among the Peruvian Quechua when contraception leads to a cessation of menstruation and women fear that "little monsters"—which Irons names *necro-techno-sapiens*—can grow in their wombs from what they perceive as the coagulating blood fed by male semen. Quechua birth control options are heavily racialized and stratified—these Indigenous women are only offered hormonal injections of Depo-Provera, instead of the full range of options that should include technologies under their own control, such as diaphragms—probably under the colonialist assumption that they are too uneducated and irresponsible to use such technologies properly. Their general suspicion of techno-medical family planning measures reflects the fact that they were subjected to mass sterilization programs some decades ago. On the "darker side" of techno-sapiens reproduction, Irons asks, can her concept of necro-techno-sapiens also be applied to the "waste products" of ARTs, such as unused eggs and embryos, and/or to fetuses devastatingly miscarried as a result of technologies like amniocentesis and radiography?

Part II: Imagining Techno-Holistic Reproductive Futures

Just as the manipulation of fertility is heavily affected by technological development, so also is perinatal care. As many of our chapters point out, obstetric care has long been dominated by technological surveillance and manipulation, much for good but also much for worse. In Chapter 11, Kelly Kara and Suzanne Miller analyze water immersion as a technology that protects women from unnecessary intervention, allowing them a sense of safety, privacy, and support. They point out that telemetry—electronic fetal monitoring—can now be done underwater; thus, under the technocratic model of birth, there is no logical reason not to allow women to labor and birth in water, as they can still be technologically surveilled, only far less intrusively. These authors show that water immersion allows for an ideal combination of technology and humanism in birth, and argue that it should be an available option wherever possible.

In Chapter 12, Anna Ozhiganova describes how some Soviet thinking, initiated by Igor Charkovsky, built an entire utopian project based on the value of water birth, ideally in the ocean with dolphins, and mother and infant water training to create the "(meta)human dolphin" able to swim for many hours, even sleeping in the water, and imbued with psychic abilities. This vision was not fully realized: such babies were no doubt great swimmers as they grew, but showed no signs of supernatural or psychic abilities. Yet such fantasies do create tantalizing imageries of superheroes with meta-human abilities, including super-strength, clairvoyance, and telepathy as well as outstanding intelligence and superior health—Superman, Supergirl, Batman, Spiderman, Wonder Woman, and other contemporary superheroes may find some commonality in these ideas, along with the Vulcan and Martian "mind melds" of *Star Trek* and the character J'on J'onnz of *The Flash*.

Integrating Humanistic and Holistic Care into Techno-Sapiens Reproduction

On a much more holistic note, in Chapter 13 Sarah Melancon uses Polyvagal Theory to argue that fear during labor and birth—described in Chapter 9 as a major source of the global cesarean epidemic—is detrimental to outcomes as mediated by the vagus nerve (which regulates the uterus and the cervix) and the autonomic nervous system, while an emotionally supportive environment for birth can relieve this pressure. Melancon describes the internal mechanisms by which fear can trigger a "fight, flight, or freeze" reaction that impedes the birth process, while a sense of safety can allow the endogenous hormones that facilitate that process to flow. Through processes called "neuroception" and "co-regulation," the autonomic nervous system can subconsciously attune to others' internal states, serving the human need for safe labor support, which Melancon demonstrates through a birth in which an anxious woman is calmed via attunement to a midwife. Relatively little attention has been paid to the autonomic nervous system in childbirth research and education, which Melancon describes as the "missing link" in our understanding of birth outcomes and experiences, and thus deserves further research.

Beverley Chalmers's Chapter 14 addresses the conflicts between technology and humanism with an integrated ideology for perinatal care that combines biological, psycho-social, cultural, and spiritual levels of care into a single approach. In her dream, much can and should be done to integrate humanistic and holistic perinatal care for the benefit of our immediate future as techno-sapiens. This futuristic, integrated ideology involves keeping the family at the center of care and utilizing technology only when essential and always in a humane and respectful manner, in what, in Chapter 1, Cheyney and Davis-Floyd call RARTRW care—the "right amount at the right time in the right way." Thus Chalmers questions birth activists' and midwives' focus on "woman-centered care," suggesting instead that the focus should be on *family*-centered care.

To Chalmers' criticism of this concept, in Chapter 15, Annekatrin Skeide adds that a focus on *woman*-centered care makes midwives into service providers whose affectivities do not matter. Skeide argues for a more all-encompassing approach that centers *midwife-woman-family* relationships. She also suggests framing a midwifery model of care as a technology for better birth, just as Noémie Merleau-Ponty argues in Chapter 4 that sociology is a technology for democratizing reproductive research, and points to Sarah Franklin's notion that "biology is a technology" of sex and social reproduction. All three arguments provocatively ask us to extend our concepts of exactly what a "technology" is and can be.

In her chapter, Skeide elides the binaries of good (humanistic/holistic) and bad (technocratic) care. Refusing to code obstetric technologies as inherently negative and harmful, as many birth activists do, Skeide calls such technologies "flexible helpers" and shows how their meanings cannot be separated from their actual uses, and how those meanings vary according to the ideals and values of the practitioner and the social relationship created between practitioner and childbearer via those flexible helpers. Skeide shows that the diagnostic and social meanings of CTG, Pinard horn, and Doptone technologies used to monitor the fetal heart rate become inseparable in their "praxiographic" use, as the diagnostic meanings inform the social meanings and vice-versa. Skeide's views about the malleability and suggestiveness of such technologies constitute a productive re-thinking and retheorizing of the role of technologies in childbirth, as does Kara's and Miller's analysis of water immersion as a humanistic technology.

In Chapter 16, George Parker and Suzanne Miller present a dystopian/uto-pian (depending on your perspective) future for our world, where birth in hospi-tals becomes so dangerous that we will, inevitably, need to return to homebirth settings as the only environments in which women can give birth safely, with the skilled attendance of midwives. These authors stand the current technocratic framing of risk and safety in childbirth on its head in their forward-thinking and satirical critique of hospital birth.

In the final chapter in this book, Dana Solomon and Beverley Chalmers describe reproduction in the multiple *Star Trek* TV series and movies. Serving as a stimulus for some of the most prominent genetic engineers of today, *Star Trek* has, over the past 5 decades, both predicted and illustrated similar issues to those being discussed in this book. It simply does birth better, both technologi-cally and humanistically. And it makes a strong case for not eliminating people with disabilities, clearly illustrating the value of such individuals and making the point that we should not try to eugenically and genetically construct an "ableist" society.

What Do Childbearers Want?

Most of our chapters in Part II seem to be based on the assumption that women *want* physiologic birth options and resent not receiving them. Yet Robbie reminds our readers here that in her study of 100 US white, middle-class, heterosexual women carried out during the late 1980s and early 1990s—and also in a fol-low-up study of multiple types of childbearers conducted by herself and Melissa Cheyney 2017–2019 for an ongoing revision and update of Robbie's first book, *Birth as an American Rite of Passage* (2003 [1992])—the majority of women both expected and wanted particular interventions in birth, most especially electronic fetal monitoring, as it made them feel safe, and epidurals, as they did not wish to feel pain. Active participants in their own cyborgification, these women were relatively happy to birth themselves and their babies as techno-sapiens (though of course they did not use that language). Only around 15% of women in both studies actively sought physiologic, intervention-free birth in the hospital or in homes and freestanding birth centers. Yet all childbearers in these two studies wanted compassionate, humanistic care; their deepest complaints were not about interventions but rather about obstetric disrespect, violence, and abuse (see Liese et al. 2021).

In contrast, the Canadian Maternity Experiences Survey of over 6,000 randomly selected women giving birth across Canada, co-chaired by Chalmers and Dzakpasu (2015), showed that for Canadian women having a vaginal delivery, the more interventions they received, the less their satisfaction with their birth experiences. In this survey, 75% of women having no interventions in labor and birth rated their experience as "very positive" while only 45% of women experiencing 8 or more interventions did so. The same pattern was observed for women's perceptions of their caregiver's respect, concern for dignity, compassion shown to them, the information given to them, their involvement in decision making, and their caregiver's competence. Alternately, for women having unplanned cesareans following attempted vaginal births, the number of interventions was not associated with satisfaction with birth; however, satisfaction ratings were consistently lower than among women giving birth vaginally. It is possible that the interventions associated with more positive ratings were perceived by women as attempts to assist them to achieve a vaginal birth prior to the cesarean. This large cross-cultural difference between US and Canadian women is worthy of further study: why do many US women seem so comfortable with technocratic birth, while most Canadian women do not?

Understanding women's cross-cultural experiences of techno-birth is a complex issue, well-covered in Davis-Floyd and Cheyney's *Birth in Eight Cultures* (2019) (though not including Canada). For example, women in Greece live under what author Eugenia Georges calls the "symbolic domination of modernity" and therefore may tend to prefer cesareans as the most modern way to birth (Georges and Daellenbach 2019), whereas Japanese women tend to value normal, physiologic birth, seeing the process as "metamorphic"—essential for transforming a woman into a mother (Williamson and Matsuoka 2019).

And returning to the question of what childbearers want, which this section addresses, we re-emphasize Chalmers's stress in Chapter 14 on the importance of including perinatal psychologists in reproductive care, as has been implemented on a national scale in all maternity care centers in the Republic of Moldova with her guidance (Chalmers 2017). A further example of how well that can work comes from Turkey, where obstetrician Hakan Çoker, birth psychologist Neşe Karabekir, and midwife/doula Serpil Varlik (2015, 2021) have created a model called "Birth with No Regret," so named because so many Turkish women were exiting birth with a great deal of regret, and what they wanted was to have no regrets about their births. In this model, the birth psychologist processes the desires and emotions of the birthing family *and* the birth practitioners, before, during, and after birth, thereby working to ensure that all exit the birth with no regrets. So effective is this model that it has spread around Turkey and is being widely implemented, with excellent outcomes, and is helping to lower Turkey's very high cesarean rate of 52%. *We strongly recommend the inclusion of birth psychologists in all obstetric teams,* as their presence would likely prevent or at least greatly diminish the obstetric disrespect, violence, and abuse so prevalent around the world (Sadler et al. 2016; Liese et al. 2021). (See Melancon's Chapter 13 and Davis-Floyd 2018 for a discussion of the significant roles stress plays in obstetric violence and abuse and how it can be reduced.)

How Culture Shapes Biology: ARTs and Missing Girls

In relation to Franklin's above-mentioned notion that "biology is a technology" of sex and social reproduction, here we note as well that culture—far from being a tapestry of diversity overlaid on a universal biology—can *shape* human biology (High 2019) via multiple means, including via culturally determined notions of what should and should not be eaten, whom one should or should not reproduce with, how the environment should or should not be shaped by human hands, and so on. Extreme forms of culture shaping biology included in our chapters are egg freezing, embryo selection, in-vitro fertilization, gametogenesis, and more. *Just as biology, evolution, and the physical environment shape culture, so culture shapes biology and the physical environment,* and has been a primary means of shaping our evolution into techno-sapiens—as the chapters in this book clearly show.

The societal and cultural issues that shape, overlay, and underlie biological issues have resulted in another topic not covered in our chapters—the current devastating effects of technological sex-selection for male gender offspring. The "natural" global sex ratio at birth has long been 105 boys per 100 girls. Yet in countries where boys are culturally more valued than girls—such as Albania, Armenia, Azerbaijan, China, Georgia, Hong Kong, India, Montenegro, South Korea, Taiwan, Tunisia, and Vietnam—due to sex selection via ultrasound technology, neglect after birth, malnourishment, or outright infanticide, girls are far more frequently "disappeared" than boys (Ritchie and Roser 2019). In some of these countries, this has resulted in a seriously skewed sex ratio of up to 120–140 boys per 100 girls. It is estimated that today there are over 136 million "missing women" in the world as a result of selective abortion and excess female deaths (Bongaarts and Guillimoto 2015)—more than the population of Mexico. Although some countries have now banned gender-selective abortion, its skewed results will haunt the next generations in those countries and others.

Negative consequences for men, especially those of lower socioeconomic and educational status, can include lack of ability to marry; social marginalization, loneliness, and psychological problems; delayed marriage; and competition for brides (Hesketh 2011). Negative consequences for women can include increased cultural valuation of their roles as wives and mothers, with negative impacts on career pathways; increased pressure to marry and have children earlier in life; and, most devastatingly, increased risk of commodification, as in bride-kidnapping and selling and sex trafficking (Hudson and Den Boer 2005). For society more broadly, results may include increased crime, violence, and disorder in communities (ibid.). Certainly, this cultural shaping of (the lack of) biological reproduction will carry demographic consequences for many decades to come (Ritchie and Roser 2019).

Techno-Sapiens and Pandemics

The rapidly changed, and changing, clinical care of all people and especially of childbearing families during the 2020 coronavirus pandemic raised a sudden need to address the impact of such health crises for the future evolution of technology and humanism in birth. This pandemic, which will surely be followed by others due to increasing globalization and the Climate Crisis (discussed below), has revealed the systemic structural flaws in the healthcare systems of many nations, with the greatest disease burden falling, as usual, on the poor and structurally marginalized (Davis-Floyd and Gutschow 2021). It has also revealed our lack of pandemic preparedness—if all countries initially had sufficient stores of personal protective equipment (PPE), disease-testing and tracking systems in place, etc., the pandemic could have been stopped before it became one and many thousands of people would not have died. Certainly, the pandemic turned many care providers into a previously rare but now-familiar form of techno-sapiens via the necessary wearing of N-95 masks and often full hazmat suits as they cared for the multiplying numbers of those infected.

Ironically, according to Justin Worland (2020), the COVID-19 pandemic has opened up new possibilities for coping with the Climate Crisis. As citizens of large and polluted cities, including Beijing, watched their air growing cleaner during lockdowns, they began to want that in the future as well. The disruptions of economies now allow new possibilities for green technologies to be widely used in economic and infrastructural rebuilding efforts, potentially creating millions of new jobs. Major global business ventures are turning to home-based employment that will reduce if not eliminate traffic commutes, crowded central city workplaces, and their environmental contamination: life for many could become office-free, paperless, and therefore less carbon-intensive. Some North American and European leaders are actively designing such plans. Yet China continues to build carbon-intensive, highly polluting coal-fired plants in its own country and in Africa, and the US under Trump seemed to be in a state of climate-change denial. His opponent President-Elect Joe Biden plans to sign on to the Kyoto Accords and has a massive plan for green re-structuring that will address the Climate Catastrophe at its roots. Perhaps Biden and his like-minded colleagues in other countries bring hope.

Alarmingly, the coronavirus pandemic has highlighted some of the very concerns that the dystopian predictions of Chapter 16 posit. During this pandemic, many women in many countries sought to avoid hospital contagion and hospital policies preventing them from bringing no, or no more than one, birth companions into hospitals by seeking to give birth at home or in freestanding birth centers (Davis-Floyd, Gutschow, and Schwartz 2020). Even more egregious were the attempts by some hospitals to force inductions and cesareans on women birthing during COVID-19 to speed up the birth process and control its environment, and the practice of separating COVID+ mothers from their newborns. Though community midwives around the world did take on as many new clients as they could—some in the very late stage of pregnancy—there were simply not enough of them to meet the demand in countries where homebirth rates are low (ibid.). Thus, unknown numbers of families chose unassisted births at home, or accepted hospital birth with the accompanying psychological trauma for some of having to choose between their partner and their doula or, in some hospitals, to labor alone (see Davis-Floyd and Gutschow 2021).

Birthing Techno-Sapiens during the Climate Crisis

As Joe Dumit and Robbie Davis-Floyd noted in *Cyborg Babies: From Techno-Sex to Techo-Tots* (1998:14):

> The cyborg seems progressive, exciting, ambiguous—a future-oriented direction for our evolution that both scorns and transcends its earth-based past. And yet we must ask, can our civilization sustain its cyborgian evolution? Will the earth provide us with enough resources to stay this course? Or will we be forced to abandon our high-tech trajectory when we have finally depleted the planet beyond technological redemption?

And indeed, as discussed in Chapter 17, the Climate Crisis is upon us. Regarding reproduction, we stress that climate change will likely necessitate the *decentralization of birth and maternity care and a revaluation of community midwives*, both traditional and professional, as strongly recommended in "Effective Maternity Care in Disaster Zones: Low-Tech, Skilled Touch" (Davis-Floyd et al. 2021). In this essay, midwives Robin Lim of Bumi Sehat and Vicki Penwell of Mercy in Action describe their and their teams' effective provision of care in the immediate aftermaths of disasters—including the Aceh tsunami of 2004, Hurricane Haiyan (2013) in the Philippines, and more recent disasters on Bali and other Indonesian islands—showing statistical outcomes that were as good as or better than national outcomes in normal times (see also Lim and Davis-Floyd 2021). When "energy-intensive health care becomes both unsustainable and unjustifiable" (Chapter 17), and when carbon-intensive hospitals are overcrowded, damaged, destroyed, inaccessible, or dangerous sites of contagion, it is the community midwives with their "low-tech, skilled touch" midwifery model of care—which itself can be framed as an *eco-technology*, as noted in Chapter 16—who will be most needed.

Of course, the Climate Crisis could change *everything* about the world as we know it. In *The Uninhabitable Earth: Life after Warming*, David Wallace-Wells (2020) takes his readers on a journey through the possibilities—some inevitable, some still up to us and our future actions—posed by the Climate Crisis—as some are suggesting, better termed the Climate Catastrophe. We are presently at 1.1 degrees of warming since the Industrial Revolution and are already seeing the effects—which include, among many others, an increasing number of wildfires, droughts, and superstorms. (Infuriatingly, the major causes of global warming and environmental pollution were generated not by the Industrial Revolution but *over the last 30 years—three decades in which the dangers of climate change were already recognized, yet few acted* [Wallace-Wells 2020].) At 2 degrees (which according to some we will inevitably reach no matter what we do now, and according to others is still avoidable, if we act quickly enough), we will reach several tipping points "where the effects of climate change go from advancing gradually to changing dramatically overnight, reshaping the planet" (Worland 2020:36). We will see even more rapid glacier melting and rising sea levels (already in motion), which will displace millions or perhaps billions of people from flooded land, resulting in mass poverty and malnutrition, even "genocide," as the Foreign Minister of the Marshall Islands named it (Wallace-Wells 2020:10). A new and massive influx of climate refugees will move from the Global South toward the Global North, which itself will be in trouble from those same rising sea levels.

What roles will our efforts to continue to re-create ourselves as techno-sapiens play during this oncoming Climate Catastrophe? Should we reach 3 or more degrees of warming (quite likely, *if* we continue on our current trajectory), most of the Earth will become uninhabitable (Wallace-Wells 2020). Will we cope by building large biospheres—techno-bubbles in which hundreds or thousands of people will either choose or be forced to live? Will such biospheres be reserved for only the 1% who can afford to pay for their construction, with others pounding on their walls and windows demanding entry, or dying because they can't get in? So far this is the stuff of science fiction, yet it could become very, very real. In the summer of 2020, the temperatures in some regions of the far North of Siberia reached and stayed for months at an uncharacteristic 30 degrees Celsius, 86 degrees Fahrenheit. The world as we know it may literally be turned upside-down.

Despite the many climate-change deniers still out there, we believe that most people do understand, or at least can glimpse, what is coming. What sustains us, lets us sleep at night, is what Robbie has long called *the myth of technological transcendence*—the "1-2 Punch" notion (see Introduction) that any problems created with technology can and will be fixed with more technology. Will we develop nanites that can clean up the increasingly polluted oceans—the source of all life on this planet? When many of our fresh-water sources dry up, will we become able to quench our thirst and to irrigate our new or remaining farmlands from de-salinated seawater—of which there will be plenty as the glaciers all melt? Or grow all our food in hydroponic gardens? Or will some or all of us degenerate into carbon-intensive wars over increasingly scarce resources? Ironically, the myth of technological transcendence may well come true—we may be able to save some of ourselves as a species due to that 1-2 Punch of technological mutilation and prosthesis that caused the Climate Crisis in the first place. As predicted in the movie *Wall-E*, will we have to move what remains of us into spaceships (or space stations, which we can already build) to wait for 700 years for the Earth to regenerate itself in our absence? We must note here that not only are we humans co-evolving ourselves with our technologies, but also our planet, which we have turned into a cyborgian system by surrounding it with thousands of satellites constantly beaming information via radio waves up from the planet, around to each other, and back down. We all should be taking stock of the environmental, physiologic, and reproductive effects of this electromagnetic radiation now permeating all planetary species, Earth itself, and our atmosphere.

As we face and deal with the onrushing Climate Catastrophe and the other effects of our climb "up" the evolutionary ladder as techno-sapiens, may we, as suggested in the Introduction, continue our search for "a prosperous way down." May we combine the best of our technologies with the best of ourselves to generate a just, humane, and ecologically sustainable future for all of the species and techno-citizens of our Cyborg Spaceship Earth.

Acknowledgment

We thank Marcia Inhorn for her careful reading of these Conclusions and for her helpful suggestions for their improvement.

References

BBC NEWS. August 2020. "Elon Musk to Show off Working Brain-Hacking Device." https://www.bbc.com/news/technology-53921596.

Bongaarts J, Guilmoto CZ. 2015. "How Many More Missing Women? Excess Female Mortality and Prenatal Sex Selection, 1970–2050."*Population and Development Review* 41(2):241–269.

Chalmers B. 2017. *Family-Centred Perinatal Care: Improving Pregnancy, Birth and Postpartum Care.* Cambridge: Cambridge University Press.

Chalmers B, Dzakpasu S. 2015. "Interventions in Labour and Birth and Satisfaction with Care: The Canadian Maternity Experiences Survey Findings." *Journal of Reproductive and Infant Psychology* 33(4):374–387. doi:10.1080/0264656838.2015.1042964.

Çoker H, Karabekir N, Varlik S. 2015. "Birth with No Regret Birth Model and Team." *Journal of Obstetrics and Women's Health and Disease* 1(3):27–34.

Çoker H, Karabekir N, Varlik S. 2021. "Birth with No Regret in Turkey." In: *Birthing Models on the Human Rights Frontier: Speaking Truth to Power*, eds. Daviss BA, Davis-Floyd R. London: Routledge, in press.

Davis-Floyd R. 2003. *Birth as an American Rite of Passage.* Berkeley: University of California Press.

Davis-Floyd R. 2018. "Open and Closed Knowledge Systems, the 4 Stages of Cognition, and the Cultural Management of Birth. " *Frontiers in Sociology* 3:23. doi:10.3389/fsoc2018.2018.0023.

Davis-Floyd R, Gutschow K, eds. 2021. *The Global Impact of COVID-19 on Maternity Care Practices*, a special issue of *Frontiers in Sociology*, in press.

Davis-Floyd R, Gutschow K, Schwartz DA. 2020. "Pregnancy, Birth, and the COVID-19 Pandemic in the United States." *Medical Anthropology* 39(5):413–427. doi:10.1080/01459740.2020.1761804.

Davis-Floyd R, Lim R, Penwell V, Ivry T. 2021. "Effective Maternity Disaster Care: Low-Tech, Skilled Touch." In: *Sustainable Birth in Disruptive Times*, eds. Gutschow K, Davis-Floyd R, Daviss BA. Springer Publishing, in press.

Dumit J, Davis-Floyd R. 1998. "Cyborg Babies: Children of the Third Millennium." In: *Cyborg Babies: From Techno-Sex to Techno-Tots*, eds. Davis-Floyd R, Dumit J. New York: Routledge, 1–20.

Georges E, Daellenbach R. 2019. "Divergent Meanings and Practices of Childbirth in Greece and New Zealand." In: *Birth in Eight Cultures*, eds. Davis-Floyd R, Cheyney ML. Grove, IL: Waveland Press, 129–164.

Hesketh T. 2011. Selecting Sex: The Effect of Preferring Sons. *Early Human Development* 87(11):759–761.

High Holly. 2019. *Cultural Values, Birth and Parenting: Reproductive Health and Lao Socialism.* Proposal for an ARC Future Fellowships Commencing in 2020. FT200100346. Canberra: Australian Research Council.

Hudson VM, Den Boer A. 2005. "Missing Women and Bare Branches: Gender Balance and Conflict." *Environmental Change and Security Program Report* 11:20–24.

Liese K, Davis-Floyd R, Stewart K, Cheyney M. 2021. "Obstetric Iatrogenesis in the United States: The Spectrum of Disrespect, Violence, and Abuse." Special Journal Issue on "Medicine's Shadowside," eds. Varley E, Varma S, *Anthropology & Medicine*, in press.

Lim R. 2021. "Bumi Sehat Bali: Birth on the Checkered Cloth." In: *Birthing Models on the Human Rights Frontier: Speaking Truth to Power*, eds. Daviss BA, Davis-Floyd R. London: Routledge, Chapter 1, in press.

Lim R, Davis-Floyd R. 2021. "Implementing the *International Childbirth Initiative* (ICI) in Disaster Zones: Bumi Sehat's Experience in Indonesia, Haiti, the Philippines, and Nepal." In: *Birthing Models on the Human Rights Frontier: Speaking Truth to Power*, eds. Daviss BA, Davis-Floyd R. London: Routledge, Chapter 9, in press.

Ritchie H, Roser M. 2019. "Gender Ratio." *Published Online at OurWorldInData.org.* https://ourworldindata.org/gender-ratio [Online Resource].

Sadler Michelle, Santos MJDS, Ruiz-Berdún D, et al. 2016. "Moving Beyond Disrespect and Abuse: Addressing the Structural Dimensions of Obstetric Violence." *Reproductive Health Matters* 24(47):47–55.

Wallace-Wells D. 2020. *The Uninhabitable Earth: Life after Warming.* New York: Tim Duggan Books.

Williamson KE, Matsuoka E. 2019. "Comparing Childbirth in Brazil and Japan: Social Hierarchies, Cultural Values, and the Meaning of Place." In: *Birth in Eight Cultures*, eds. Davis-Floyd R, Cheyney M. Long Grove, IL: Waveland Press, 129–164.

Worland J. "The Defining Year." *Time*, July 20–27:36–43.

INDEX

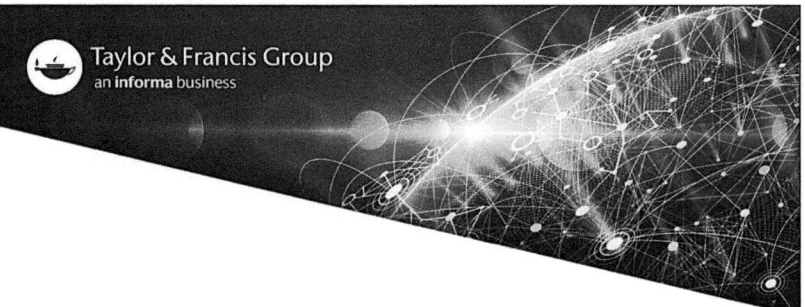
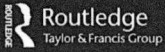
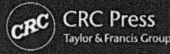